DEDICATION

*To my husband Robert,
for his constant love and encouragement*

COUNCIL OF ORIENTAL MEDICAL PUBLISHERS

DESIGNATION

This text is a whole-text translation of 从 病 例 谈 辨 证 论 治 *Cóng Bìng Lì Tán Biàn Zhèng Lùn Zhì* (Case Studies on Pattern Identification to Determine Treatment) by Jiāo Shù-Dé, published by People's Medical Publishing House (Běijīng).

The terminology used in the translation of the original text is found in *A Practical Dictionary of Chinese Medicine* (Wiseman and Féng, Paradigm Publications, 1998). Any unfamiliar terms found in the text may also be easily accessed in the *Practical Dictionary*.

TABLE OF CONTENTS

Chapter Five
When treating diseases diagnosed by Western medicine, use pattern identification
as a basis for determining treatment 129

Chapter Six
A brief discussion on the Chinese medical statement, "Treating different diseases with
the same method and treating same diseases with different methods." 167

Chapter Seven
Important issues when applying pattern identification to determine treatment 191

Chapter Eight
Constantly improve and develop pattern identification skills to determine treatment 247

Index

TRANSLATOR'S FOREWORD

Case Studies on Pattern Identification from the Personal Experience of Jiāo Shù-Dé is the final volume in a series that presents the lifelong experience and work of a great contemporary master of Chinese medicine.

The first volume, *Ten Lectures on the Use of Chinese Medicinals from the Personal Experience of Jiāo Shù-Dé*, was first published by Paradigm Publications in 2003, and it serves as a straightforward and comprehensive introduction to the clinical rigor of Chinese medicinal therapy. The second volume, *Ten Lectures on the Use of Formulas from the Personal Experience of Jiāo Shù-Dé*, is more extensive in its discussions of Chinese medicine and includes some case studies as illustrations in prescribing formulas.

This final work, *Case Studies on Pattern Identification from the Personal Experience of Jiāo Shù-Dé*, is an in-depth presentation of 40 case studies used by Jiāo Shù-Dé as an educational tool for both students and seasoned practitioners alike. He has not only presented the reader with interesting case studies, but has also compared and contrasted many of the studies, thus providing a rich and clinically relevant reading experience.

Case Studies on Pattern Identification represents a more advanced level of clinical knowledge and culminates in the practical application of the material from the first two volumes. As all three volumes have enjoyed lasting popularity in China, it is our privilege to present English readers with this final and most clinically detailed volume. It comprises a complete translation of the original work, and also contains indexes for all the formulas and book titles referenced in all three volumes, adding a powerful reference tool heretofore unavailable to Chinese readers.

It is my sincere hope that this book—written by a clinician, translated by a clinician, and presented to clinicians—will lead to the enhanced clinical effectiveness of Chinese medicine practitioners.

Lynn Kuchinski

Albuquerque, New Mexico

March, 2006

CHAPTER ONE

Pattern identification as a basis for determining treatment requires skilled mastery of the four examinations.

In clinic, when conducting pattern identification to determine treatment, the physician must skillfully and accurately utilize the principles of the four examinations: inspection, listening and smelling, inquiry, and palpation. Physicians also need to be able to collect accurate and useful information so as to develop a comprehensive understanding of the patient's illness. Only then can a good foundation be laid for treatment based on pattern identification. Proficiency in conducting the four examinations is essential. To illustrate this point, I present here five case studies together with short discussions based on my personal experience.

CASE STUDIES

CASE ONE
CONCRETION AND CONGLOMERATION MOUNTING PAIN (TWISTED OVARIAN CYST)
癥瘕疝痛(卵巢囊肿蒂扭转)

The patient was a 67-year-old woman whose first examination date was April 17, 1961.

CHIEF COMPLAINT

Severe pain in the lower abdomen that had persisted for ten days.

INQUIRY EXAMINATION

The patient had a large swelling on the right side of her abdomen that was painful and resisted pressure. Five days earlier, she had gone to her local hospital, where she received a diagnosis of "twisted ovarian cyst" and was told that her condition needed surgery. Refusing this option, she came to my hospital for diagnosis and treatment.

Her chief complaint was severe lower abdominal pain and swelling that resisted pressure. She exhibited fidgetiness when sitting or lying down and experienced disquieted sleep. Her food and drink intake were reduced, she experienced oppression and distention in her stomach duct after eating, and her mouth was dry but she was unable to drink much. She had dry bound stool and experienced vexing heat in the five hearts at night.

INSPECTION EXAMINATION

The patient appeared to be in a state of acute pain and suffering. Although she was fidgety while sitting and lying down, she did not move freely. Her tongue was red with white fur.

LISTENING AND SMELLING EXAMINATION

She exhibited subtle groaning and a low voice, and her breathing was relatively weak.

PALPATION EXAMINATION

The lower abdomen was bulging and distended, and slightly to the right below the umbilicus was an eggplant-shaped lump the size of a child's head. The lump was painful, resisted pressure, and was relatively hard. The pressure pain was (+++); abdominal muscle tension was (++); rebound pain was (+). All six pulses were slightly rapid and stringlike, especially in the bar and cubit positions. Her body temperature was 37.8 C.

PATTERN IDENTIFICATION

I knew that the illness was located in both the liver and kidney channels because her chief complaint was pain in the lower abdomen and the swelling affected the right side below the umbilicus. As for the tension of the abdominal flesh, Chinese medicine calls this abdominal sinew tension. The liver governs the sinews, and disharmony of the sinews results in tension. The *Huáng Dì Nèi Jīng* ("The Yellow Emperor's Inner Canon") states:

"Disease arises when foot reverting yīn liver [channel] is stirred… In men this causes mounting [pain], in women lesser-abdominal swelling… In severe cases, dry throat is present."

The *Jīn Guì Yì* ("The Wings of the Golden Coffer") further explains:

"Women also suffer from mounting qì; whenever there are symptoms such as blood desiccation with absence of menstruation and clots in the lesser-abdomen, this surely indicates disease in the liver channel."

According to this explanation, the liver channel was the primary location of this disease. The *Zhèng Zhì Huì Bǔ* ("Collected Supplement to Patterns and Treatments") elaborates:

"Whenever mounting endures, it can form accumulations shaped like a dish that attach above, below, and to the left and right of the umbilicus. These can be either concretions or conglomerations and cause endless pain."

On the basis of this, in conjunction with the fact that the onset of abdominal pain was rapid, I knew that this illness belonged to the category of concretion and conglomeration mounting disease. The stringlike pulse in both hands indicated liver channel disease, as well as mounting-conglomeration, accumulation, and gathering with tension and pain in the abdomen. The *Mài Jīng* ("The Pulse Canon") says: "In the diagnosis of mounting-conglomeration, accumulations, and gatherings in women, the pulse will be stringlike and urgent." The correlation of the four examinations supported the diagnosis of concretion and conglomeration mounting pain.

TREATMENT METHOD

The swelling in the abdomen that refused pressure indicated repletion evil, but the patient was over sixty years of age, the illness had continued for ten days, and eating and sleeping were irregular. The patient also demonstrated qì timidity, low voice, and a long history of fatigue, so there were symptoms of vacuity within the repletion. Consequently, the treatment used the method of moving qì and quickening the blood while regulating the liver and relaxing tension to alleviate pain. After right qì had been gradually restored, a prescription was given to disperse the lump and eliminate the concretion.

PRESCRIPTION

The patient received two packets of the following prescription:

wū yào (乌药 lindera, Linderae Radix) 12.5 g
dāng guī (当归 Chinese angelica, Angelicae Sinensis Radix) 12.5 g

bái sháo yào (白芍药 white peony, Paeoniae Radix Alba) 25 g

wú zhū yú (吴茱萸 evodia, Evodiae Fructus) 3.5 g

chǎo chuān liàn zǐ (川楝子 stir-fried toosendan, Toosendan Fructus Frictus) 12.5 g

lì zhī hé (荔枝核 litchee pit, Litchi Semen) 9 g, crushed

chǎo jú hé (橘核 stir-fried tangerine seed, Citri Reticulatae Semen Frictum) 9 g

hú lú bā (胡芦巴 fenugreek, Trigonellae Semen) 6 g

chǎo xiǎo huí xiāng (炒小茴香 stir-fried fennel, Foeniculi Fructus Frictus) 9 g

qīng pí (青皮 unripe tangerine peel, Citri Reticulatae Pericarpium Viride) 6 g

mù xiāng (木香 costusroot, Aucklandiae Radix) 4.5 g

rǔ xiāng (乳香 frankincense, Olibanum) 6 g

mò yào (没药 myrrh, Myrrha) 6 g

yán hú suǒ mò (延胡索 powdered corydalis, Corydalis Rhizoma Pulveratum) 4.5 g (divided into two portions and taken drenched)

FORMULA EXPLANATION

This formula is a modification of *wū líng tōng qì tāng* (Lindera and Poria Free the Qì Decoction) in combination with *huí xiāng jú hé wán* (Fennel and Tangerine Pill). In this formula, *wū yào* (lindera) acts as the chief medicinal by moving stagnant qì in the abdomen, normalizing counterflow qì in the kidney channel, and treating mounting pain by moving qì.

The support medicinals, *dāng guī* (Chinese angelica) and *bái sháo yào* (white peony), nourish the liver, quicken the blood, relax the sinews, and relieve tension.

Acting as the assistant medicinals, *jú hé* (tangerine seed), *xiǎo huí xiāng* (fennel), *lì zhī hé* (litchee pit), *hú lú bā* (fenugreek), and *mù xiāng* (costus root) warm and dissipate stagnant qì in both the liver and kidney channels, for when the qì moves, the blood also moves. *Rǔ xiāng* (frankincense), *mò yào* (myrrh), and *yán hú suǒ* (corydalis) quicken stasis and soothe the sinews, and disperse swelling and settle pain. By regulating the physiological functions, the assistant medicinals enhance the treatment effect.

As couriers, *wú zhū yú* (evodia) and *qīng pí* (unripe tangerine peel) primarily enter the liver channel to course the liver and open depression and to rectify qì and break binds. *Chuān liàn zǐ* (toosendan) soothes the sinews and moves qì, which makes it an important medicinal for treating mounting pain. Since its nature is bitter and cold, it can clear heat from the small intestine, the urinary bladder, the liver, and the kidney. Therefore, it is a useful medicinal in the treatment of mounting pain in this formula and is a paradoxical support medicinal to prevent overheating from warm medicinals.

FOLLOWUP TREATMENT

Second visit, April 19: The abdominal pain was alleviated, urine and bowels were uninhibited, and the patient was able to sleep at night for more than a hour at a time. The abdominal wall had already softened, and the tenderness of the concretion lump was also relieved. She was still unable to eat or drink much; she had weakness in the entire body and a low voice, and she demonstrated qì timidity. Her tongue appeared unchanged, and the pulse was slightly stringlike. The diagnostic tests had revealed a leukocyte count of 19,700/mm^3, 82% neutrophil granulocytes, 16% lymphocytes, and 2% basophils.

Keeping with the original method, I removed *wú zhū yú* from the previous formula and added *xī yáng shēn* (American ginseng, decocted separately and then added) 4.5 g and *zhì huáng qí* (mix-fried astragalus) 9 g to assist the right qì. The patient received two more prescription packets.

Third visit, April 24: The patient experienced very good results after taking the above-mentioned formula and had taken two more preparations of this formula in the meantime. By now, the abdominal pain was completely gone; she was sleeping well and her food intake had increased. Her essence-spirit had improved, and she could sit, lie down, and walk with a cane. Urination was normal, but her bowels had not moved in five days. Palpation of the abdomen revealed that the abdominal wall had softened, and there was a distinguishable, slightly moveable swelling approximately the size of a child's head in the lower abdomen on the right side. The pain with pressure was (+). The six pulses were slightly rapid, stringlike, and slippery. The tongue fur was white and thick. The diagnostic tests revealed a leukocyte count of 9,200/mm^3, 79% neutrophil granulocytes, 20% lymphocytes, and 1% basophils. A routine urinalysis revealed a glucose level of (++), and further inquiry into her health history showed that she was diabetic. Therefore, the previous formula was modified, and two packets were given as follows:

rén shēn (人参 ginseng, Ginseng Radix) 6 g

bái zhú (白术 white atractylodes, Atractylodis Macrocephalae Rhizoma) 6 g

fú líng (茯苓 poria, Poria) 6 g

zhì gān cǎo (炙甘草 mix-fried licorice, Glycyrrhizae Radix cum Liquido Fricta) 4.5 g

chén pí (陈皮 tangerine peel, Citri Reticulatae Pericarpium) 6 g

chuān liàn zǐ (川楝子 toosendan, Toosendan Fructus) 9 g

chǎo xiǎo huí xiāng (炒小茴香 stir-fried fennel, Foeniculi Fructus Frictus) 6 g *lì zhī hé* (荔枝核 litchee pit, Litchi Semen) 9 g

xiāng fù (香附 cyperus, Cyperi Rhizoma) 9 g

zhì huáng qí (炙黄芪 mix-fried astragalus, Astragali Radix cum Liquido Fricta) 12 g

rǔ xiāng (乳香 frankincense, Olibanum) 3 g

mò yào (没药 myrrh, Myrrha) 3 g

guā dì (瓜蒂 melon stalk, Melonis Pedicellus) 19 *g* (mixed with *yuán míng fěn* (元明粉 refined mirabilite, Natrii Sulfas Exsiccatus) 1.5 g)

yán hú suǒ mò (延胡索 powdered corydalis, Corydalis Rhizoma Pulveratum) 3.5 *g* (divided into two portions and taken drenched)

Fourth visit, April 26, and fifth visit, May 3: All symptoms were alleviated, and the bowels were unobstructed. The patient was moving without impediment, food and drink intake had doubled, and her complexion was lively and lustrous. The urinary glucose level was still at (++). *Guā dì* (melon stalk) and *yuán míng fěn* (refined mirabilite) were removed from the formula, and the following medicinals were added to clear heat from the qì and blood and to disperse the center:

zhī mǔ (知母 anemarrhena, Anemarrhenae Rhizoma)

shēng shí gāo (生石膏 raw gypsum, Gypsum Crudum)

huáng qín (黄芩 scutellaria, Scutellariae Radix)

dān shēn (丹参 salvia, Salviae Miltiorrhizae Radix)

qīng pí (青皮 unripe tangerine peel, Citri Reticulatae Pericarpium Viride)

Sixth visit, May 8: The patient was symptom-free. Her complexion had luster and her essence-spirit was good. Palpation of the abdomen revealed a swelling the size of an apple on the right side of the lower abdomen, but she reported no pain during her daily activities and no tenderness when her abdomen was pressed. Both the bar and cubit pulses were still slightly stringlike, and the tongue fur was thin and white. Accordingly, I changed the prescription to support the right qì and to disperse the accumulation at the same time. This was a method of concurrent attack and supplementation. The prescription was administered in pill form. *Huáng qí* (astragalus) was removed from the formula and the following medicinals were added:

sān léng (三棱 sparganium, Sparganii Rhizoma)

é zhú (莪术 curcuma rhizome, Curcumae Rhizoma)

táo rén (桃仁 peach kernel, Persicae Semen)

hóng huā (红花 carthamus, Carthami Flos)

bīng láng (槟榔 areca, Arecae Semen)

wū yào (乌药 lindera, Linderae Radix)

bái sháo yào (白芍药 white peony, Paeoniae Radix Alba)

jiāo shān zhā (焦山楂 scorch-fried crataegus, Crataegi Fructus Ustus)

jiāo shén qū (焦神曲 scorch-fried medicated leaven, Massa Medicata Fermentata Usta)

jiāo mài yá (焦麦芽 scorch-fried barley sprout, Hordei Fructus Germinatus Ustus)

These medicinals were ground into a fine powder and then formed into water pills the size of mung beans. The dosage was 3–6 g taken twice a day with warm boiled water.

<u>Sixth visit, September 19, 1961</u>: The complexion of the patient was still lustrous, her daily activities were normal, and she could manage her own household activities. The urinary glucose tests were negative. Palpation of the abdomen revealed a small swollen mass on the right side which was the size of an apricot. She was advised to continue with the prescription pill.

<u>Seventh visit, May 17, 1962</u>: The patient was in good health, and the urinary glucose test was still negative. The abdominal swelling had completely disappeared.

Case Two

Cough and panting (chronic geriatric bronchitis, pulmonary emphysema, cardiopulmonary disease, and cardiac functional insufficiency [Level II–III])
咳喘(老年慢性支气管炎；肺气肿；肺心病；心功能不全 II–III 度)

The patient was a 67-year-old woman whose first examination date was December 12, 1969.

Chief complaint

Cough, panting, and inability to lie flat for the last two weeks.

Inquiry examination

The patient had suffered from cough and panting for many years, but with the recent onset of cold weather her complaint had worsened. She had gone to the local hospital for examination, and she had received a diagnosis of chronic geriatric bronchitis, pulmonary emphysema, cardio-pulmonary disease, and cardiac functional insufficiency (Level II-III). Since her biomedical treatment had not brought good results, she requested treatment with Chinese medicine. At the time of the examination, the coughing and panting were quite obvious, and she also presented with the following symptoms: flusteredness and short-ness of breath, inability to lie flat and difficulty going to sleep, profuse clear thin phlegm that was easy to expectorate and contained white froth, and puffy swelling in the lower limbs. Urine was scant, bowels were still regular, but her food intake had diminished and she had no desire for liquids. She suffered from blockage in the stomach duct, slight pain, and nausea and retching.

INSPECTION EXAMINATION

Her complexion was yellowish-white without luster, and her lower eyelids were slightly puffy and swollen. She leaned back when sitting. The phlegm was like clear water and contained white froth. The tongue fur was white and glossy.

LISTENING AND SMELLING EXAMINATION

She was repeatedly coughing with urgent panting; she spoke in a low voice and had intermittent shortness of breath.

PALPATION EXAMINATION

There was glomus and oppression below the heart that resisted heavy pressure, and puffy swelling in both lower limbs that pitted when pressure was applied. All six pulses were slippery and rapid; the inch pulses were fine, slippery, and somewhat stringlike, the right bar pulse was slippery, the left bar stringlike and slippery, and both cubit pulses were sunken, slippery, and slightly stringlike.

PATTERN IDENTIFICATION

I knew that yáng qì was insufficient because her complexion was yellow-ish-white and lacked luster, her voice was low, and the illness was exacerbated by seasonal cold weather. In this elderly patient, yáng became vacuous; the spleen and lung function was depleted, the spleen failed to transform, and the depurative downbearing of the lung was impaired. When damp-cold was not transformed, it engendered phlegm-rheum. Rheum evil ascended and intimidated the heart and lungs; thus, there were symptoms such as cough and panting, hasty breathing, and flusteredness. The patient could not lie flat and had difficulty falling asleep at night. When rheum evil was present, it presented in phlegm that was clear and thin, easy to expectorate, profuse, and contained white froth. When damp evil stagnated, the center burner did not transform; thus, the stomach duct was blocked, and the patient had no desire for fluids. The tongue fur was white and glossy. When damp evil poured downward, it caused water swelling in the lower limbs. Furthermore, when water-rheum intimidated the heart at the same time that chest yáng was devitalized, the water-rheum shot into the lung, and the lung had difficulty with its functions of depurating and downbearing, spreading and transforming. As a result, the lung could not "govern regulation of the waterways or the downward transportation of water to the urinary bladder." Therefore, urine was scant, but water swelling increased daily.

Because both inch pulses appeared fine, slippery, and slightly stringlike, I knew that water-rheum was ascending and intimidating the heart and lung. The stringlike and slippery bar pulses indicated stagnant water-rheum that was not transformed. From the sunken, slippery, and slightly stringlike cubit pulse I knew that water-rheum was amassing in the lower burner and causing water swelling in the lower limbs. The correlation of all four examinations resulted in the diagnosis of phlegm-rheum intimidating the heart and lung.

TREATMENT METHOD

The method of downbearing qì and eliminating phlegm while assisting yáng and transforming rheum to treat root and tip simultaneously is based on these principles: "In acute conditions, treat the tip; in moderate conditions, treat the root"; and "In phlegm-rheum disease, harmonize with warming medicinals."

PRESCRIPTION

The patient received three packets of the following prescription:

chǎo sū zǐ (炒苏子 stir-fried perilla fruit, Perillae Fructus Frictus) 10 g

chǎo lái fú zǐ (炒莱菔子 stir-fried radish seed, Raphani Semen Frictum) 9 g

zhì bàn xià (制半夏 processed pinellia, Pinelliae Rhizoma) 10 g

huà jú hóng (化橘红 Huazhou pomelo rind, Citri Grandis Exocarpium Rubrum) 10 g

zhì gān cǎo (炙甘草 mix-fried licorice, Glycyrrhizae Radix cum Liquido Fricta) 6 g

fú líng (茯苓 poria, Poria) 15 g

zhū líng (猪苓 polyporus, Polyporus) 15 g

guì zhī (桂枝 cinnamon twig, Cinnamomi Ramulus) 8 g

zé xiè (泽泻 alisma, Alismatis Rhizoma) 10 g

zhēn zhū mǔ (珍珠母 mother-of-pearl, Margarita) 30 g (pre-decocted)

huò xiāng (藿香 patchouli, Pogostemonis Herba) 10 g

yán hú suǒ (延胡索 corydalis, Corydalis Rhizoma) 9 g

FORMULA EXPLANATION

This prescription modified three classical formulas: *sān zǐ yǎng qīn tāng* (Three-Seed Filial Devotion Decoction), *èr chén tāng* (Two Matured Ingredients Decoction), and *wǔ líng sǎn* (Poria Five Powder). The chief medicinals are *zǐ sū zǐ* (perilla fruit), which downbears qì and disinhibits the lung to disperse phlegm, and *bàn xià* (pinellia), which fortifies the spleen and dries dampness to transform phlegm.

As support medicinals, *lái fú zǐ* (radish seed) and *jú hóng* (red tangerine peel) regulate qì and eliminate phlegm, and *guì zhī* (cinnamon twig) and *fú líng* (poria) warm yáng and transform rheum.

As assistant medicinals, *zhū líng* (polyporus) and *zé xiè* (alisma) combine with *guì zhī* to transform qì and disinhibit water and thereby reduce swelling; *gān cǎo* (licorice) combines with *bàn xià*, *jú hóng*, and *fú líng* to eliminate phlegm and transform dampness while fortifying and moving the center burner. *Huò xiāng* (patchouli) and *yán hú suǒ* (corydalis) combine with *lái fú zǐ* to regulate the center and transform stagnation and thereby eliminate fullness and dispel pain.

As the courier, *zhēn zhū mǔ* (mother-of-pearl) benefits the heart and subdues yáng; it also settles timidity and quiets the spirit.

Since the stomach duct was blocked and slightly painful, *bái zhú* (white atractylodes) was removed from *wǔ líng sǎn* and *bái jiè zǐ* (white mustard) was removed from *sān zǐ yǎng qīn tāng*. *Huò xiāng* and *yán hú suǒ* were the substitutions. Each of these three formulas has its own particular emphasis, and when combined, they complement each other. Together they are able to downbear qì, eliminate phlegm, assist yáng, and transform rheum; in addition, they are effective for benefiting the heart and quieting the spirit.

FOLLOWUP TREATMENT

<u>Second visit on December 15</u>: After taking the above prescription, the cough and panting were clearly alleviated, phlegm was reduced, urine had increased, and the swelling had dispersed. She was able to lie flat and sleep well. The tongue fur had become thin, and the pulses were slightly slippery and moderate. After taking three more prepared packets of the above-mentioned prescription, her daughter came to inform me that the patient had clearly recovered, but I advised her to take another three packets to strengthen the therapeutic effect. Two weeks later on a follow-up visit, the patient had experienced no recurrence of symptoms.

CASE THREE
DIZZINESS AND INSOMNIA (LOW BLOOD PRESSURE)
眩晕；失眠(低血压)

The patient was a 47-year-old woman whose first examination date was June 8, 1973.

CHIEF COMPLAINT

Dizzy head, insomnia, and low blood pressure for the past two or three years.

INQUIRY EXAMINATION

During this period the patient had often suffered from dizzy head, insomnia, no pleasure in eating, scant food intake, and dry stools, with bowel movements only once every few days.. She had been to several hospitals for treatment, but without results. Her diagnosis was low blood pressure (78/50 mmHg). She had turned to Chinese medicine for diagnosis and treatment and had received and taken many prescription packets of *bǔ zhōng yì qì tāng* (Center-Supplementing Qì-Boosting Decoction), but the symptoms were not relieved and the blood pressure did not rise.

INSPECTION EXAMINATION

She had poor essence-spirit, fatigue, and lack of strength. Moreover, she was agitated. Her development was normal, but she was slightly undernourished, and she had a yellowish facial complexion without luster. The tongue fur was normal; the tongue body was moist without any abnormalities.

LISTENING AND SMELLING EXAMINATION

Her speech and voice were basically normal and her breathing was regular.

PALPATION EXAMINATION

The pulses all appeared slightly fine, but there were no other abnormalities.

PATTERN IDENTIFICATION

"All wind with shaking and dizzy vision is ascribed to the liver." From the symptom of enduring dizziness, I knew that the disease was in the liver. Seeing the yellow complexion, fine pulse, and tendency to agitation, I knew that she suffered from blood vacuity yáng effulgence with liver wind harassing the upper body. Because her blood was vacuous and unable to nourish the heart, the heart spirit could not keep its composure, and insomnia resulted. Liver effulgence damaged the stomach, and the center failed to move and transform, thereby devitalizing the appetite and causing bowel elimination to become dry and scant. The correlation of the four examinations resulted in a diagnosis of dizziness and insomnia due to blood vacuity with liver effulgence.

TREATMENT METHOD

Nourish blood and subdue yáng, emolliate the liver and extinguish wind, and foster the heart and quiet the spirit.

The patient received six to ten packets of the following prescription:

bái sháo yào (白芍药 white peony, Paeoniae Radix Alba) 12 g
shēng lóng gǔ (生龙骨 crude dragon bone, Mastodi Ossis Fossilia Cruda) 24 g (pre-decocted)
shēng mǔ lì (生牡蛎 raw oyster shell, Ostreae Concha Cruda) 24 *g* (pre-decocted)

dāng guī (当归 Chinese angelica, Angelicae Sinensis Radix) 9 g

gōu téng (钩藤 uncaria, Uncariae Ramulus cum Uncis) 21 g

zhēn zhū mǔ (珍珠母 mother-of-pearl, Margarita) 24 g (pre-decocted)

lóng chǐ (龙齿 dragon tooth, Mastodi Dentis Fossilia) 21 g (pre-decocted)

xiāng fù (香附 cyperus, Cyperi Rhizoma) 9 g

chǎo huáng qín (炒黄芩 stir-fried scutellaria, Scutellariae Radix Fricta) 9 g

yuǎn zhì (远志 polygala, Polygalae Radix) 9 g

chái hú (柴胡 bupleurum, Bupleuri Radix) 3 g

gān cǎo (甘草 licorice, Glycyrrhizae Radix) 4.5 g

quán guā lóu (栝楼 whole trichosanthes, Trichosanthis Fructus Totus) 30 g

FORMULA EXPLANATION

The chief medicinals are *bái sháo yào* (white peony), which nourishes the blood and emolliates the liver, and *shēng lóng gǔ* (crude dragon bone) and *shēng mǔ lì* (raw oyster shell), which constrain, absorb, and subdue yáng.

Acting as support medicinals, *dāng guī* (Chinese angelica) supplements blood and nourishes the liver; *gōu téng* (uncaria) calms the liver and extinguishes wind; *xiāng fù* (cyperus) courses the liver and rectifies qì; and *huáng qín* (scutellaria) clears the liver and eliminates heat.

As assistant medicinals, *zhēn zhū mǔ* (mother-of-pearl) and *lóng chǐ* (dragon tooth) foster heart yīn and quiet the heart spirit; *yuǎn zhì* (polygala) promotes heart-kidney interaction; *guā lóu* (trichosanthes) downbears qì and moistens dryness, thereby freeing the intestines; and the sweet nature of *gān cǎo* (licorice) relaxes and regulates the center and harmonizes the stomach.

The courier medicinal, *chái hú* (bupleurum), enters the liver and gallbladder channels and upbears clear qì in the lesser yáng.

FOLLOWUP TREATMENT

<u>Second visit on July 30, 1973</u>: After taking six packets of the above-mentioned prescription, the patient was able to restfully repose at night and the dizziness had disappeared. She continued with the formula and found that her appetite increased and her bowels became normal. After taking 20 more packets, her blood pressure was 100/70 mmHg and her body weight had increased by 9 kilograms. If her work was demanding and she had trouble falling asleep, she would buy several packets of the original formula and take a dose. As soon as she ingested the medicine she was able to sleep normally. Now her essence-spirit was good, and her efficiency at work was clearly enhanced. Her complexion was red and moist, her blood pressure normal, and she seemed to be a different person altogether.

CASE FOUR
LESSER YÁNG (*SHÀO YÁNG*) HEAT DEPRESSION (FEVER OF UNDETERMINED CAUSE)
少阳郁热（发热，原因待查）

The patient was a 30-year-old male, an outpatient from a hospital in Héběi Province; his first examination date was May 29, 1972.

CHIEF COMPLAINT

Frequent recurrence of a body temperature of more than 39 °C, which had lasted for close to two years.

INQUIRY EXAMINATION

For almost two years now, the patient had suffered frequent fever that was always accompanied by coughing of bloody phlegm and a temperature of more than 39 °C. Antibiotic treatment would bring the fever down after two or three days, but seven to ten days later, the fever and coughing of bloody phlegm would return. He would resort to antibiotics again for relief, only to have the cycle repeat itself. This had been his condition for almost two years, and even though he had sought help at the hospital for diagnosis and treatment several times, he still had not recovered. At the time of the first examination he had experienced relief for six to seven days, but had the feeling that the fever was about to return. Each time before the fever occurred, the patient had a slightly cold sensation followed immediately by the onset of the fever which lasted three to four days or sometimes a week. With the exception of the concurrent coughing of bloody phlegm, the patient had few other symptoms. He had been through many chest examinations, but his heart and lungs appeared normal.

INSPECTION EXAMINATION

His development was normal and his nutrition was average, but he had a slightly anxious expression. The tongue body and fur were normal.

LISTENING AND SMELLING EXAMINATION

His speech, voice, and breathing showed no obvious abnormalities.

PALPATION EXAMINATION

The abdominal examination was normal, the liver and spleen were not enlarged, and the pulses were stringlike.

PATTERN IDENTIFICATION

From observing that all six pulses were stringlike and that the fever occurred at set times, I knew that it was a pathocondition of evil seizing lesser yáng. When enduring disease entered the blood, evil was depressed in the blood aspect, where it was blocked and not resolved. During every fever attack, heat evil harassed the blood, and the blood failed to stay in the channels. Because of this, it ascended counterflow, resulting in coughing of blood. The correlation of all four examinations led to a diagnosis of heat depressed in the lesser yáng.

TREATMENT METHOD

Harmonize and resolve lesser yáng, clear heat and cool the blood.

PRESCRIPTION

The patient received three packets of the following prescription, to be taken as a decoction:

> *chái hú* (柴胡 bupleurum, Bupleuri Radix) 22 g
>
> *huáng qín* (黄芩 scutellaria, Scutellariae Radix) 12 g
>
> *bàn xià* (半夏 pinellia, Pinelliae Rhizoma) 9 g
>
> *dǎng shēn* (党参 codonopsis, Codonopsis Radix) 12 g
>
> *dì gǔ pí* (地骨皮 lycium root bark, Lycii Cortex) 12 g
>
> *qīng hāo* (青蒿 sweet wormwood, Artemisiae Annuae Herba) 12 g
>
> *bái wēi* (白薇 black swallowwort, Cynanchi Atrati Radix) 12 g
>
> *shēng dì huáng* (生地黄 dried rehmannia, Rehmanniae Radix Exsiccata) 12 g
>
> *bái jí* (白及 bletilla, Bletillae Rhizoma) 9 g

FORMULA EXPLANATION

This formula uses *chái hú* (bupleurum) to mildly clear, course, and outthrust and to harmonize and resolve lesser yáng. It uses *huáng qín* (scutellaria) to clear heat from the lesser yáng. These two are the chief medicinals.

As support medicinals, *bàn xià* (pinellia) opens binds and downbears counterflow; *dǎng shēn* (codonopsis) supports right qì and thereby assists in expelling evil outwards.

As assistant medicinals, *qīng hāo* (sweet wormwood) clears evil that has already penetrated deeply into the bones and the yīn aspect, and conducts evil to the exterior. *Bái wēi* (black swallowwort) treats fever that occurs at set periods of time. *Dì gǔ pí* (lycium root bark) clears heat, drains lung fire, and suppresses bloody cough. *Shēng dì huáng* (dried rehmannia) cools the blood and boosts yīn, and clears heat and stanches bleeding.

As the courier medicinal, *bái jí* (bletilla) stops lung bleeding and quickens stasis. The entire formula harmonizes and resolves lesser yáng, clears heat, cools blood, and stanches bleeding.

After taking the first packet of medicinals on the morning of May 31, the patient had several bouts of diarrhea. He inquired whether he should continue with the formula. I told him that the medicinals were causing an internal adjustment, that the prescription was not meant as a laxative, and that he should continue with the packets and finish all three of them.

FOLLOWUP TREATMENT

Second visit on June 2:   The patient had finished the three medicinal packets. After taking the medicine he felt that his body was lively. His condition was much improved and the diarrhea had stopped. His essence-spirit had improved, and there had been no further fever attacks for over 10 days. The tongue appeared normal; the stringlike quality of the pulse was abating gradually. I prescribed three more packets of the original formula, with the dosage of *chái hú* reduced to 12 g.

On June 10th, I saw him on the street and inquired about his condition. He said that he had recovered and no longer had the fever.

Third visit on June 27: I went to his home for a follow-up visit. The patient said there had been no recurrence of the fever, and he had no sense that it would return; he went to work as usual and he was healthy and vigorous.

CASE FIVE

MENSTRUAL BLOCK WITH BLOOD STASIS ENGENDERING MACULES (SUBACUTE LUPUS ERYTHEMATOSUS)
经闭, 血瘀生斑(亚急性红斑狼疮)

The patient was a 24-year-old woman whose first examination date was April 15, 1968.

CHIEF COMPLAINT

Butterfly-shaped red macules on her face and a low-grade generalized fever, both of which had continued for more than a year.

INQUIRY EXAMINATION

In the previous year, during her menstrual period, the menses had abruptly stopped when the patient became very angry. Subsequently, butterfly-shaped red macules gradually appeared on her face, and red maculopapular eruptions appeared on top of her nose. The palms of her hands and her elbows were also covered with red macules. At night she experienced vexing heat, heat in the heart of the soles and palms, and a constant low-grade fever (37.2–37.8 °C). She sought diagnosis and treatment at a hospital in Hārbīn where she was diagnosed with lupus erythematosus. She was informed that no effective cure existed, and was given hormones. When she experienced no noticeable results, she sought treatment at another hospital, the Běijīng Chinese Medical Research Institute, where she again received the diagnosis of lupus erythematosus and was given hormone treatment. She returned to Hārbīn and requested a consultation with a Chinese medical doctor. Even though she had been treated many times by both Chinese and Western medical doctors, she had obtained no effective cure. Finally, she came to my hospital in Běijīng for treatment. In addition to the symptoms mentioned above, I found out through inquiry that her menses commonly arrived only once in several months and was extremely scant. Currently, her menstruation was already delayed by seven or eight months.

INSPECTION EXAMINATION

Her face, tip of the nose, and elbows were covered with red macules as described above, and the palms of her hands were red. Her face and the back of her hands had an aversion to sunlight; the macules worsened if she was exposed to sunlight. She had to use an umbrella to block the sun whenever she went outdoors, and in the summertime she did not dare to wear short-sleeved clothing. Her body development and nutrition were both normal.

LISTENING AND SMELLING EXAMINATION

Examination revealed nothing abnormal.

PALPATION EXAMINATION

The pulses were stringlike, fine, and rapid.

PATTERN IDENTIFICATION

The liver governs the storage of blood. Because her episode of anger caused binding depression of liver qì, stored blood failed to descend, and as a result the menses became blocked. Superabundant qì formed fire, and enduring blood stasis formed heat. When the blood contracted heat, it moved frenetically and spilled into and stagnated in the face, nose, and elbows, where it produced red macules. The macules appeared on the yáng brightness (*yáng míng*) area of the body. Yáng brightness governs the flesh, and its channels travel to the face; thus the majority of the red macules appeared on the flesh of the face and elbows. Enduring depressed fire damaged yīn, and yīn vacuity engendered internal heat; thus, at night there was vexing heat in the heart, and the palms and soles generated heat (vexing heat in the five hearts). Yáng brightness is hot in nature; when the flesh was exposed to sunshine, heat existed both internally and externally and the macules worsened. From palpating her stringlike pulse, I knew that she suffered from liver depression. The fine pulse indicated yīn vacuity, and the fine rapid pulse indicated yīn vacuity with internal heat. The correlation of all four examinations led me to diagnose liver depression menstrual block, yīn vacuity with internal heat, and blood stasis producing macules.

TREATMENT METHOD

Nourish yīn and cool the blood, quicken stasis and transform macules, and soothe depression and free the menses.

PRESCRIPTION

> shēng dì huáng (生地黄 dried rehmannia, Rehmanniae Radix Exsiccata) 24 g
>
> xuán shēn (玄参 scrophularia, Scrophulariae Radix) 12 g
>
> chì sháo yào (赤芍药 red peony, Paeoniae Radix Rubra) 15 g
>
> hóng huā (红花 carthamus, Carthami Flos) 9 g
>
> kǔ shēn (苦参 flavescent sophora, Sophorae Flavescentis Radix) 12 g
>
> bái xiān pí (白鲜皮 dictamnus, Dictamni Cortex) 15 g
>
> lián qiáo (连翘 forsythia, Forsythiae Fructus) 15 g
>
> rěn dōng téng (忍冬藤 lonicera stem, Lonicerae Caulis) 24 g
>
> xiāng fù (香附 cyperus, Cyperi Rhizoma) 12 g
>
> qiàn cǎo (茜草 madder, Rubiae Radix) 9 g
>
> liú jì nú (刘寄奴 anomalous artemisia, Artemisiae Anomalae Herba) 5 g
>
> shēng lóng gǔ (生龙骨 crude dragon bone, Mastodi Ossis Fossilia Cruda) 15 g (pre-decocted)
>
> shēng mǔ lì (生牡蛎 raw oyster shell, Ostreae Concha Cruda) 15 g (pre-decocted)
>
> chán tuì (蝉蜕 cicada molting, Cicadae Periostracum) 6 g
>
> shé tuì (蛇蜕 snake slough, Serpentis Periostracum) 2.4 g

The patient was instructed to take one packet per day, decocted in water. If she experienced no side effects, she was to continue, taking 20–30 packets overall. At the same time, she was to take *fáng fēng tōng shèng wán* (Saposhnikovia Sage-Inspired Pill) in an amount sufficient to free her bowel movements but not cause diarrhea, and to course and clear heat and dispel the toxin in the sores.

FORMULA EXPLANATION

The yīn-nourishing blood-cooling medicinals *shēng dì huáng* (dried rehmannia) and *xuán shēn* (scrophularia) are the chief medicinals.

As support medicinals, *chì sháo yào* (red peony), *hóng huā* (carthamus), and *liú jì nú* (anomalous artemisia) quicken stasis and transform macules, and *rěn dōng téng* (lonicera stem) and *lián qiáo* (forsythia) clear heat, resolve toxins, and transform macules and papules.

As assistant medicinals, *xiāng fù* (cyperus) soothes liver depression. *Qiàn cǎo* (madder), together with *hóng huā* and *chì sháo yào*, frees the menses. *Kǔ shēn* (flavescent sophora) and *bái xiān pí* (dictamnus) dispel damp heat that is depressed in the skin. *Lóng gǔ* (dragon bone) and *mǔ lì* (oyster shell) subdue yáng caused by vacuity, thereby treating the vexing heat.

Lastly, *chán tuì* (cicada molting) and *shé tuì* (snake slough) act as courier medicinals by dispersing wind heat and wind toxin from the skin.

FOLLOWUP TREATMENT

All the symptoms were alleviated after the patient took the formula, so she continued with an additional 40 packets. After taking the remaining packets, she went through two menstrual cycles, and the volume and color of the menses were normal. The red macules on the face, hands, and elbows abated. Moreover, the patient was again able to dress in short-sleeved clothing and did not use an umbrella; even when exposed to sunshine the macules on the face and arms did not reappear. She felt that all of the symptoms had completely disappeared. She had discontinued the hormone treatments while taking the Chinese medicinals. I advised her to take six more preparations of the earlier prescription and afterwards take a pill medicine. This pill prescription was the same as the decoction, but with the addition of:

> *qí shé* (蕲蛇 agkistrodon, Agkistrodon) 1.5 g
> *dāng guī* (当归 Chinese angelica, Angelicae Sinensis Radix) 9 g
> *wū zéi gǔ* (乌贼骨 cuttlefish bone, Sepiae Endoconcha) 6 g
> *zhì shān jiǎ* (炙山甲 mix-fried pangolin scales, Manis Squama cum
>   Liquido Fricta) 6 g

The dosage was tripled, and the ingredients were ground into a fine powder and mixed with honey to form pills that weighed 9 grams each. I instructed her to take one pill twice a day with warm boiled water. The patient was pleased and returned to Hārbīn.

In the beginning of February 1969, the patient sent a letter saying that she had finished the pill formula after returning from Běijīng. She said that her periods were arriving regularly every month, and the color and volume were normal. The red macules had not returned. Her life had resumed without problems.

EMPIRICAL KNOWLEDGE

During inspection, pay attention to physical form, spirit, color, tongue, substances, and environment.

"Physical form" refers to the physical appearance and physical condition. "Spirit" refers to the spirit-mind or spirit-affect. "Color" refers to the color of the face, color of the eyes, and the color of macules and rashes. "Tongue" refers to tongue shape (physical appearance), tongue body, and tongue fur. "Substances" refers to any material that is discharged from the body, such as phlegm, urine and excrement, blood, or vomitus. "Environment" refers to the living environment surrounding the patient, such as living conditions, or their physical location (whether they live in the southern or northern regions of the country, for instance).

For example, in the inspection examination in Case 1, "physical form" and "spirit" refer to the appearance of acute pain. In this case, although the patient was fidgety, she did not move freely due to the pain and the severe sub-umbilical swelling. Accordingly, I knew that the abdominal pain was very intense. I also observed exhaustion of the spirit-mind, qì timidity, and low voice, and thus concluded that her condition was severe.

As far as "color" is concerned, I observed in Case 2 that the patient had a yellowish-white complexion without luster. I knew that this was caused by old age, severe illness, and generalized vacuity, and that it tended to cause disease during the cold season. This provided the basis for my diagnosis of yáng vacuity. In Case 5, the patient had red macules that were aggravated by exposure to sunshine, and red macules that appeared on her hands, allowing me to understand that blood heat was involved with the pattern of blood stasis.

Concerning the "tongue," in Case 1 a red tongue indicated that the disease had already influenced the blood aspect. This alerted me to include medicinals such as *dāng guī* (Chinese angelica) and *bái sháo yào* (white peony) in the prescription. From the white tongue fur I also knew that although the disease had lasted ten days, it had not transformed into heat; therefore, I used warm dispersing medicinals as the assistants.

Concerning "substance," I observed white-colored, thin, and slightly foamy phlegm in Case 2. When I combined this knowledge with the inspection of the "physical body," I knew that the disease was caused by cold phlegm water-rheum.

Finally, when looking at the "environment" of the patients, I learned in Case 2 that the patient fell ill during the winter, but lived in the north and had a stove heater that kept the interior of his home warm. So, although the pattern was yáng vacuity phlegm-rheum, it was not necessary to use very acrid or very hot medicinals, but rather it was enough to use acrid warming medicinals such as *zǐ sū zǐ* (perilla fruit), *bàn xià* (pinellia), *jú hóng* (red tangerine peel), and *huò xiāng* (patchouli). Moreover, the use of *guì zhī* (cinnamon twig) assisted yáng and transformed qì. This approach obtained good results.

In listening and smelling examination, pay attention to breathing, sound, odor, and speech.

"Breathing" refers to the way in which the patient breathes, and whether the breath is rough, thin, faint, or weak, and whether panting occurs. "Sound" refers to the quality of the voice, and the sounds made during speaking, breathing, coughing, and groaning. "Odor" refers to flavor, not the flavor of food, but rather the quality of odors. For instance, pay attention to whether the patient's body, nose, mouth, or discharged substances have any peculiar odor. "Speech" refers to speaking; consider whether the speech is distinct and without delirium, stuttering, or incoherence. Also note if the patient talks to himself or speaks not at all.

For example, in Case 1, I knew from the qì timidity and low voice, together with groaning, that the condition of the patient was acute and severe. In Case 2, the patient presented with shortness of breath and panting, and the voice and speech were shallow; therefore, her illness revealed a vacuity pattern.

Of the four examinations, the inquiry examination is especially important.

Clinicians should pay attention to the basic characteristics of Chinese medical diagnosis, which focus on the chief complaint, the presentation of symptoms, and the medical history, constitution, and life-style of the patient. Detailed inquiry into these topics provides substance to analyze when determining treatment based on pattern identification.

In Case 1, the chief complaint was severe pain in the lower abdomen, but I also inquired whether she liked or disliked pressure there and determined whether any concretions, conglomerations, or other pathologic lumps were present. In addition, it was important to inquire whether the patient's dry mouth was accompanied by a desire for liquids, whether she had vexing heat in the five hearts at night, what her bowel movements or food and drink were like, and whether she experienced distention and oppression in the stomach duct after eating. Obtaining this information was relevant to differentiate between vacuity and repletion and between cold and heat.

In Case 2, I inquired into the nature of the chief complaint and found that the phlegm was clear, thin, not sticky, and easy to expectorate. Urine was scant, the stomach duct was blocked and oppressed, and the patient had no desire to drink water. She had experienced nausea and counterflow retching at times, and she had a tendency to contract disease during the cold season. All this information provided a strong basis for identifying patterns to determine treatment and for selecting the appropriate Chinese formula and medicinals. In Case 3, inquiry revealed that the patient had used *bǔ zhōng yì qì tāng* (Center-Supplementing Qì-Boosting Decoction) frequently for a long period of time without results. Moreover, inquiry concerning the bowels revealed that she had infrequent bowel movements and dry stools. Thus, I knew that this was not a case of qì vacuity, but rather one of blood vacuity. In Case 4, I found out that the patient suffered from a slight sensation of cold before the onset of a fever, and that the fever occurred at a set time, with first the cold sensation and then the fever. This information pointed to a diagnosis of depressed heat in the lesser yàng.

In addition to performing diagnostic inquiry according to the specifics of Chinese medicine, you should also understand how to diagnose and treat with modern medicine. Thereby, you will be able to refer to determining treatment on the basis of pattern identification, while at the same time exploring the partial information gained from integrating Chinese and Western medicine. For instance, in Case 1, the patient was diagnosed with "twisted ovarian cyst" and was advised to have surgery, yet by taking Chinese medicinals internally, she recovered. This can provide accumulated experience for non-surgical treatments in the future. At the same time, it can also demonstrate that Chinese medicine is capable not only of treating functional diseases, but can also obtain excellent results when treating organic diseases.

Palpation of the pulse, the head and feet, and the abdomen

In studying diagnostic palpation, we need to pay attention to all the information on palpation found in the basic theory of Chinese medicine. In addition, I think that attention must be paid to two aspects of palpation examination: "head, foot, and abdominal palpation" which means using the hands to examine the entire body by knocking, touching, pressing, and pushing, and "pulse palpation." In the examination of inch, bar, and cubit positions on both hands, it is important to pay attention to the three positions and nine indicators. At each indicator you should wait for more than 50 beats. The duration of time should not be cut short since it is important to diagnose in combination (such as the quality of the left pulse, the quality of the right pulse, or the overall quality of all six pulses), as well as separately (such as the quality of the left inch, left bar, and left cubit pulses, or the quality of the right inch, bar, and cubit pulses).

Generally speaking, you should be proficient in diagnosing the twenty-eight pulses, and among these you should accurately master those pulses most often seen in clinic: floating, sunken, slow, rapid, vacuous, weak, surging, soggy, stringlike, slippery, fine, large, bound, skipping, and intermittent. The remaining pulses can be gradually mastered by practice. To study palpation examination, you must emphasize extensive practical experience and repetition. Only then can you accomplish the ideal of "completing bamboo in the mind" (editor's note: this is a reference to an artist's ability to visualize a complete picture of bamboo in the mind before being able to draw it) and obtain accurate distinction beneath the finger. Furthermore, each pulse finding should be combined with the results of the other three methods of diagnosis; palpation of the pulse alone is not a recommended diagnostic technique.

In Case 2, the patient had a rapid pulse, yet I treated her with warming medicinals. Even though in this analysis the pulse seemed "rapid," it was due to blockage caused by water-rheum affecting the heart and lung, not due to a heat pattern. The patient in Case 1 also had a slightly rapid pulse, which was caused by the severe pain and disquietude in sitting and lying. Here I used a warming and freeing preparation. A further important point is that when the condition of the patient is extremely serious, the physician should not only palpate both hand pulses at the inch, bar, and cubit, but also palpate BL-59 (*fū yáng*) and KI-3 (*tài xī*).

The *fū yáng* pulse (located at the highest point on the instep of the foot) reveals the condition of the stomach qì, and the *tài xī* pulse (located on the foot posterior and slightly inferior to the medial portion of the ankle) reveals the condition of kidney qì. People in ancient times called these the root pulses; when these two pulses were interrupted, the condition was critical and difficult to treat. In the cases mentioned above, the palpation examination provided a very strong basis for determining treatment by pattern identification. For example, abdominal palpation in Case 1 revealed a concretion lump the size of a child's head in the lower abdomen, which was accompanied by aching pain that refused pressure. Thus, I considered this a repletion pattern of qì and blood stoppage. Since the location of the concretion was in the lesser abdomen (the area below the umbilicus), and the pulses were stringlike, I knew that the condition was associated with the liver channel. Since the stringlike quality was especially pronounced in the bar and cubit pulses, I knew that there was severe pain in the lower abdominal area. Also, in Case 2, the puffy swelling in the lower limbs, which pitted when pressure was applied, illustrated the severity of the water-rheum blockage.

During pulse examination, pay careful attention to examination of the pulse "spirit."

Palpation of the pulse is a special characteristic of Chinese medicine. Physicians of the past certainly accumulated an abundance of valuable experience concerning pulse palpation; this experience is vastly supportive when identifying patterns to determine treatment. For this reason physicians should not only carefully differentiate the various pulse images such as floating, sunken, slow, rapid, slippery, rough, vacuous, and replete, but also carefully examine the pulse spirit. Pulse manifestation refers to the image of the pulse beat, its form and structure. Pulse spirit, on the other hand, refers to the spirit-qì, atmosphere, and spirit-affect within the pulse manifestation. For instance, one person may be tall and have a large body, but the essence-spirit might be listless and the eyes without luster. Another person may be short, but the eyes are bright and shining, and the essence-spirit is very good. This is an indication that the essence-spirit or spirit-qì for these two individuals is different. To clearly distinguish the pulse manifestation, just examine the image of the pulse beat, then very carefully investigate the spirit of the pulse manifestation. When this is understood, you can carefully observe and identify the severity of disease and its current condition. When people in ancient times discussed pulse examination, they emphasized that "the pulse is valuable because it has spirit," and "the one who has a lifelike pulse will prosper, the one who has a pulse without spirit will die."

There are two aspects concerning the examination of the pulse spirit that I can discuss from my experience. The first aspect concerns the beat of the pulse manifestation. This should be orderly and not chaotic and feel more or less even in size; it should be strong, but yielding, and soft, but have a root; it should be orderly; it should gently rise and fall and be relaxed; and it should vary in accordance with the climate of the four seasons (for example, in spring it should be stringlike; in summer, surging; in autumn, hair-like; in winter, stone-like). A pulse manifestation such as this is said to have spirit and stomach qì. In a discussion of pulse differentiation, Sūn Guāng-Yù explained it as follows:

> "What is called spirit is the spirit that enriches and engenders stomach qì. Within floating or sunken, slow or rapid pulses, there is a portion that is mixed with spirit qì. This is neither too fast nor too slow. Although disease is unpredictable, all the myriad diseases in the four seasons take stomach qì as their root. In general the pulse is neither large nor small, neither long nor short, neither floating nor sunken, neither rough nor slippery; it moves along smoothly and harmoniously, has a thriving purpose, and is nameless because it is [the same as] stomach qì."

Quoting the *Biàn Zhèng Lù* ("The Record of Pattern Identifications"), the *Mài Xué Jí Yāo* ("Complied Essentials of Pulse Theory") explains:

"When examining the pulse, you must observe whether it has spirit or not; this is the true secret to success. How do you distinguish whether or not the pulse has spirit? Regardless of whether a pulse is floating or sunken, slow or rapid, rough or slippery, large or small, when you press down, if it is arranged neatly and follows an orderly sequence, this indicates utmost spiritedness. If you press and it is full and has force, this is next in spiritedness. As for other pulses, if the pulse is very lightly agitated when pressed, this also means that it has spirit. A pulse that lacks spirit may be scattered and chaotic when pressed. It may be sometimes present and sometimes not, or may arrive with force, but leave without force. It may be present with light touch but expired and absent with heavy touch. A pulse that lacks spirit may be continuous, then interrupted, or verging on continuity but unable [to be continuous]. It may verge on being palpable yet [its quality] cannot be obtained. A sunken fine pulse may suddenly manifests as vague, or a surging large [pulse may become] dimly discernible. When a pulse gets to the point where it has no spirit, this is a condition to be dreaded."

The second aspect refers to the tranquility (yīn) or agitation (yáng) of the spirit qì and the atmosphere within the pulse. Generally speaking, if the spirit qì is agitated and disquieted when the pulse arrives, continue to carefully monitor the treatment because the condition of the patient is not yet stabilized, and the illness may continue to pass to the next channel or to the interior, or may relapse or recur. Consider, for example, the patient with a high fever. Even if the body temperature has dropped from 39 °C to 36 °C, as long as the pulse spirit is still agitated, rapid, urgent, tense, and not tranquil, the high fever will most likely return in the afternoon or on the next day. If the high fever has abated, and the examination reveals that the pulse spirit is also peaceful and tranquil, then there is little chance that the fever will recur. The famous Hàn Dynasty physician, Zhāng Zhòng-Jǐng pointed this out long ago in the *Shāng Hán Lùn* ("On Cold Damage"):

"On the first day of cold damage, greater yáng (*tài yáng*) contracts [the disease]. If the pulse is tranquil, this means no passage [to the interior]. A strong desire to vomit, agitation and vexation, and a rapid and urgent pulse [agitation and not tranquility] indicate passage."

Later generations of physicians commonly used the saying, "tranquil pulse and cool body" to describe the condition of heat disease moving toward recovery. So, we can see that very careful examination of the pulse spirit greatly assists the diagnosis, treatment, prognosis, and prevention of disease. To be truly able to identify patterns when determining treatment, the clinician must carefully differentiate the pulse manifestations and carefully examine the changes of the pulse spirit simultaneously. The understanding and mastery of the pulse spirit can only be grasped firmly over time on the basis of long-term personal experience.

Pay attention to the correlation of all four examinations.

Although palpation of the pulse is a unique characteristic of Chinese medicine, it will not lead to comprehensive pattern identification for determining treatment when it is used alone. There are times when the pulse manifestation and the condition of the patient coincide, and other times when they do not. Take the information obtained from inspection, listening and smelling, inquiry, and palpation (the four examinations) and use it as mutual reference or support to carefully identify symptoms. Only then can you clearly identify patterns, and on the basis of this, determine the correct treatment method, select the correct formulas and medicinals, and obtain prompt recovery from illness. It is exactly as the Míng dynasty physician, Zhāng Jǐng-Yuè, explained:

> "Whenever you encounter something doubtful that is difficult to bring into the light, you must use the method of the four examinations. Inquire in detail about the disease cause, while at the same time identify the sound and complexion of the patient. If you just rectify the order between root and tip, and earlier and later conditions, everything else will fall into place. But if you do not observe this and only use one diagnosis as evidence, you will act spontaneously and will treat in confusion. How could you know which of the pulse signs are most true or false? When you observe some that are not true, how can you verify that they are not false? For a person who constantly practices diagnosis, knowing this is extremely easy, but for a beginner, determining this is of utmost difficulty. This is the reason you should not disregard the four examinations. In the *Nàn Jīng* ("Classic of Difficult Issues"), palpation occupies the final place in the four examinations since its meaning is profound."

In clinic, the four examinations must confirm each other as a precondition for identifying symptoms and patterns comprehensively; then you are able to compare the results to comprehensively identify the disease. Physicians in the past have referred to this kind of diagnosis as "the correlation of the four examinations," "the mutual reference of the four examinations," and "the correlation of pulse and disease." This is very important in identifying patterns to determine treatment. Sometimes in clinic when examining and treating illness, the pulse takes precedence over the pathocondition, but typically this occurs only under special circumstances and is decided only after first proceeding with the correlation of the four examinations. Do not ever emphasize the precedence of the pulse over the pathocondition, or use it as a pretext for disregarding the correlation of the four examinations. In summary, when studying the four examinations, they can be learned separately, but when they are applied in clinic, you must always correlate the proof from each of the four examinations and integrate them tightly. This is extremely important when identifying patterns to determine treatment in clinic.

CHAPTER TWO

Chinese medical theory is the solid foundation of "pattern identification as the basis for determining treatment."

The concrete actualization of pattern identification as a basis for determining treatment in the clinic involves four aspects: principles, methods, formulas, and medicinals. The most important of these is principle. "Principle" means the application of Chinese medical theory to the relevant information that has been obtained through the four examinations, in order to draw analytical conclusions and identify disease patterns. This lays the foundation for the next steps of establishing a method, determining a formula, and selecting medicinals. When discussed separately, principle refers to Chinese medicine theory, but when discussed in context, it penetrates through these other three aspects; namely, establishing methods, determining formulas, and selecting medicinals. Thus principles, methods, formulas, and medicinals are not completely separate issues. You must study and scrutinize Chinese medical theory in depth to improve your proficiency of identifying patterns when determining treatment. To illustrate this point, I present my personal experience with five case studies.

CASE STUDIES

CASE ONE
ENURESIS DURING SLEEP
睡中遗尿

The patient was a 22-year-old male who was a driver in a factory in Běijīng. The date of his first examination was March 7, 1975.

CHIEF COMPLAINT

Enuresis occurring every night during sleep.

INQUIRY EXAMINATION

For 20 years, he had been wetting his bed every night during sleep, in extreme cases even twice a night. Since he hung the soiled bedding out to dry in the courtyard every day, all the neighbors had nicknamed him "Mr. Urine-Stink." He often slept on a board to avoid soiling the bed sheets. He had tried Chinese medicinals and Western drugs numerous times, as well as therapies like acupuncture and moxibustion, but all methods of treatment had been ineffective. At the time of the initial examination, besides the nocturnal enuresis once or twice a night, he experienced aching lumbus, fear of wind, and a liking for warmth.

INSPECTION EXAMINATION

His development was average; his spirit-mind was clear. His complexion as well as tongue body and fur showed no abnormalities.

LISTENING AND SMELLING EXAMINATION

His speech was clear and his breathing was normal.

PALPATION EXAMINATION

His head and face, abdomen, and limbs appeared normal. The left cubit pulse was slightly sunken and the right cubit pulse was relatively weak. Neurological examination revealed no particular results; knee, heel, and anal reflexes were normal, and the buttocks had no feeling of obstruction.

PATTERN IDENTIFICATION

The urinary bladder is the receptacle that holds urine. The kidney stands in interior-exterior relationship with the urinary bladder and is in charge of the opening and closing of the urinary and bowel passages. When the kidney is vacuous, the urinary bladder loses its control over opening and closing. Thus, during sleep, enuresis occurs. For this patient, the left cubit pulse was sunken and the right cubit weak. Considering this in conjunction with his symptoms of lumbar pain, fear of wind, liking of warmth, and fear of cold, I diagnosed kidney channel vacuity cold and urinary bladder loss of control over opening and closing.

TREATMENT METHOD

Warm and supplement kidney yáng, and secure and contain the lower origin.

PRESCRIPTION

The prescription was a modified combination of two formulas: *jīn guì shèn qì wán* (Golden Coffer Kidney Qì Pill) and *suō quán wán* (Stream-Reducing Pill) as follows:

shú dì huáng (熟地黄 cooked rehmannia, Rehmanniae Radix Praeparata)
   25 g

sāng piāo xiāo (桑螵蛸 mantis egg-case, Mantidis Ootheca) 12 g

zhì fù piàn (制附片 sliced processed aconite, Aconiti Radix Lateralis
   Praeparata Secta) 6 g

ròu guì (肉桂 cinnamon bark, Cinnamomi Cortex) 5 g

yín yáng huò (淫羊藿 epimedium, Epimedii Herba) 12 g

yì zhì rén (益智仁 alpinia, Alpiniae Oxyphyllae Fructus) 9 g

wū yào (乌药 lindera, Linderae Radix) 12 g

fù pén zǐ (覆盆子 rubus, Rubi Fructus) 12 g

xù duàn (续断 dipsacus, Dipsaci Radix) 12 g

suǒ yáng (锁阳 cynomorium, Cynomorii Herba) 12 g

sāng jì shēng (桑寄生 mistletoe, Loranthi seu Visci Ramus) 30 g

jī nèi jīn (鸡内金 gizzard lining, Galli Gigeriae Endothelium Corneum)
   12 g

FORMULA EXPLANATION

As chief medicinals, this prescription used *shú dì huáng* (cooked rehmannia), *fù piàn* (sliced processed aconite), and *ròu guì* (cinnamon bark), from *jīn guì shèn qì wán* (Golden Coffer Kidney Qì Pill) to warm and supplement kidney yáng, and *sāng piāo xiāo* (mantis egg-case) from *suō quán wán* (Stream-Reducing Pill) to supplement the kidney and reduce urine.

As support medicinals, *yín yáng huò* (epimedium) warms and assists kidney yáng, and *wū yào* (lindera) and *fù pén zǐ* (rubus) warm and normalize the urinary bladder cold qì and supplement the kidney to reduce urine.

The assistant medicinals, *xù duàn* (dipsacus), *yì zhì rén* (alpinia), *sāng jì shēng* (mistletoe), and *suǒ yáng* (cynomorium) supplement the liver and kidney, dry spleen dampness, invigorate the sinews and bones, and secure the lower origin.

The courier medicinal, *jī nèi jīn* (gizzard lining), enters the urinary bladder and checks enuresis.

FOLLOWUP TREATMENT

<u>Second visit on March 31</u>: For some reason, the patient had not been able to take all the medicine that I had prescribed on the previous visit, and up to this time he had only taken six packets. The frequency of the bedwetting episodes had lessened, but enuresis still occurred once or twice a week. The aching pain in the lumbus was still present, and the tongue and pulse signs remained unchanged. I again gave him the above-mentioned prescription and advised him to continue to take the packets according to my instructions.

Third visit on July 3: Altogether, the patient had taken 48 packets of the above prescription. He had not experienced any bed-wetting incidences for almost three months. The lumbar pain was alleviated and occurred only during cloudy weather or when lifting a heavy load. When he was excessively overworked or tired, the enuresis would recur. He was vigorous and healthy, and full of self-confidence. Since he and his parents had not seen any results after undergoing so many treatments, they had lost all hope that this condition could be treated. With his recovery his entire family was overjoyed. He slept very well without incident on the bedding, but sometimes had many dreams. His stomach was also more comfortable than before and his appetite was good. The tongue tip was a little red and the pulse was slightly stringlike, more pronounced on the left side than on the right. Given the many years that he had been assailed by dampness from the urine (i.e., sleeping in wet bedding), I added *bái zhú* (white atractylodes) and *wēi líng xiān* (clematis) to the basic prescription to dispel damp evil. The patient received 10–20 packets of this prescription:

> *shú dì huáng* (熟地黄 cooked rehmannia, Rehmanniae Radix Praeparata) 25 g
>
> *sāng piāo xiāo* (桑螵蛸 mantis egg-case, Mantidis Ootheca) 12 g
>
> *zhì fù piàn* (制附片 sliced processed aconite, Aconiti Radix Lateralis Praeparata Secta) 6 g
>
> *ròu guì* (肉桂 cinnamon bark, Cinnamomi Cortex) 5 g
>
> *yín yáng huò* (淫羊藿 epimedium, Epimedii Herba) 12 g
>
> *xù duàn* (续断 dipsacus, Dipsaci Radix) 15 g
>
> *fù pén zǐ* (覆盆子 rubus, Rubi Fructus) 12 g
>
> *wū yào* (乌药 lindera, Linderae Radix) 12 g
>
> *suǒ yáng* (锁阳 cynomorium, Cynomorii Herba) 12 g
>
> *yì zhì rén* (益智仁 alpinia, Alpiniae Oxyphyllae Fructus) 9 g
>
> *sāng jì shēng* (桑寄生 mistletoe, Loranthi seu Visci Ramus) 30 g
>
> *jī nèi jīn* (鸡内金 gizzard lining, Galli Gigeriae Endothelium Corneum) 12 g
>
> *bái zhú* (白朮 white atractylodes, Atractylodis Macrocephalae Rhizoma) 6 g
>
> *wēi líng xiān* (威灵仙 clematis, Clematidis Radix) 9 g

Fourth visit, October 1975: He had completely recovered from his illness after taking 10 packets of the above prescription. His body was healthy and strong, he had returned to work as usual, and he had experienced no relapse.

CASE TWO
COUGHING BLOOD (HEMOPTYSIS) (BRONCHIECTASIS)
咳血(支气管扩张)

The patient was a 41-year-old male whose first examination date was June 14, 1968.

CHIEF COMPLAINT

Coughing of blood for the last seven to eight days.

INQUIRY EXAMINATION

The patient had been suffering from cough and expectoration of phlegm for more than ten years and had visited several hospitals during that time. In each case, he had received the diagnosis of bronchiectasis, without ever having undergone a bronchography. During the last seven to eight days, the coughing and expectoration of phlegm had not only worsened, but had developed into coughing of blood. Every morning the phlegm was streaked with blood, and every evening the patient coughed up a great amount of bright red blood. Each time he coughed up blood, the amount would fill half a spittoon, and sometimes he fainted afterwards. Even though he had undergone numerous treatments, none of them had been able to stop the bleeding.

Since the onset of the hemoptysis, he had been forced to go to the emergency room of the local hospital and had stayed there overnight. Every time he had coughed a large amount of blood, the hospital had administered an adrenosin injection (a drug to stop bleeding) and an intravenous hormone drip to the posterior lobe of the pituitary gland. After the coughing spell, he had vacuity sweating, but later was able to fall asleep. However, on the next morning upon awakening there would again be blood present in the phlegm. During the daytime he experienced no particular problem with coughing blood, but when evening came, he again coughed up a large amount of blood and had to go to the emergency room for the pituitary hormone injection and other drugs before he was able to sleep calmly. In this way, he had been forced to spend the past 7-8 days in the emergency room of the hospital.

Finally, he admitted himself to the outpatient clinic at my hospital for consultation. At the time of the initial examination, the patient complained that his body was limp and aching and that his mouth was numb. He had no appetite and suffered from abnormally dry stools.

INSPECTION EXAMINATION

His physical development was excellent, and his nutrition was normal. He was quick-tempered and appeared anxious, but his posture and movements appeared normal. The tongue fur was thick and white, but yellow on the surface. The phlegm color was yellowish-white.

LISTENING AND SMELLING EXAMINATION

His speech was clear, his voice normal, and the cough was loud and sonorous.

PALPATION EXAMINATION

His neck and chest appeared normal. The pulse on the left was stringlike and rapid; the right inch pulse was surging, large and rapid, and the right bar and cubit pulses were stringlike and rapid.

PATTERN IDENTIFICATION

Zhū Dān-Xī proposed, "If coughing with phlegm comes first and you see blood afterwards, then usually [it is a pattern of] phlegm accumulating heat." Relating this to the patient at hand, he suffered from a constitutional cough and had recently begun coughing blood incessantly. The expectorated blood was bright red in color, the phlegm was slightly yellowish, the tongue fur was yellow, the stools were dry, the cough itself was loud and sonorous, and the pulse was stringlike, rapid, and forceful. From this, I knew that this was a pattern of repletion heat. The fact that the patient suffered every evening from a severe attack of coughing blood was a sign of heat in the blood aspect and blood heat engendering fire. Since fire by nature flames upward, it distressed the upper body and affected the lung, so the lung lost its ability to depurate. Lung heat and qì counterflow caused blood to follow the qì upward, and frenetic movement of hot blood led to the bloody cough. The surging, large, and rapid inch pulse on the right hand indeed indicated a lung heat pattern. The correlation of the four examinations supported the diagnosis of frenetic movement of hot blood, blood spillage distressing the lung, and impaired depurative downbearing of the lung.

TREATMENT METHOD

Cool blood, clear heat, and downbear qì, assisted by quickening stasis and stanching bleeding.

PRESCRIPTION

I gave the patient three packets of the following prescription to be decocted in water:

> shēng dì huáng (生地黄 dried rehmannia, Rehmanniae Radix Exsiccata) 13 g
> shēng dà huáng (生大黄 raw rhubarb, Rhei Radix et Rhizoma Crudi) 6 g
> shēng shí gāo (生石膏 raw gypsum, Gypsum Crudum) 47 g (pre-decocted)

chǎo huáng qín (炒黄芩 stir-fried scutellaria, Scutellariae Radix Fricta)
    12 g

zhī zǐ tàn (栀子炭 charred gardenia, Gardeniae Fructus Carbonisatus) 9 g

xuán fù huā (旋覆花 inula flower, Inulae Flos) 9 g (wrapped in cloth)

jiāo bīng láng (焦槟榔 scorch-fried areca, Arecae Semen Ustum) 12 g

tiān mén dōng (天门冬 asparagus, Asparagi Radix) 12 g

máo gēn tàn (茅根炭 charred imperata, Imperatae Rhizoma) 15 g

ǒu jié tàn (藕节炭 charred lotus root node, Nelumbinis Rhizomatis
    Nodus Carbonisatus) 15 g

bái jí (白及 bletilla, Bletillae Rhizoma) 9 g

hé yè tàn (荷叶炭 charred lotus leaf, Nelumbinis Folium Carbonisatum)
    12 g

dāng guī tàn (当归炭 charred tangkuei, Angelicae Sinensis Radix
    Carbonisata) 9 g

hóng huā (红花 carthamus, Carthami Flos) 6 g

mǔ dān pí (牡丹皮 moutan, Moutan Cortex) 6 g

niú xī (牛膝 achyranthes, Achyranthis Bidentatae Radix) 9 g

FORMULA EXPLANATION

The chief medicinals in the formula are *shēng dì huáng* (dried rehmannia), which is sweet and cold and cools the blood, and *shēng dà huáng* (raw rhubarb), which, being bitter and cold, drains fire and heat from the blood aspect.

As support medicinals, *shēng shí gāo* (raw gypsum), stir-fried *huáng qín* (scutellaria), and charred *shān zhī zǐ* (gardenia) clear both qì and blood.

Acting as assistant medicinals, *xuán fù huā* (inula flower) and *jiāo bīng láng* (scorch-fried areca) downbear qì and cause phlegm-fire to follow qì downward. *Tiān mén dōng* (asparagus) enriches yīn, clears heat, and down-bears fire. *Ǒu jié tàn* (charred lotus root node), *hé yè tàn* (charred lotus leaf), *máo gēn tàn* (charred imperata), and *dāng guī tàn* (charred tangkuei) are medicinals that stanch bleeding and thereby treat the tip of the disease. *Hóng huā* (carthamus) and *mǔ dān pí* (moutan) dispel stasis and engender new blood, while simultaneously preventing the blood-stanching medicinals from engendering blood stasis.

As couriers, *bái jí* (bletilla) enters the lung, dispels stasis, and stanches bleeding while simultaneously being able to engender flesh and astringe, and *niú xī* (achyranthes) enters the blood aspect and drives counterflow ascending blood downward.

Followup treatment

Second visit, June 17: After the previous visit, on the very day of starting the Chinese medicinals, the patient went to the local hospital emergency room as had become his custom to spend the night. However, on that particular night he did not present with the bloody cough and therefore did not receive the drug injections. For three days after that, he did not suffer a single attack of hemoptysis, and he did not spend another night at the hospital. At the time of the second visit, he said that there were only occasionally small flecks of blood in the phlegm. The tongue fur was still yellow on the surface, and the pulse was still stringlike and rapid, but the right inch pulse was no longer surging and large. The medicinals had already produced results, so I gave him an only slightly modified prescription.

I added 9 g of *shēng dì huáng* (dried rehmannia) and 12 g of charred *shān zhī zǐ* (gardenia) to the original formula to strengthen the effect of clearing and draining blood heat. I removed *dāng guī tàn* (charred tangkuei) to avoid promoting heat with an acrid warm medicinal. I also added 12 grams each of *xuán shēn* (scrophularia) and *mài mén dōng* (ophiopogon) to enhance the yīn-enriching, blood-cooling, and fire-draining ability of the formula. In combination with *shēng dì huáng* (dried rehmannia) and *tiān mén dōng* (asparagus), these medicinals not only cool blood, but also supplement yīn that has sustained damage from coughing blood. In this way, the prescription not only dispels evil but supports right. I gave the patient three to five additional packets.

Third visit, June 22: By the time the patient had finished three packets, the coughing of blood had completely stopped. After taking two more packets, the patient's spirit and physical strength had clearly improved and the cough was also clearly alleviated. He had been able to return to work. The patient himself felt that he had recovered and intended to take several more packets of the prescription, but now was engaged in business travel; thus, he requested a pill form of the prescription instead of the decoction so that he could maintain his dosage while traveling. At this time he still had some throat pain. The tongue fur was no longer yellow and had changed to thin white, but the pulse was still rather rapid. I continued with the blood-cooling, heat-clearing, and yīn-nourishing method and prepared the following prescription for him:

> *shēng dì huáng* (生地黄 dried rehmannia, Rehmanniae Radix Exsiccata)
>   21 g
>
> *xuán shēn* (玄参 scrophularia, Scrophulariae Radix) 15 g
>
> *tiān mén dōng* (天门冬 asparagus, Asparagi Radix) 9 g
>
> *mài mén dōng* (麦门冬 ophiopogon, Ophiopogonis Radix) 9 g
>
> *shēng shí gāo* (生石膏 raw gypsum, Gypsum Crudum) 60 g (pre-decocted)
>
> *zhī mǔ* (知母 anemarrhena, Anemarrhenae Rhizoma) 9 g

huáng qín (黄芩 scutellaria, Scutellariae Radix) 12 g

zhī zǐ tàn (栀子炭 charred gardenia, Gardeniae Fructus Carbonisatus) 12 g

bǎn lán gēn (板蓝根 isatis root, Isatidis Radix) 9 g

sāng bái pí (桑白皮 mulberry root bark, Mori Cortex) 9 g

dì gǔ pí (地骨皮 lycium root bark, Lycii Cortex) 9 g

bái jí (白及 bletilla, Bletillae Rhizoma) 9 g

ǒu jié (藕节 lotus root node, Nelumbinis Rhizomatis Nodus) 15 g

chì sháo yào (赤芍药 red peony, Paeoniae Radix Rubra) 9 g

mǔ dān pí (牡丹皮 moutan, Moutan Cortex) 6 g

The patient received three to five packets of this prescription. In addition, he received 14 pills of *hé yè wān* (Lotus Leaf Pill) and was instructed to take one pill twice a day in warm, boiled water after taking the decoction. The patient had a follow-up visit in September 1968. He had long ago recovered, he was working regularly, and no relapse of coughing blood had occurred.

CASE THREE

INVERTED MENSTRUATION (CEREBRAL ARTERIO-VENOUS DEFORMITY)
倒经（脑动、静脉血管畸型）

The patient was a 16-year-old female student who was an in-patient at a Běijīng hospital. The consultation date was August 10, 1973.

CHIEF COMPLAINT

Headache, nosebleed, and stupor (subarachnoid hemorrhage), from which she had been resuscitated through emergency measures.

INQUIRY EXAMINATION

Earlier in the year on February 9, when the patient got up in the morning, she had experienced a sudden headache and unclear mental state. She was admitted to the emergency room of the hospital where a lumbar puncture was performed to examine the cerebrospinal fluid. The diagnosis was subarachnoid hemorrhage and intracranial vascular deformity with an unknown etiology. Because of concerns about the results of the cerebral angiography, she remained in the hospital for 54 days. After her subjective symptoms were eliminated, she was released on April 4. She appeared to be doing well at that time. At the end of May, the patient experienced emotional excitement, too much activity, and not enough rest, and on June 1 suffered a fever of 37.5-38°C. An examination at a neighborhood hospital revealed no unusual findings. Then during afternoon naps on June 2 and 3, she experienced distention and pain in the head and vomiting, which became progressively worse. She again came to the emergency room on June 4, where she received another lumbar puncture. The diagnosis was "relapse of subarachnoid hemorrhage," and the patient was admitted to the hospital for the second time.

During her hospitalization, she twice underwent a cerebral angiography; the diagnosis was cerebral arterio-venous deformity located at the temporo-parietal and occipital regions on the right side and at the occipital region on the left. The surgeon with the department of cerebral surgery said that performing surgery would be too dangerous because the venous deformity affected both sides of the head, the affected area was deeply set on the midline in the area of the cerebral ganglion, and the artery in question was located in the cerebrum. Such a procedure therefore could critically disable the patient, especially by impacting the cerebral ganglionic region. Under these circumstances, he refused to perform the surgery. He recommended to emphasize prevention and to avoid further bleeding by controlling blood pressure levels. Nevertheless, he stated that even with precautions, bleeding might recur anyway, and that she could possibly develop epilepsy or paralysis of the body and limbs in the future. The physician related the seriousness of the condition to the family members, who in turn requested a Chinese medical consultation.

At this time, she was completely bed-ridden. Her condition had stabilized more than two months ago, and, although her spirit-mind was clear, she was still unable to sit up, take nourishment, get out of bed, or move around or engage in physical activities. According to her mother, her menses had been overdue both times the illness had erupted, and she had in the past experienced nosebleeds when her menses were supposed to arrive. At the time of the last occurrence in June, her menses had not arrived for two months. Also at that time, the patient had complained of a cold sensation at the back of her brain that had caused stiffness in her neck, a cold sensation in her spine and back, followed by a headache (in the back of the head and to the left side of the head and neck), vomiting, and nosebleed. This had gradually led to unconsciousness, so they had taken her to the hospital for diagnosis and treatment.

INSPECTION EXAMINATION

Her facial complexion was blue-greenish white, she was completely bed-ridden, and her essence-spirit was devitalized. The tongue body was red and the tongue fur was normal.

LISTENING AND SMELLING EXAMINATION

Her speech was clear and distinct, but her voice was low.

PALPATION EXAMINATION

The left inch pulse was weak and the remaining pulses were sunken. There were no other abnormalities.

PATTERN IDENTIFICATION

The back of the head is associated with the foot greater yáng (*tài yáng*) urinary bladder channel. The foot greater yáng urinary bladder channel stands in interior-exterior relationship with the lesser yīn (*shào yīn*) kidney channel. The back of the head is also associated with the governing vessel (*dū mài*). The governing vessel and the kidney channel are connected to each other, as well as to the thoroughfare (*chōng*) and controlling (*rèn*) vessels. The *Huáng Dì Nèi Jīng* ("The Yellow Emperor's Inner Canon") states, "When a woman is two times seven (fourteen years of age), the menarche occurs. The controlling vessel is free and the great thoroughfare vessel becomes exuberant. The menses descend at their time, and she can bear children."

This patient's menses had not been able to descend at the correct time. Moreover, the headache, vomiting, and nosebleed were caused by qì ascending counterflow in the thoroughfare (*chōng*) and controlling (*rèn*) vessels with failed downbearing of turbid yīn. All these factors indicated a pattern of inverted menstruation.

TREATMENT METHOD

Free the menses and quicken the blood, assisted by boosting the liver and kidney.

PRESCRIPTION

The patient received six packets of the following prescription:

dāng guī (当归 Chinese angelica, Angelicae Sinensis Radix) 12 g

chuān xiōng (川芎 chuanxiong, Chuanxiong Rhizoma) 9 g

chì sháo yào (赤芍药 red peony, Paeoniae Radix Rubra) 15 g

shēng dì huáng (生地黄 dried rehmannia, Rehmanniae Radix Exsiccata) 15 g

qiàn cǎo (茜草 madder, Rubiae Radix) 12 g

qiāng huó (羌活 notopterygium, Notopterygii Rhizoma et Radix) 3 g

niú xī (牛膝 achyranthes, Achyranthis Bidentatae Radix) 9 g

táo rén (桃仁 peach kernel, Persicae Semen) 9 g

xiāng fù (香附 cyperus, Cyperi Rhizoma) 9 g

hóng huā (红花 carthamus, Carthami Flos) 6 g

liú jì nú (刘寄奴 anomalous artemisia, Artemisiae Anomalae Herba) 9 g

bái máo gēn (白茅根 imperata, Imperatae Rhizoma) 24 g

The patient also received 14 pills of *dà huáng zhè chóng wán* (Rhubarb and Ground Beetle Pill) and was instructed to take one pill twice a day.

FORMULA EXPLANATION

Dāng guī (Chinese angelica) and *chuān xiōng* (chuanxiong) are the chief medicinals in this prescription; they nourish the blood and free the menses.

As support medicinals, *chì sháo yào* (red peony), *qiàn cǎo* (madder), *táo rén* (peach kernel), and *hóng huā* (carthamus) quicken stasis and move the blood, thereby helping the chief medicinals to free the menses.

As an assistant medicinal, *shēng dì huáng* (dried rehmannia) matches chief medicinal *dāng guī* (Chinese angelica) in nourishing the liver and kidney, thereby transforming and engendering essence and blood. Moreover, in combination with *chuān xiōng* (chuanxiong) and *chì sháo yào* (red peony), it regulates the thoroughfare (*chōng*) and controlling (*rèn*) vessels and consequently frees the menses. Together with *niú xī* (achyranthes), it frees the menses by conducting blood downward. *Xiāng fù* (cyperus) moves the qì of the twelve channels while simultaneously entering the blood aspect, thus moving qì and quickening blood. *Liú jì nú* (anomalous artemisia) quickens stasis and moves blood; *bái máo gēn* (imperata) cools blood and stops nosebleed.

As the courier, *qiāng huó* (notopterygium) enters the greater yáng channel and governing vessel and works in combination with *niú xī* (achyranthes); because *qiāng huó* has an upbearing effect and *niú xi* has a downbearing effect, the former ascends the clear and the latter downbears the turbid.

Together, all these medicinals create a formula that frees the menses and quickens the blood, and nourishes the liver and boosts the kidney. I also added *dà huáng zhè chóng wán* as a supplement to flush away the amassed and static dry bound blood and to dispel phlegm and engender new blood, thereby further freeing the menses.

FOLLOWUP TREATMENT

<u>Second visit, August 17</u>: After taking the prescribed medicinals, the patient could already sit up and talk with her ward mate in the hospital room. She was able to sit very well and to get up and stand for a while. The menses had still not arrived. The tongue fur and tongue body appeared normal, but the pulse was sunken, slippery, and rapid. I made modifications to the original prescription as follows:

dāng guī wěi (当归尾 tangkuei tail, Angelicae Sinensis Radicis
  Extremitas) 12 g
chuān xiōng (川芎 chuanxiong, Chuanxiong Rhizoma) 9 g
chì sháo yào (赤芍药 red peony, Paeoniae Radix Rubra) 15 g

táo rén (桃仁 peach kernel, Persicae Semen) 9 g

hóng huā (红花 carthamus, Carthami Flos) 9 g

niú xī (牛膝 achyranthes, Achyranthis Bidentatae Radix) 15 g

qiàn cǎo (茜草 madder, Rubiae Radix) 30 g

hǎi piāo xiāo (海螵蛸 cuttlefish bone, Sepiae Endoconcha) 9 g

jiǔ dà huáng (酒大黄 wine-processed rhubarb, Rhei Radix et Rhizoma
  cum Vino Preparati) 6 g

sū mù (苏木 sappan, Sappan Lignum) 30 g

zé lán (泽兰 lycopus, Lycopi Herba) 12 g

xiāng fù (香附 cyperus, Cyperi Rhizoma) 12 g

The patient received six packets of this prescription. I also gave her twelve pills of *dà huáng zhè chóng wán* to be taken in the same dosage as before.

<u>Third visit, August 24</u>: Her menses had arrived on the day after starting the above-mentioned formula. All the subjective symptoms were relieved, but I again modified the prescription and gave her six more packets:

dāng guī wěi (当归尾 tangkuei tail, Angelicae Sinensis Radicis
  Extremitas) 12 g

chuān xiōng (川芎 chuanxiong, Chuanxiong Rhizoma) 4.5 g

bái sháo yào (白芍药 white peony, Paeoniae Radix Alba) 12 g

shēng dì huáng (生地黄 dried rehmannia, Rehmanniae Radix Exsiccata)
  12 g

qiàn cǎo (茜草 madder, Rubiae Radix) 6 g

hóng huā (红花 carthamus, Carthami Flos) 4.5 g

táo rén (桃仁 peach kernel, Persicae Semen) 6 g

xiāng fù (香附 cyperus, Cyperi Rhizoma) 9 g

bái máo gēn (白茅根 imperata, Imperatae Rhizoma) 15 g

shí chāng pú (石菖蒲 acorus, Acori Tatarinowii Rhizoma) 6 g

niú xī (牛膝 achyranthes, Achyranthis Bidentatae Radix) 9 g

zhǐ qiào (ké) (枳壳 bitter orange, Aurantii Fructus) 9 g

qiāng huó (羌活 notopterygium, Notopterygii Rhizoma et Radix) 4.5 g

<u>Fourth visit, August 31</u>: The menses had arrived smoothly and without inhibition and concluded normally after seven days. The patient had no headache or dizziness; in general her condition was very good. By August 25th and 26th, she could get up from bed and walk about 3–6 meters. Now her condition was even better, and she could walk a distance of about 12–15 meters without any difficulty. The neurological examination revealed no focal evidence. I prepared the same prescription that I gave her on August 10th and advised her to take this formula long-term. Whenever menstruation was delayed, I told her

to take the prescription that she had received on August 17th. The patient was
discharged from the hospital on September 1st.

Fifth visit, September 18: The patient came to the outpatient service of the
Internal Medicine Department of the Dōng Zhí Mén Institute of the Academy
of Traditional Chinese Medicine and asked to see me again for diagnosis and
treatment. Recently, she had experienced dizziness and pulsating on both
sides of her head, with disturbed sleep, a poor appetite, clear drool flowing
from her mouth, and rumbling intestines and diarrhea. The tongue body was
red and thin with scant fur; the pulse was sunken and stringlike. I treated her
by quickening stasis and moving blood, and wrote out the following prescription, of which she should take six packets:

> *dāng guī* (当归 Chinese angelica, Angelicae Sinensis Radix) 9 g
>
> *chuān xiōng* (川芎 chuanxiong, Chuanxiong Rhizoma) 9 g
>
> *táo rén* (桃仁 peach kernel, Persicae Semen) 9 g
>
> *hóng huā* (红花 carthamus, Carthami Flos) 9 g
>
> *shēng dì huáng* (生地黄 dried rehmannia, Rehmanniae Radix Exsiccata)
>   15 g
>
> *shú dì huáng* (熟地黄 cooked rehmannia, Rehmanniae Radix Praeparata)
>   15 g
>
> *chì sháo yào* (赤芍药 red peony, Paeoniae Radix Rubra) 12 g
>
> *bái sháo yào* (白芍药 white peony, Paeoniae Radix Alba) 12 g
>
> *shēng máo gēn* (生茅根 raw imperata, Imperatae Rhizoma Crudum) 30 g
>
> *mǔ dān pí* (牡丹皮 moutan, Moutan Cortex) 9 g
>
> *niú xī* (牛膝 achyranthes, Achyranthis Bidentatae Radix) 12 g
>
> *liú jì nú* (刘寄奴 anomalous artemisia, Artemisiae Anomalae Herba) 9 g
>
> *xiāng fù* (香附 cyperus, Cyperi Rhizoma) 9 g
>
> *tǔ chǎo bái zhú* (土炒白术 earth-fried white atractylodes, Atractylodis
>   Macrocephalae Rhizoma cum Terra Frictum) 9 g

Sixth visit, September 28: All symptoms had been alleviated. I modified
the prescription once again by removing *liú jì nú* (anomalous artemisia), *mǔ
dān pí* (moutan), and *niú xī* (achyranthes), and by adding:

> *shēng zhě shí* (生赭石 crude hematite, Haematitum Crudum) 24 g (pre-
>   decocted)
>
> *chén pí* (陈皮 tangerine peel, Citri Reticulatae Pericarpium) 9 g
>
> *yì mǔ cǎo* (益母草 leonurus, Leonuri Herba) 12 g

I gave the patient 6–10 packets. Hereafter, I modified this formula only
slightly; she took the medicinals daily, and altogether I prescribed approximately
60 packets. Additionally, she received 40–50 pills of *dà huáng zhè chóng wán*.

Seventh visit, December 4: The headache and the pulsating sensation in the head were alleviated. The menses either arrived on time or, when they were late, immediately after she took a few doses of the decoction. Her complexion had become excellent, and the tongue and pulse were normal. At this time, I again changed the prescription to pill form. The pill prescription was as follows:

> *dāng guī* (当归 Chinese angelica, Angelicae Sinensis Radix) 45 g
>
> *chuān xiōng* (川芎 chuanxiong, Chuanxiong Rhizoma) 21 g
>
> *shēng dì huáng* (生地黄 dried rehmannia, Rehmanniae Radix Exsiccata) 30 g
>
> *shú dì huáng* (熟地黄 cooked rehmannia, Rehmanniae Radix Praeparata) 30 g
>
> *chì sháo yào* (赤芍药 red peony, Paeoniae Radix Rubra) 30 g
>
> *hóng huā* (红花 carthamus, Carthami Flos) 30 g
>
> *táo rén* (桃仁 peach kernel, Persicae Semen) 30 g
>
> *niú xī* (牛膝 achyranthes, Achyranthis Bidentatae Radix) 24 g
>
> *huáng qín* (黄芩 scutellaria, Scutellariae Radix) 30 g
>
> *xià kū cǎo* (夏枯草 prunella, Prunellae Spica) 30 g
>
> *jīng jiè* (荆芥 schizonepeta, Schizonepetae Herba) 24 g
>
> *shēng dà huáng* (生大黄 raw rhubarb, Rhei Radix et Rhizoma Crudi) 12 g
>
> *xiāng fù* (香附 cyperus, Cyperi Rhizoma) 30 g
>
> *wǔ líng zhī* (五灵脂 squirrel's droppings, Trogopteri Faeces) 30 g
>
> *pú huáng* (蒲黄 typha pollen, Typhae Pollen) 30 g
>
> *yuǎn zhì* (远志 polygala, Polygalae Radix) 30 g
>
> *bái jí lí* (白蒺藜 tribulus, Tribuli Fructus) 30 g

The ingredients were all ground into a fine powder, then thoroughly mixed with 3 g of separately ground *shè xiāng* (musk). All were combined with refined honey to form pills that weighed 9 g each. The dosage was 1–2 pills twice a day taken with plain boiled water. I also advised her to take several packets of the decocted prescription and 6–10 pills of *dà huáng zhè chóng wán* every month before the menses were scheduled to arrive.

Eighth visit, November 8, 1974: The patient had taken the pill prescription mentioned above three times now. Due to a heavy load of homework, she had recently suffered occasional headaches and overdue menses. The tongue fur was thin and white, and the pulse was slightly slippery. Once more I prescribed a decoction:

shēng shí jué míng (生石决明 raw abalone shell, Haliotidis Concha
    Cruda) 30 g (pre-decocted)

shēng mǔ lì (生牡蛎 raw oyster shell, Ostreae Concha Cruda) 30 g (pre-
    decocted)

xià kū cǎo (夏枯草 prunella, Prunellae Spica) 12 g

dāng guī (当归 Chinese angelica, Angelicae Sinensis Radix) 9 g

chuān xiōng (川芎 chuanxiong, Chuanxiong Rhizoma) 9 g

jú huā (菊花 chrysanthemum, Chrysanthemi Flos) 9 g

màn jīng zǐ (蔓荆子 vitex, Viticis Fructus) 9 g

niú xī (牛膝 achyranthes, Achyranthis Bidentatae Radix) 9 g

zé lán (泽兰 lycopus, Lycopi Herba) 9 g

shēng dà huáng (生大黄 raw rhubarb, Rhei Radix et Rhizoma Crudi) 1.5 g

hóng huā (红花 carthamus, Carthami Flos) 9 g

táo rén (桃仁 peach kernel, Persicae Semen) 9 g

qiàn cǎo (茜草 madder, Rubiae Radix) 12 g

chì sháo yào (赤芍药 red peony, Paeoniae Radix Rubra) 12 g

This decoction was combined with *dà huáng zhè chóng wán*, 10 pills; the
dosage method was the same as before.

Ninth visit, August 22, 1975: At this time, the patient attended regular
class and had successfully passed her school examinations. She continued to
take her pill prescription. Her complexion was lustrous, her essence-spirit
good, and her development normal. Only when she worked too much did her
head feel unwell. The tongue and pulse were all close to normal. I once again
changed the decoction prescription and advised her to take several packets
whenever she felt discomfort in her head. The ingredients were:

màn jīng zǐ (蔓荆子 vitex, Viticis Fructus) 9 g

shēng shí jué míng (生石决明 raw abalone shell, Haliotidis Concha
    Cruda) 21 g (pre-decocted)

dāng guī (当归 Chinese angelica, Angelicae Sinensis Radix) 12 g

chì sháo yào (赤芍药 red peony, Paeoniae Radix Rubra) 15 g

hóng huā (红花 carthamus, Carthami Flos) 9 g

táo rén (桃仁 peach kernel, Persicae Semen) 9 g

chuān xiōng (川芎 chuanxiong, Chuanxiong Rhizoma) 12 g

shú dì huáng (熟地黄 cooked rehmannia, Rehmanniae Radix Praeparata)
    12 g

xiāng fù (香附 cyperus, Cyperi Rhizoma) 9 g

qiàn cǎo (茜草 madder, Rubiae Radix) 30 g

hǎi piāo xiāo (海螵蛸 cuttlefish bone, Sepiae Endoconcha) 12 g *niú xī* (牛膝 achyranthes, Achyranthis Bidentatae Radix) 12 g

gǎo běn (藁本 Chinese lovage, Ligustici Rhizoma) 3 g

In addition, I slightly changed the pill prescription from here on in accordance with the pattern, by sometimes adding *shēng shí jué míng* (raw abalone shell), *xuán shēn* (scrophularia), *màn jīng zǐ* (vitex), *dì gǔ pí* (lycium root bark), or *qiàn cǎo* (madder), or by omitting *shú dì huáng* (cooked rehmannia). I used either 1 or 1.2 grams of *shè xiāng* (musk), but mostly 1.2 g. Other times, I omitted such medicinals as *jú huā* (chrysanthemum), *xuán shēn* (scrophularia), or *shēng shí jué míng* (raw abalone shell).

Tenth visit, May 10, 1976: Her essence-spirit and complexion had both clearly improved. The subjective symptoms had almost completely subsided. I prescribed the pills again, this time with a higher dosage of *shè xiāng* (musk) (1.8 g).

Eleventh visit, October 25, 1976: The patient had successfully graduated from high school and her studies were going smoothly. The symptoms in her head were no longer apparent. I still gave her the pill prescription, to be taken intermittently.

Twelfth visit, October 17, 1978: She had been working for almost two years as a staff member at an English language night school, and in general, her health was good. She suffered slight insomnia only when she was exhausted from work, and this was immediately relieved when she took a few packages of the decocted medicine. It had been 4–5 years since the illness had passed, and she was extremely happy. The tongue tip was red and the pulse was sunken and fine. Ordinarily, she was not taking any medicine at all, and the illness had not relapsed.

On a follow-up visit in October 1980, her complexion was rosy. Compared to before, she had gained weight and grown taller, and she was lively. She was now working full-time at a technical training school as an English language translator. There had been no relapse at all of the headaches, pulsing sensation in the head, or nosebleeds. Since having started the Chinese medicinals, more than seven years had passed without relapse of the cerebral angiopathy, and in addition to this, her memory was very good.

CASE FOUR
URINARY INCONTINENCE AND TOOTHACHE
小便失禁，牙痛

The patient was a 50-year-old male whose first examination date was April 4, 1961.

CHIEF COMPLAINT

Urinary incontinence and an aching pain in the upper and lower molars on the left side of his face, which had already lasted for more than twenty days.

INQUIRY EXAMINATION

For over 20 days, the patient had suffered from urinary incontinence, frequent urination with clear urine and no pain, and occasional bedwetting and wetting himself during the day. He also had an aching pain in the upper and lower molars on the left side, the gums were swollen and painful, and when he chewed, he had the feeling that his teeth moved, so he was only able to eat soft foods. Both legs had become weak but his food intake was still acceptable, and he was thirsty and could drink. The day before, he had discovered that the heels of his feet were puffy and swollen. In the past he had often taken heat-clearing and fire-draining medicinals such as *shí gāo* (gypsum), *huáng lián* (coptis), and *huáng qín* (scutellaria) and formulas such as *niú huáng jiě dú wán* (Bovine Bezoar Toxin-Resolving Pill), but none of these had been effective.

INSPECTION EXAMINATION

His development was normal, but he was somewhat nervous and agitated. The gums were swollen at the molar area on the left side, but not very red. The tongue fur was thin and white, and the root area was thick and slimy.

LISTENING AND SMELLING EXAMINATION

His speech and voice were both normal.

PALPATION EXAMINATION

His right wrist pulse was stringlike fine and rapid. The left wrist pulse was vacuous and rapid. Both cubit pulses were forceless when pressed.

PATTERN IDENTIFICATION

The kidney governs hibernation and is the root of storage. It also controls the opening and closing of the urine and stool. I knew that this was a pattern of kidney vacuity from the symptoms of urinary incontinence, weak legs, and a forceless cubit pulse when pressed. The kidney governs the bones, and the teeth are the surplus of the bones. When kidney water is insufficient, vacuity fire floats upward; this caused the toothache. The kidney governs water; when the kidney was vacuous and therefore could not warm and transform water-damp, water-damp poured downward and caused puffy swelling of the heels. The correlation of the four examinations supported the diagnosis of enuresis and toothache due to kidney vacuity, with inability to contain and secure the lower origin and upward floating of vacuity fire.

TREATMENT METHOD

Supplement the kidney to promote securing and continence, and return fire to the origin.

PRESCRIPTION

I gave the patient three packets of the following prescription, to be decocted in water:

> *shēng dì huáng* (生地黄 dried rehmannia, Rehmanniae Radix Exsiccata) 9 g
>
> *shú dì huáng* (熟地黄 cooked rehmannia, Rehmanniae Radix Praeparata) 9 g
>
> *shān yào* (山药 dioscorea, Dioscoreae Rhizoma) 12 g
>
> *shān zhū yú* (山茱萸 cornus, Corni Fructus) 9 g
>
> *yì zhì rén* (益智仁 alpinia, Alpiniae Oxyphyllae Fructus) 9 g
>
> *sāng piāo xiāo* (桑螵蛸 mantis egg-case, Mantidis Ootheca) 9 g
>
> *fù pén zǐ* (覆盆子 rubus, Rubi Fructus) 9 g
>
> *jīn yīng ròu* (金樱肉 Cherokee rose fruit flesh, Rosae Laevigatae Pericarpium) 6 g
>
> *duàn lóng gǔ* (煅龙骨 calcined dragon bone, Mastodi Ossis Fossilia Calcinata) 12 g (pre-decocted)
>
> *wū yào* (乌药 lindera, Linderae Radix) 6 g
>
> *wǔ wèi zǐ* (五味子 schisandra, Schisandrae Fructus) 3 g
>
> *zé xiè* (泽泻 alisma, Alismatis Rhizoma) 6 g
>
> *zhī mǔ* (知母 anemarrhena, Anemarrhenae Rhizoma) [salt-processed] 5 g
>
> *huáng bǎi* (黄柏 phellodendron, Phellodendri Cortex) [salt-processed] 5 g
>
> *ròu guì* (肉桂 cinnamon bark, Cinnamomi Cortex) 3 g

FORMULA EXPLANATION

The principle of this prescription follows classical formulas such as *zhī bǎi dì huáng wán* (Anemarrhena, Phellodendron, and Rehmannia Pill), *suō quán wán* (Stream-Reducing Pill), and *dū qì wán* (Metropolis Qì Pill). It uses *shēng dì huáng* (dried rehmannia) and *shú dì huáng* (cooked rehmannia) as the chief medicinals to enrich yīn and supplement the kidney.

These are matched by the following support medicinals: *Shān zhū yú* (cornus) supplements the kidney and astringes essence, thereby alleviating frequent urination. *Shān yào* (dioscorea) strengthens the kidney, secures essence, and boosts the spleen. *Wǔ wèi zǐ* (schisandra) supplements the kidney by sour contraction and thereby checks enuresis.

Acting as assistant medicinals, *sāng piāo xiāo* (mantis egg-case), *yì zhì rén* (alpinia), *wū yào* (lindera), *fù pén zǐ* (rubus), *jīn yīng zǐ* (Cherokee rose fruit), and *lóng gǔ* (dragon bone) supplement the kidney to promote contraction and containment; they reduce urine and check enuresis. *Zé xiè* (alisma) percolates and drains kidney dampness, disinhibits dampness, and disperses swelling. *Zhī mǔ* (anemarrhena) and *huáng bǎi* (phellodendron) consolidate the kidney and clear heat, while at the same time preventing the warm-natured medicinals from engendering heat.

The courier medicinal *ròu guì* (cinnamon bark) returns fire to its origin.

Altogether, the prescription supplements the kidney and secures containment, and returns fire to the origin.

Followup treatment

Second visit, May 10: The patient had taken just two packets of the decoction, and it was already particularly effective. He could control his own urination, the gum swelling had disappeared, and the toothache stopped. He could chew hard food without having the feeling that his teeth were moving. The physical strength of his legs had also improved. Due to his work schedule, he had only taken two of the three packets of medicinals, and today his teeth seemed to be about to start hurting again, so he came in for another examination. The tongue presentation was the same as before, and the pulse was not rapid any more. So, I stayed with the original prescription, only adding 9 g of *bā jǐ tiān* (morinda), and gave him five more packets.

Third visit, May 15: All the symptoms had completely disappeared after taking the medicinals; moreover, his impotence, which he had had for one to two years, had now also been treated. The tongue fur had become thin and white; the pulse was more forceful than before. I gave the patient another 3–6 packets of the original prescription to strengthen the healing effect and to eliminate the disease root.

The patient made two follow-up visits: on June 19, 1961 and on November 6, 1962. He had been attending to his job without any interruptions, and the illness had not recurred.

Case Five

Bladder cough (cough with urinary incontinence) 膀胱咳

The patient was a 55-year-old woman retired from a Běijīng factory. Her first examination date was January 29, 1981.

CHIEF COMPLAINT

Coughing and wetting herself for more than three months.

INQUIRY EXAMINATION

In the winter after the 1976 earthquake, the patient had caught a cold, with a cough persisting for more than a month. Every year in winter the cough had recurred and was sometimes so severe that she urinated spontaneously after a coughing spell, even wetting her pants. The cough always lasted for a little over a month, after which the patient gradually recovered. This condition recurred every winter.

In the winter of 1980, the cough had again occurred, gradually worsening day-by-day, and the patient had not been able to recover since. She was now coughing up white phlegm, and also suffered from shortness of breath and a subjective feeling of having no stamina. Inhalation had become more difficult than exhalation and even a slight coughing episode was followed by wetting her pants. She experienced profuse flatulence after urination. For over two months now, she had been unable to pass even a single drop of urine when squatting over the toilet unless she coughed, in which case it came out immediately. She wore a padded diaper in her pants and suffered greatly. In the past, she had tried Chinese and Western medicines and had even spent one month in the local hospital to receive a desensitization injection, but these measures had proven ineffective.

INSPECTION EXAMINATION

Her development and nutrition were normal, but she was slightly anxious. The tongue body was normal and the tongue fur thin and white.

LISTENING AND SMELLING EXAMINATION

The sound of the cough was not loud; her breathing was slightly fast, but her speech was normal.

PALPATION EXAMINATION

Examination of her chest, abdomen, and limbs revealed nothing abnormal. The pulse was slightly slippery and was sunken in the cubit position.

PATTERN IDENTIFICATION

The *Huáng Dì Nèi Jīng* ("The Yellow Emperor's Inner Canon") chapter "Treatise on Cough" says:

> "All five viscera and six bowels can cause a person to cough; a cough is not merely caused by the lung.
>
> "There is a mutual connection between humans, heaven, and earth; therefore, a person may become ill if any of the five viscera contract cold. If the illness is mild, cough occurs; if the

illness is severe, then painful diarrhea occurs. If the illness occurs in autumn, the lung first contracts the evil; if it occurs in
winter, the kidney first contracts it."

This patient had a cough that was due to contraction of cold during winter. Not only did she have a cough and shortness of breath, she also experienced lack of stamina and difficulty with inhalation. Physicians of the past have said the following about exhalation and inhalation: "Exhalation is discharged from the heart and lungs; inhalation enters the kidney and liver," as well as "the kidney governs qì absorption." Moreover, since her cubit pulse was sunken, I knew that this cough was due to contraction of cold in the kidney channel. The chapter "Treatise on Cough" states further, "Enduring cough of the five viscera will shift to the six bowels. When kidney cough endures, the urinary bladder will contract it. Bladder cough presents as coughing with urinary incontinence." This patient had been ill for the past five years, so I knew that the kidney cough had already affected the urinary bladder and coughing therefore resulted in incontinence. The correlation of the four examinations supported the diagnosis of bladder cough.

TREATMENT METHOD

Warm the lung and dispel cold while boosting the kidney and securing the bladder, assisted by downbearing qì and transforming phlegm.

PRESCRIPTION

I gave the patient seven packets of the following prescription:

zhì má huáng (炙麻黄 mix-fried ephedra, Ephedrae Herba cum Liquido
    Fricta) 6 g
xìng rén (杏仁 apricot kernel, Armeniacae Semen) 10 g
jié gěng (桔梗 platycodon, Platycodonis Radix) 6 g
zǐ wǎn (紫菀 aster, Asteris Radix) 15 g
sāng piāo xiāo (桑螵蛸 mantis egg-case, Mantidis Ootheca) 10 g
fù pén zǐ (覆盆子 rubus, Rubi Fructus) 10 g
wū yào (乌药 lindera, Linderae Radix) 12 g
chǎo sū zǐ (炒苏子 stir-fried perilla fruit, Perillae Fructus Frictus) 10 g
chǎo lái fú zǐ (炒莱菔子 stir-fried radish seed, Raphani Semen Frictum)
    10 g
chǎo bái jiè zǐ (炒白芥子 stir-fried white mustard, Sinapis Albae Semen
    Frictum) 3 g
bàn xià (半夏 pinellia, Pinelliae Rhizoma) 10 g
huà jú hóng (化橘红 Huazhou pomelo rind, Citri Grandis Exocarpium
    Rubrum) 12 g

wǔ wèi zǐ (五味子 schisandra, Schisandrae Fructus) 5 g
chǎo jī nèi jīn (炒鸡内金 stir-fried gizzard lining, Galli Gigeriae
   Endothelium Corneum Frictum) 10 g

FORMULA EXPLANATION

I created this prescription on the basis of my own formula *má xìng èr sān tāng* (Ephedra and Apricot Kernel Two-Three Decoction) and *suō quán wán* (Stream-Reducing Pill) with modifications.

The chief medicinals are *má huáng* (ephedra), which warms the lung and dispels cold, and *sāng piāo xiāo* (mantis egg-case), which supplements the kidney and reduces urine.

As support medicinals, *xìng rén* (apricot kernel) downbears qì and disinhibits the lung; *zǐ wǎn* (aster) warms the lung and dispels cold; *fù pén zǐ* (rubus) warms the kidney and reduces urine; *wū yào* (lindera) warms the kidney and rectifies qì; and *wǔ wèi zǐ* (schisandra) draws together the qì of the lung and kidney.

The assistant medicinals *lái fú zǐ* (radish seed), *zǐ sū zǐ* (perilla fruit), *bái jiè zǐ* (white mustard), *bàn xià* (pinellia), and *huà jú hóng* (Huazhou pomelo rind) downbear qì and transform phlegm.

As the courier medicinal, *jī nèi jīn* (gizzard lining) secures urinary bladder qì and stops incontinence.

FOLLOWUP TREATMENT

<u>Second visit, February 19</u>: The patient had already recovered from the cough and urinary incontinence. The symptoms had been clearly relieved after seven packets of the decoction, and she was able to urinate normally in the bathroom. By the time she finished the eighth packet, the cough had completely disappeared, the incontinence had stopped, and several months of suffering were resolved. To strengthen the effect, I gave her three more packets. After she had taken a total of eleven packets, she was again a normal person and she therefore discontinued the prescription. Since then there has been no recurrence of the cough, and the patient has been completely normal.

EMPIRICAL KNOWLEDGE

Concerning the seriousness of nocturnal enuresis

The kidney governs hibernation and is the root of storage. It stands in interior-exterior relationship with the urinary bladder and it governs water. Urine is the surplus of water-humor and is stored in the urinary bladder. The urinary bladder is regularly restrained and loosened as a result of being managed by kidney qì. When kidney yáng vacuity occurs, kidney yīn is exuberant. Thus, the urinary bladder also suffers vacuity cold. At night, the human body is characterized by yáng vacuity and yīn exuberance. When a person sleeps, yáng qì is debilitated and hidden and is not able to restrain yīn. Consequently, yīn qì acts independently and the urinary bladder loses its retentive ability. The descent of water is not arrested, urine is discharged unconsciously, and bed-wetting occurs.

In Case 1, the patient had a sunken left cubit pulse, a weak right cubit pulse, and lumbar pain, so I knew the pattern was kidney vacuity. Furthermore, I observed that his knees feared wind and cold and liked warmth, and combined this with the fact that at night yīn tends to be exuberant and yáng tends to be vacuous. Thus, I was able to diagnose the pattern as kidney vacuity cold. This had to be treated by warming and supplementing kidney yáng as a precondition to restraining yīn. For it is only when yīn is calm and yáng secure that the body is able to store, to hibernate and secure, and to constrain the urinary bladder, thereby stopping enuresis.

According to a principle stated in the *Huáng Dì Nèi Jīng* ("The Yellow Emperor's Inner Canon"): "To treat yáng well, seek yáng within yīn." In the previous case I used *shú dì huáng* (cooked rehmannia) as the basis of the formula to warm and supplement yīn-blood within the kidney, and I used *fù zǐ* (aconite), *ròu guì* (cinnamon bark), and *yín yáng huò* (epimedium) to greatly supplement kidney yáng. With *chuān xiōng* (chuanxiong), *sāng jì shēng* (mistletoe), *suǒ yáng* (cynomorium), and *yì zhì rén* (alpinia), I secured the lower origin; this followed the method of treating the root. In addition, I took into consideration that the patient had already suffered from bed-wetting for nearly twenty years. Thus, I also used urine-reducing and kidney-supplementing medicinals to simultaneously treat the root. By attending to both the root and the tip, the treatment effect was both speedy and stable. Therefore, I also used *sāng piāo xiāo* (mantis egg-case), *fù pén zǐ* (rubus), and *wū yào* (lindera) both to warm and supplement kidney and bladder qì as well as to restrain and reduce urine. If I had only used restraining and astringing medicinals such as *lóng gǔ* (dragon bone), *mǔ lì* (oyster shell), *wū méi* (mume), and *hē zǐ* (chebule), but not kidney-supplementing medicinals, it would have been difficult to achieve a good result. *Jī nèi jīn* (gizzard lining) entered the small intestine to separate the clear and turbid, while also entering the urinary bladder to secure bladder qì and to stop enuresis; thus, this channel conducting medicinal assisted the therapeutic effect of the treatment.

The patient in Case 4 had a diagnosis of enuresis due to kidney vacuity, with vacuity fire floating upwards and insecurity of the lower origin. In Case 5, the cough with enuresis was due to incessant kidney cough that had shifted to the urinary bladder. In both cases, I obtained results by securing and containing the lower origin.

The kidney governs bone and the teeth are the surplus of bone. The kidney and the urinary bladder stand in interior-exterior relationship. The kidney is in charge of the urine and the stool and governs the lower origin. The cubit pulse is the chief indicator of kidney disease. Thus, theories such as cold damage to the kidneys are able to guide clinical practice.

The application of Chinese medical theory is discussed above in the disease conditions of Cases 1, 4, and 5. However, enuresis is not entirely due to a kidney vacuity cold pattern. Some cases are due to qì vacuity or to lung vacuity with inability to control the lower body. Other cases are associated with heat exuberance and stirring fire or insecurity of bladder qì. Each pattern has its own special characteristics. In summary, the application of Chinese medicine theory requires careful synthesis of specific situations and cannot be applied mechanically.

Concerning the coughing of a great amount of blood every evening

Although physicians of the past differentiated the coughing of blood into patterns such as internal damage, external contraction, yīn and yáng, and vacuity and repletion, they also believed that most cases belonged to the category of lung heat. The *Chì Shuǐ Xuán Zhū* ("Mysterious/Black Pearl of Red Water") states, "Coughing blood is usually due to fire depression within the lung; clearing the lung and downbearing fire is the appropriate treatment." Zhū Dān-Xī said, "Spitting up blood is a fire disease." Chén Xiū-Yuán agreed, "In any treatment of a bleeding pattern, you should first treat fire."

The experience of these physicians tells us that diseases characterized by a great amount of bleeding are mostly diseases due to fire-heat patterns. Of course, we must pay attention and differentiate between different types of fire such as vacuity fire, repletion fire, dragon thunder fire, or rootless fire (identified by physicians of the past as resembling the fire of lamps and candles that self-extinguish when the lamp-oil or wax is consumed). They believed that the evil of fire-heat caused blood to contract heat, and to boil, soar, and move frenetically. Thus, blood failed to stay in the channels and instead spilled out from the upper body, discharging through coughing, vomiting, and nosebleed; and spilled out from the lower body, discharging via the stool, urine, and vaginal flooding.

From another perspective, blood is yīn and qì is yáng. There is yáng within yīn and yīn within yáng; there is blood within qì and qì within blood. Blood is the mother of qì and qì is the commander of blood. Qì is the root for the movement of blood. Physicians of the past treated bleeding in the upper body with the principle of "downbearing qì to downbear fire. When fire is borne down, qì does not ascend. Since blood follows the movement of qì, no spillage of blood occurs in the upper orifices."

When I combined these theories, I knew from the pulse manifestation of the patient in Case 2 that the pattern was lung and stomach repletion fire with frenetic movement of hot blood. In treatment, I did not select large quantities of blood-stanching medicinals to stop bleeding. Instead, I primarily used the blood-cooling, fire-clearing, and qì-downbearing method that complied with the idea of *yù nǚ jiān* (Jade Lady Brew) for dual clearing of qì and blood. I combined this with the notion of "raking firewood from beneath the cauldron" from the *Qiān Jīn Fāng* ("Essential Thousand Gold Formulary") by using *shēng dì huáng* (dried rehmannia) and *dà huáng* (rhubarb) to treat blood ejection, which I modified according to the pattern. In this formula, I used *shēng dì huáng* (dried rehmannia) to cool the blood and calm the heat boiling within the blood, and *shēng dà huáng* (raw rhubarb) to drain repletion heat from the blood aspect and rake the firewood from beneath the cauldron. As support medicinals, I used *shēng shí gāo* (raw gypsum) to greatly drain fire-heat from the qì aspect, and *shān zhī zǐ* (gardenia) and *huáng qín* (scutellaria) to clear and drain fire-heat from the center and upper burners.

Moreover, according to the theory of downbearing qì to downbear fire, I chose *xuán fù huā* (inula flower) to downbear qì and eliminate phlegm. I chose *bīng láng* (areca) for its special characteristic of "downbearing like a heavy stone," for the purpose of downbearing fire by moving qì downward. Then I chose *tiān mén dōng* (asparagus) and *xuán shēn* (scrophularia) to enrich yīn and downbear fire. I also took into consideration that the patient had been coughing a great amount of blood every evening and that this had continued for seven to eight days without ceasing, so I complied with the urgency of the situation and treated the tip of the illness. I selected charred *bái máo gēn* (imperata), *hé yè tàn* (charred lotus leaf), *ǒu jié tàn* (charred lotus root node), *dāng guī tàn* (charred tangkuei), and *bái jí* (bletilla) to stanch bleeding. I also feared that since the blood was moving frenetically and outside the channels, this could easily engender static blood, in addition to the fact that several charcoaled medicinals in a formula can cause static blood. I matched them with small amounts of *mǔ dān pí* (moutan) and *hóng huā* (carthamus) because these medicinals remove stasis and engender the new (when there is new blood, bleeding quickly stops). *Niú xī* (achyranthes) enters the blood aspect and can conduct blood that is ascending counterflow back downward. Downbearing qì dispersed fire, and downbearing blood calmed heat, so the coughing of blood stopped spontaneously.

Physicians of the past have readily warned us, "If you see blood, do not just treat blood; if you see phlegm, do not just treat phlegm." Instead they urge us to comply with the principle, "To treat disease, seek its root." Thus, you should identify the pattern to determine the treatment and not just treat the head for headache or treat the foot for foot pain. In other words, do not just treat the symptoms. I hope that everyone learns from my experience through these examples.

"To treat disease seek the root"

The *Huáng Dì Nèi Jīng* ("The Yellow Emperor's Inner Canon") states:

> "Yīn and yáng are the way of heaven and earth; they are the guiding principle of the universe, the parents of transmutation and transformation, the root and beginning of life and death, and the residence of the "spirit light." To treat disease, one must seek the root."

Chinese medical theory is also subject to the laws of yīn and yáng and applies these notions to the human body. The viscera and bowels and qì and blood of the human body; wind, cold, summerheat, and dampness of the weather; the interior and exterior and the upper and lower locations of disease; the slow and rapid, floating and sunken qualities of the pulse; the warming, balanced, cold, and hot natures of medicinals—these are all, without exception, subject to the laws of yīn and yáng. Hence, to treat disease you must have a firm grasp of the transformational laws of yīn and yáng, inquire into the origin and development of disease, and understand the reasons for transformation and change. Understanding this is called "treating disease by seeking the root." This "root" refers to the laws of yīn and yáng. For example, the *Huáng Dì Nèi Jīng* ("The Yellow Emperor's Inner Canon") says, "Good examination first observes the complexion and takes the pulse to distinguish yīn from yáng."

All the various theories in Chinese medicine equally touch on the doctrine of yīn and yáng. When identifying patterns to determine treatment, you must integrate the reasons behind exuberance or debilitation, waxing or waning, or transmutations and transformations of yīn and yáng, to be able to analyze the condition of the patient. By grasping the intrinsic nature of the transformations and transmutations of the disease, you can then provide the most appropriate treatment. Only this can heighten the effectiveness of the treatment.

For instance, in Case 1, I grasped the intrinsic nature of the disease as being kidney yáng vacuity, and I knew that the chief medicinal must warm and invigorate kidney yáng so that health would be restored. In Case 2, however, the pattern was yáng exuberance fire and heat, so I achieved results with blood-cooling and fire-draining medicinals as chief medicinals. In Case 4, I grasped that the condition was rooted in a dual vacuity of yīn and yáng and in vacuity fire flaming upward, so to restore health I used the method of returning fire to its origin. In all these cases, the approach was to observe the disease dynamically on the basis of yīn and yáng, to apply a holistic analysis, and to differentiate patterns by understanding the dynamics of the exuberance and debilitation of yīn and yáng, the strengthening and weakening of evil and right qì, the upbearing and downbearing of qì and blood, and the conversions between tip and root.

I use "tip and root" to explain the primary and secondary treatment concerns and to elucidate the idea of mutual relationship. For example, when speaking of right qì and evil qì, right qì is the root while evil qì is the tip. When speaking of the onset of disease and disease subsequent to onset, the disease at onset is considered the root, and the disease subsequent to onset is the tip. When speaking of disease cause and symptoms, then disease cause is the root, and the symptoms are the tip. As the *Huáng Dì Nèi Jīng* ("The Yellow Emperor's Inner Canon") says, "When you know the root and the tip, then all your actions will be appropriate; when you do not know them, then any action will be reckless." Thus, we see how the meaning of "tip and root" is also derived from yīn-yáng theory. When performing pattern identification to determine treatment in the clinic, we must skillfully master all these theories to improve the standard.

Observing pathomechanical changes from the holistic viewpoint

Through the theories of yīn and yáng, viscera and bowels, channels and network vessels, qì and blood, and the five phases, Chinese medicine integrates the physiology and pathology of the human body, the interior-exterior and upper-lower locations, the organic functions, and the essence-spirit into one complete whole. Thus, the five viscera of Chinese medicine should not by any means be classified simply as morphology. Through the visceral manifestation theory, Chinese medicine summarily categorizes the organs of the human body and their functions into five great types, thereby integrating the interior of the human body and the human body in relationship to its environment into one system. Chinese medicine considers the human body as an integrated whole when using pattern identification as a basis for determining treatment.

In Case 3, for example, Western medicine diagnosed the patient with cerebral arterio-venous deformity and recommended a procedure to resection the deformed blood vessels. Chinese medicine, however, coming from the viewpoint of holism, considered the integrated whole and noted that while the disease was located in the upper body, this was closely related to the lower body, and that the blood inappropriately discharging from the upper body should have been discharged from the lower body. On the basis of this notion, I diagnosed the condition as menstrual block with inverted menstruation, and I chose a method to treat the upper body disease through the lower body and to free the menses and quicken the network vessels; this achieved satisfactory results.

Another example was Case 4. According to the theories that the teeth are the surplus of bone and that the kidney governs bone, I reasoned on the basis of the holistic approach that the pattern was caused by lower origin vacuity and vacuity fire floating upward; therefore, by selecting a holistic treatment method, I treated the toothache without ever specifically treating the teeth. I also considered Case 5 from a holistic standpoint and adopted the method of combined treatment for the lung, kidney, and urinary bladder. Not only did the cough disappear, but the patient also recovered quickly from the cough-induced urinary incontinence. In this last case, if I had treated only the cough or only the urinary incontinence, I would have failed to achieve results either way; however, the results appeared extraordinarily fast with the holistic approach.

When applying pattern identification to determine treatment in clinic, whether you treat specific local symptoms, essence-spirit symptoms, viscera-bowel symptoms, or specific functional disorders, all treatments should proceed from a holistic perspective. We must integrate the relationship between the physiology and pathology of the entire body to observe pathomechanical changes, and from there proceed to identify patterns to determine treatment.

Regulating dynamic equilibrium on the basis of movement and change

There is another important idea in Chinese medicine—the belief that the manifestations of life in the human body and the manifestations of disease are all unceasingly moving, transmuting, and transforming. The *Huáng Dì Nèi Jīng* ("The Yellow Emperor's Inner Canon") says:

> "Movement and tranquility summon each other, the upper and the lower relate to each other, yīn and yáng make use of each other, and the changes come from life itself."

The *Nèi Jīng* ("Inner Canon") also states:

> "The life of things comes about by transformation, the end of things comes from transmutation. Transmutation and transformation weaken each other and are the cause of success or failure. … Where there is no life, there is no transformation; there

is only a time of tranquility. ... Where there is no inward and outward movement, there is no birth, growth, prime, aging, and death; where there is no upward movement or downward movement, there is no growth, transformation, withdrawal, and storage."

Such movement, transmutation, and transformation is mutually restraining, mutually stimulating, continuously moving, transmuting, and transforming, and continuously developing and progressing; this is the meaning of transmuting, moving, restraining, and transforming. The manifestations of life and of pathology in the human body both exist within the process of restraining and engendering transformation. This dynamic equilibrium has requirements fixed within a certain range. The Chinese medical treatment of disease quite correctly balances this dynamic equilibrium. As it says in the *Huáng Dì Nèi Jīng* ("The Yellow Emperor's Inner Canon"), "when you cautiously observe yīn and yáng and regulate them, then balance endures." Moreover, the *Nèi Jīng* ("Inner Canon") explains that "when yīn is calm and yáng is sound, then the essence-spirit is well."

On the basis of this notion of restraining and engendering transformation, we can now consider Case 3. In spite of the fact that the cerebral arteriovenous deformity had already arisen, it existed because it had encountered factors in the process of restraining and engendering transformation that gave rise to a functional disturbance. If I could cause these factors to change, I could also change the environment that had produced the functional disturbance and thereby obtain a change to improve the patient's condition. Thus, I chose the method of regulating the thoroughfare (*chōng*) and controlling (*rèn*) vessels, treating upper body disease through the lower body, regulating the menses, and quickening the network vessels. Within the process of restraining and engendering transformation, a change occurred gradually, leading to recovery, to the principle of "calm yīn and sound yáng," and to the dynamic equilibrium of emotional and mental well-being or "well-being of essence-spirit."

I believe that the process of restraining and engendering transformation is a way of looking at the occurrence and development of disease. Timely use of medicinals, together with acupuncture and moxibustion, can holistically balance the human body and cause the process of transformation to occur. This process advantageously changes the condition of the patient; it promotes the process of transformation to correct itself, and the patient then recovers his proper dynamic equilibrium. When you conduct pattern identification to determine treatment, you should keep this concept constantly in mind. With these ideas, I am just presenting a few personal views for your consideration.

CHAPTER THREE

Using a treatment method according to the pattern is a vital link in treatment based on pattern identification.

In applying Chinese medical theory to treat disease, the physician first analyzes and determines the illness and its symptoms through pattern identification. He determines whether the condition is vacuous or replete, hot or cold, and then decides the treatment method. Then the physician chooses a formula and medicinals and organizes the prescription, determining the treatment principle and applying it according to the specific conditions by following the pattern. Flexible use of the treatment method according to the pattern is the vital link when determining treatment based on pattern identification. If this process is not followed, then even though the pattern identification is correct, optimal treatment results will not be achieved. The condition of the patient may even be harmed and all previous work undone. Here are five case studies together with brief discussions from my experience that illustrate this point.

CASE STUDIES

CASE ONE
MALARIA (HEAT EFFUSION OR FEVER, ETIOLOGY UNKNOWN)
疟疾(发热，原因待查)

The patient was a 65-year-old male whose initial examination date was April 15, 1974.

CHIEF COMPLAINT
Recurring bouts of high fever for more than two years.

INQUIRY EXAMINATION

Approximately every three to seven days in the evening the patient had a high fever and a body temperature from 38.5–40 °C. After onset, the fever persisted for three to four days, then gradually resolved itself and finally abated. Previously during the onset stage of the fever, the patient had tried various kinds of medicines, but nothing was able to alter the regular pattern of the attacks. Occasionally a fever occurred consecutively every few days, and then would self-abate, or an interval of twenty days occurred between one attack and the next. However, these conditions were rare, and usually the fever occurred weekly. Just prior to the onset of the fever, the patient first had a sensation of cold then the fever would follow, sometimes accompanied by vomiting. Finally he had come from Húnán Province to Běijīng and had spent more than a month in the hospital undergoing various diagnostic examinations and receiving antibiotics and even Chinese medical treatment, all in an attempt to stop the fever attacks. Besides the usual examinations, the patient also underwent diagnostic testing including a radioisotope scan, ultrasonic wave, gastroscope, and cholecystography, but these tests were unable to help determine a diagnosis. When the hospital had recommended a peritoneoscopy the patient did not agree and had left the hospital. He came to my outpatient clinic.

Four to five days had already passed by the time of the initial visit, so the fever was on the verge of recurrence. The patient felt discomfort and fullness on the right side of his body in the area of the gallbladder. He also had symptoms of nausea, a bitter taste in the mouth, thirst, poor food intake, nasal congestion, a cough that produced yellowish-white sticky phlegm, weak aching lumbus, and a devitalized essence-spirit.

INSPECTION EXAMINATION

His development was normal, but he was relatively thin; he had the appearance of one with an enduring and serious illness, and a complexion without luster. The tongue fur was thin and slightly yellow.

LISTENING AND SMELLING EXAMINATION

His speech and voice were relatively low; sometimes he was short of breath, and he had a cough that was resonant.

PALPATION EXAMINATION

The head, neck, chest, and abdomen showed no abnormalities. The left pulse was sunken and fine and the right stringlike and fine.

PATTERN IDENTIFICATION

I knew that the disease evil was in the lesser yáng (*shào yáng*), half-exterior and half-interior, because of symptoms such as alternating cold and heat, fixed time of the onset, bitter taste in the mouth, nausea, sometimes vomiting, fullness in the right costal area, thin tongue fur, and a stringlike pulse. Since the patient had suffered the disease for more than two years, I knew the illness was associated with malaria. The characteristic of this disease was the greater amount of heat than of cold at the time of onset, so I diagnosed patterns of exterior-interior disharmony, constructive-defense disharmony, and enduring internal heat disease.

TREATMENT METHOD

Harmonize and resolve the lesser yáng, clear heat and outthrust evil.

PRESCRIPTION

The following prescription was a combination of *xiǎo chái hú tāng* (Minor Bupleurum Decoction) and *bái hǔ jiā guì zhī tāng* (White Tiger Decoction Plus Cinnamon Twig) with modifications; I gave the patient 4–6 packets to be decocted in water:

chái hú (柴胡 bupleurum, Bupleuri Radix) 25 g

huáng qín (黄芩 scutellaria, Scutellariae Radix) 12 g

dǎng shēn (党参 codonopsis, Codonopsis Radix) 15 g

zhì gān cǎo (炙甘草 mix-fried licorice, Glycyrrhizae Radix cum Liquido Fricta) 3 g

shēng shí gāo (生石膏 raw gypsum, Gypsum Crudum) 30 g (pre-decocted)

chì sháo yào (赤芍药 red peony, Paeoniae Radix Rubra) 12 g

bái sháo yào (白芍药 white peony, Paeoniae Radix Alba) 12 g

guì zhī (桂枝 cinnamon twig, Cinnamomi Ramulus) 6 g

shēng jiāng (生姜 fresh ginger, Zingiberis Rhizoma Recens) 3 slices

dà zǎo (大枣 jujube, Jujubae Fructus) 4 pieces

chén pí (陈皮 tangerine peel, Citri Reticulatae Pericarpium) 9 g

fú líng (茯苓 poria, Poria) 12 g

niú xī (牛膝 achyranthes, Achyranthis Bidentatae Radix) 9 g

FORMULA EXPLANATION

Chái hú (bupleurum) is the chief medicinal in this prescription; it harmonizes and resolves evil heat in the lesser yáng (half-exterior and half-interior).

As support medicinals, *huáng qín* (scutellaria) clears and drains lesser yáng fire-heat, and *shēng shí gāo* (raw gypsum) clears and resolves evil heat in the qì aspect.

As assistant medicinals, sweet and moderate *dǎng shēn* (codonopsis), *gān cǎo* (licorice), and *dà zǎo* (jujube) harmonize the center, supplement right qì, and strengthen resistance against evil. Acrid, sweet, and warming *guì zhī* (cinnamon twig) resolves the flesh and outthrusts the exterior, regulates and harmonizes the constructive-defense, and expels evil to the exterior; *chì sháo yào* (red peony) and *bái sháo yào* (white peony) benefit yīn and harmonize construction while quickening the blood and clearing heat. *Chén pí* (tangerine peel) and *fú líng* (poria) treat cough by transforming phlegm and eliminating dampness. *Shēng jiāng* (fresh ginger) frees the exterior and interior with acrid dispersing, and prevents the cold nature of *huáng qín* (scutellaria) and *shí gāo* (gypsum) from damaging the center.

Niú xī (achyranthes) disinhibits the lumbus and knees and is the courier medicinal.

In summary, I selected *xiǎo chái hú tāng* (Minor Bupleurum Decoction) to harmonize and resolve the pivot and *bái hǔ jiā guì zhī tāng* (White Tiger Decoction Plus Cinnamon Twig) to clear heat and outthrust evil. In combination, they harmonize and resolve the lesser yáng while clearing heat and outthrusting evil.

Followup Treatment

<u>Second visit on April 19</u>: The patient had taken four packets of the decoction, and it had been seven to eight days since the onset of the last fever, but there was still no new occurrence. His essence-spirit had changed for the better, and he was no longer thirsty. The rest of the symptoms remained the same. I modified the previous prescription and gave him four more packets for decoction as follows:

chái hú (柴胡 bupleurum, Bupleuri Radix) 25 g

huáng qín (黄芩 scutellaria, Scutellariae Radix) 12 g

bàn xià (半夏 pinellia, Pinelliae Rhizoma) 9 g

dǎng shēn (党参 codonopsis, Codonopsis Radix) 15 g

shēng shí gāo (生石膏 raw gypsum, Gypsum Crudum) 30 g (pre-decocted)

chì sháo yào (赤芍药 red peony, Paeoniae Radix Rubra) 12 g

bái sháo yào (白芍药 white peony, Paeoniae Radix Alba) 12 g

guì zhī (桂枝 cinnamon twig, Cinnamomi Ramulus) 6 g

chén pí (陈皮 tangerine peel, Citri Reticulatae Pericarpium) 9 g

xìng rén (杏仁 apricot kernel, Armeniacae Semen) 9 g

fú líng (茯苓 poria, Poria) 12 g

bīng láng (槟榔 areca, Arecae Semen) 9 g

cǎo guǒ (草果 tsaoko, Tsaoko Fructus) 9 g

cháng shān (常山 dichroa, Dichroae Radix) 9 g

<u>Third visit on April 22</u>: It had now been more than ten days since starting the decoction, and there had been no recurrence of fever. The discomfort in the rib-side had subsided, he had not vomited, the bitter taste in the mouth had lessened, but the tongue and pulse signs were the same as before. I gave him

three more prescription packets, which were the same as he had previously received on April 19.

Fourth visit on May 3: The patient had taken ten packets of the decoction and had experienced no recurrence of the fever. He had regained his physical strength. However, the tongue fur was slightly thick and the cough remained. Still using the previous prescription, I increased the dosage of *dǎng shēn* (codonopsis) to 18 grams, removed *cháng shān* (dichroa), and added 9 grams of *hòu pò* (official magnolia bark). I gave the patient 3–6 packets to continue the therapeutic effect.

Fifth visit on May 17: By now, the patient had taken fourteen packets of the above-mentioned prescription with no recurrence of fever. His food intake had increased, and his coughing and expectoration of phlegm had lessened. The tongue fur was the same as before, but the fineness of the pulse was abating. I gave him six packets to continue the effect, but this time I reduced the dosage of *guì zhī* (cinnamon twig) to 4.5 grams and added 9 grams of *bái jí lí* (tribulus).

Sixth visit on May 31: The patient had finished more than ten packets of the previous prescription since the last visit. His essence-spirit was vigorous, he had regained his physical strength, his complexion was ruddy and lustrous, and all other symptoms were gone. The tongue fur had become thin, and the pulse was slightly stringlike and slippery, but no longer fine. I modified the prescription from May 17th by changing the dosage of *dǎng shēn* (codonopsis) to 30 grams, removing *bái jí lí* (tribulus), and adding 12 grams of *hé shǒu wū* (flowery knotweed). I gave him 3–6 packets again to continue the effect.

Seventh visit on June 8: Now his essence-spirit, complexion, and physical strength had all greatly improved since his last visit. Eating and drinking were essentially normal, and bowels and urine were regular. His tongue fur was still thin and yellow; his pulse was slightly slippery and slow. After the last visit, he had taken altogether 40 packets and had gone 50 days without any occurrence of fever. I discontinued the medicinals for a week and observed his condition. During this period of time, he had a fever of 39°C for one day, and he immediately took a dose of Chinese medicinals. On that very day the fever abated, and thereafter, as long as he took the medicinals, the fever did not recur. On the basis of this situation and the correlation of the four examinations, I knew that right qì, although renewed, was still not fully strong and healthy and that evil qì was also not entirely resolved and cleared. Thus, while dispelling evil qì, I also had to strengthen and support right qì, so that right qì itself would recover. I gave the patient six packets of the following prescription:

chái hú (柴胡 bupleurum, Bupleuri Radix) 25 g
huáng qín (黄芩 scutellaria, Scutellariae Radix) 12 g
bàn xià (半夏 pinellia, Pinelliae Rhizoma) 9 g

dǎng shēn (党参 codonopsis, Codonopsis Radix) 30 g

hé shǒu wū (何首乌 flowery knotweed, Polygoni Multiflori Radix) 15 g

shēng shí gāo (生石膏 raw gypsum, Gypsum Crudum) 30 g (pre-decocted)

chì sháo yào (赤芍药 red peony, Paeoniae Radix Rubra) 12 g

bái sháo yào (白芍药 white peony, Paeoniae Radix Alba) 12 g

guì zhī (桂枝 cinnamon twig, Cinnamomi Ramulus) 6 g

chén pí (陈皮 tangerine peel, Citri Reticulatae Pericarpium) 9 g

cǎo guǒ (草果 tsaoko, Tsaoko Fructus) 9 g

yīn chén hāo (茵陈蒿 virgate wormwood, Artemisiae Scopariae Herba) 12 g

zé xiè (泽泻 alisma, Alismatis Rhizoma) 9 g

bīng láng (槟榔 areca, Arecae Semen) 9 g

hòu pò (厚朴 official magnolia bark, Magnoliae Officinalis Cortex) 9 g

xìng rén (杏仁 apricot kernel, Armeniacae Semen) 9 g

Eighth visit on June 15: The patient had taken seven packets of this pre-scription. His essence-spirit and his physical strength were regained and even better than before, and there was still no recurrence of fever. Not only did the persistent cough disappear, but all the rest of the symptoms were gone as well. The tongue fur was no longer yellow, and the pulse had gradually moderated. Consequently, I decreased the dosage of *chái hú* (bupleurum) and *huáng qín* (scutellaria), removed the evil-dispelling medicinals *shēng shí gāo* (raw gypsum), *yīn chén hāo* (virgate wormwood), and *zé xiè* (alisma), and shifted my focus to support right qì. I prescribed six packets of the following medicinals:

chái hú (柴胡 bupleurum, Bupleuri Radix) 18 g

huáng qín (黄芩 scutellaria, Scutellariae Radix) 9 g

bàn xià (半夏 pinellia, Pinelliae Rhizoma) 9 g

dǎng shēn (党参 codonopsis, Codonopsis Radix) 30 g

hé shǒu wū (何首乌 flowery knotweed, Polygoni Multiflori Radix) 15 g

guì zhī (桂枝 cinnamon twig, Cinnamomi Ramulus) 4.5 g

chì sháo yào (赤芍药 red peony, Paeoniae Radix Rubra) 9 g

bái sháo yào (白芍药 white peony, Paeoniae Radix Alba) 9 g

cǎo guǒ (草果 tsaoko, Tsaoko Fructus) 9 g

bīng láng (槟榔 areca, Arecae Semen) 9 g

hòu pò (厚朴 official magnolia bark, Magnoliae Officinalis Cortex) 9 g

xìng rén (杏仁 apricot kernel, Armeniacae Semen) 9 g

zǐ wǎn (紫菀 aster, Asteris Radix) 12 g

Ninth visit on June 22: By now, his essence-spirit and physical strength were very good. Throughout this time the fever had not recurred. He felt that he had completely recovered from the illness, and when he discontinued the medicinals for a week as he had once before, the fever did not return. He was preparing to return home to fully recuperate, and he requested that the prescription be changed to pill form so that he could continue to strengthen the therapeutic effect. His complexion, tongue, and pulse showed no abnormalities upon examination, so I agreed with his travel plans, but also advised him to continue with several packets of the decoction while he waited for the preparation of the pill prescription. Later, he could put the pills together with the decoction. The prescriptions were as follows:

DECOCTION PRESCRIPTION

I removed *hòu pò* (officinal magnolia bark) and added 12 grams of *fú líng* (poria) to the prescription from his last visit, and I gave him six packets.

PILL PRESCRIPTION

chái hú (柴胡 bupleurum, Bupleuri Radix) 48 g

huáng qín (黄芩 scutellaria, Scutellariae Radix) 25 g

bàn xià (半夏 pinellia, Pinelliae Rhizoma) 25 g

dǎng shēn (党参 codonopsis, Codonopsis Radix) 78 g

hé shǒu wū (何首乌 flowery knotweed, Polygoni Multiflori Radix) 46 g

guì zhī (桂枝 cinnamon twig, Cinnamomi Ramulus) 12 g

chì sháo yào (赤芍药 red peony, Paeoniae Radix Rubra) 21 g

bái sháo yào (白芍药 white peony, Paeoniae Radix Alba) 21 g

cǎo guǒ (草果 tsaoko, Tsaoko Fructus) 24 g

bīng láng (槟榔 areca, Arecae Semen) 24 g

xìng rén (杏仁 apricot kernel, Armeniacae Semen) 18 g

zǐ wǎn (紫菀 aster, Asteris Radix) 30 g

fú líng (茯苓 poria, Poria) 30 g

hòu pò (厚朴 officinal magnolia bark, Magnoliae Officinalis Cortex) 30 g

bái zhú (白术 white atractylodes, Atractylodis Macrocephalae Rhizoma) 15 g

yīn chén hāo (茵陈蒿 virgate wormwood, Artemisiae Scopariae Herba) 15 g

xiāng fù (香附 cyperus, Cyperi Rhizoma) 21 g

yán hú suǒ (延胡索 corydalis, Corydalis Rhizoma) 21 g

zé xiè (泽泻 alisma, Alismatis Rhizoma) 15 g

All the ingredients were ground together into a fine powder and mixed with refined honey to form pills weighing 9–10 grams each. The dosage was 1–2 pills twice a day, taken with boiled water. The patient happily took the prescriptions with him and returned home.

CASE TWO

CONVULSIONS (CEREBRAL TUMOR?)

瘛疭（脑肿瘤？）

The patient was a 29-year-old female who was hospitalized for consultation in Hénán Province. Her initial examination date was December 9, 1969.

CHIEF COMPLAINT

Numbness and convulsions on the left side of the body, constant convulsion of the mouth and left eye, and dull speech for seven to eight days.

INQUIRY EXAMINATION

In the last part of October 1969, while she was breast-feeding her baby, the patient suddenly felt her whole body tremble. She had been unable to speak, and soon afterward she had fainted and had fallen to the ground. White foamy spit came from her mouth, her eyes rolled upward, and her daughter, whom she was holding at the time, dropped to the ground. The patient was immediately taken to the emergency room and examination revealed that her blood pressure was 150/90 mm/Hg, but her hemogram was normal. The diagnosis was symptomatic epilepsy and hypertension. At the hospital, she was given Dilantin, verticilum, dibazole, and vitamin B_1, and she received injections of penicillin, streptomycin, folic acid, and vitamins B_6 and B_{12}. Yet, three to twelve times every day, her body and face still convulsed for 3–10 minutes each time. She transferred to Zhèngzhōu Medical Hospital in Hénán for diagnosis and treatment.

On December 3, she consulted with doctors in the internal medicine and neurology departments, where an electroencephalogram (EEG) and a lumbar puncture were performed. The diagnostic opinion was suspicious of a condition in the right hemispheric and central vertex regions of the brain. She underwent treatment for 5–6 days without any improvement and the convulsions continued. She consulted with doctors in every department of the hospital, and the diagnosis was the same: intracranial lesion (a cerebral tumor?). The doctors advised her to go to Shànghǎi or Běijīng for surgery. The patient, however, would not consent to brain surgery and returned to her hometown hospital on December 8 for treatment, and at that time, requested a consultation with a Chinese medical doctor.

I consulted with the patient on the next day. She had the following symptoms: numbness and sometimes convulsions on the left side of her body, mouth deviation to the left, mouth and eye convulsions, stiff tongue, dull speech, forgetfulness and inability to remember events. The convulsions were constant, both day and night. She was using the Dilantin and other medications, but these were ineffective for stopping the convulsions. She had gone several days and nights without sleep, and because of that had a nervous mental state and was fearful. Both of her hands pulled on the hand of her husband; day and night she was without relief.

INSPECTION EXAMINATION

Her development was normal and nutrition regular. She had an acute and serious illness, a nervous mental state, an anxious expression, and a dark and gloomy complexion without luster. She suffered deviation of the mouth and left eye with constant convulsions; her four limbs convulsed repeatedly especially the upper and lower limbs on the left side. Her tongue fur was white.

LISTENING AND SMELLING EXAMINATION

Her speech was not clear, and her voice was low. When she was not convulsing, her breathing was regular; when convulsing, her breathing was irregular.

PALPATION EXAMINATION

Palpation of the head, neck, chest, and abdomen revealed no abnormalities. Convulsions could be felt on the left side of the face, and when the convulsions occurred in the upper and lower limbs on the left side, the limbs became hypertonic with intermittent spasms. The pulses on both hands were slippery and slightly stringlike.

PATTERN IDENTIFICATION

Constant convulsions of limbs, body, mouth, and eyes and a stringlike pulse is a pattern of stirring wind. "All wind with shaking and dizzy vision is ascribed to the liver," so I knew that the disease was in the liver. The forgetfulness and the sleeplessness were caused by the spirit failing to keep to its abode. The tongue had lost its flexibility, speech was dull, tongue fur was white, and the pulse was stringlike. Phlegm-damp followed wind and invaded the upper body, and phlegm obstructed the tongue body and clouded the clear orifices. Wind is a yáng evil and by nature moves. Thus, swift and changeable, moving wind caused hypertonicity of the sinews, so the limbs and body and the mouth and eyes convulsed. By correlating the four examinations, I knew that the disease was in the liver, heart, and spleen, but primarily in the liver. Therefore, I diagnosed convulsions due to liver wind stirring internally with wind-phlegm harassing the upper body.

TREATMENT METHOD

Calm the liver and extinguish wind while transforming phlegm and quieting the spirit, assisted by opening the orifices.

PRESCRIPTION

I used an empirical formula, *píng gān xī fēng tāng* (Calm the Liver and Extinguish Wind Decoction), together with *dí tán tāng* (Phlegm-Flushing Decoction), both modified according to the pattern.

> *shēng shí jué míng* (生石决明 raw abalone shell, Haliotidis Concha Cruda) 31 g (pre-decocted)
> *shēng dài zhě shí* (生代赭石 crude hematite, Haematitum Crudum) 30 g
> *bái sháo yào* (白芍药 white peony, Paeoniae Radix Alba) 12 g
> *xiāng fù* (香附 cyperus, Cyperi Rhizoma) 12 g
> *bái jí lí* (白蒺藜 tribulus, Tribuli Fructus) 12 g
> *gōu téng* (钩藤 uncaria, Uncariae Ramulus cum Uncis) 25 g
> *quán xiē* (全蝎 scorpion, Scorpio) 9 g
> *wú gōng* (蜈蚣 centipede, Scolopendra) 2 whole
> *huà jú hóng* (化橘红 Huazhou pomelo rind, Citri Grandis Exocarpium Rubrum) 9 g
> *qīng bàn xià* (清半夏 purified pinellia, Pinelliae Tuber Depuratum) 9 g
> *tiān nán xīng* (天南星 arisaema, Arisaematis Rhizoma) 4.5 g
> *sāng zhī* (桑枝 mulberry twig, Mori Ramulus) 30 g
> *zhū yuǎn zhì* (朱远志 cinnabar polygala, Polygalae Radix et Cinnabare) 9 g

When the first three packets proved effective, I gave the patient another three.

FORMULA EXPLANATION

As chief medicinals, *shēng shí jué míng* (raw abalone shell) subdues liver yáng and *shēng dài zhě shí* (crude hematite) settles and downbears liver yáng.

As support medicinals, *bái sháo yào* (white peony) nourishes yīn and emolliates the liver; *xiāng fù* (cyperus) rectifies qì and soothes the liver; and *bái jí lí* (tribulus) and *gōu téng* (uncaria) calm the liver and extinguish wind.

As assistant medicinals, *quán xiē* (scorpion) and *wú gōng* (centipede) check tetany, stabilize convulsions, and dispel wind; *jú hóng* (red tangerine peel), *bàn xià* (pinellia), and *tiān nán xīng* (arisaema) eliminate dampness and transform phlegm; *zhū yuǎn zhì* (cinnabar polygala) opens the orifices and calms the spirit. The use of *zhū yuǎn zhì* (cinnabar polygala) with *shēng shí jué míng* (raw abalone shell) and *shēng dài zhě shí* (crude hematite) strengthens the spirit-quieting effect.

As the courier medicinal, *sāng zhī* (mulberry twig) frees and penetrates the four limbs, soothes the liver and quickens the network vessels, and at the same time dispels wind.

FOLLOWUP TREATMENT

Second visit on December 15: The prescription had been effective, so the patient took another six packets. The convulsions had stopped, speech was distinct, and the numbness on the left side of her body had lessened. She was now able to get some sleep, but she was still forgetful. The tongue fur and the pulse were the same as before. I gave the patient six more packets of this prescription, but added:

shí chāng pú (石菖蒲 acorus, Acori Tatarinowii Rhizoma) 4.5 g
zhū shā fěn (朱砂粉 cinnabar powder, Cinnabaris Pulverata) 1.2 g
   (divided and taken drenched)
hǔ pò (琥珀 amber, Succinum) 1.2 g (divided and taken drenched)

Third visit on December 22: The patient had not experienced any convulsions after taking the medicinals. The left side of the body and the limbs were no longer numb, but she still felt weak in the left upper and lower limbs. Her speech and voice had returned to normal, she was able to sleep, her forgetfulness and essence-spirit had greatly improved, and her complexion was lustrous. The tongue fur was thin and white and the pulse slightly slippery. I again prescribed the same formula as before with only minor modifications. I removed tiān nán xīng (arisaema), changed the dosage of shēng dài zhě shí (crude hematite) to 45 grams, and added:

tiān zhú huáng (天竹黄 bamboo sugar, Bambusae Concretio Silicea) 6 g
fú líng (茯苓 poria, Poria) 12 g

I also removed zhū shā (cinnabar) and hǔ pò (amber) and gave the patient six packets. I advised her to take a pill prescription after she finished the decoction packets to strengthen the effect and eliminate the disease root. The pill prescription was the same as the decoction, but with five times the amount of each medicinal; however, the amount of dài zhě shí (hematite) was slightly reduced. These ingredients were ground into a fine powder and mixed with refined honey to make pills of 9–10 grams each. The dosage was 1–2 pills, to be taken twice a day with boiled water.

Follow-up visit on July 21, 1970: The patient had taken the pill prescription for four to five months, and from the first month, the convulsions had not recurred. She had recovered and was now six months pregnant. I advised her to discontinue the pills and to get some rest to prevent miscarriage. I gave her a fetus-quieting and fetus-nourishing formula to prepare her for childbirth. On a subsequent visit in the winter of 1973, she said her illness had not relapsed and she was working again. By May 1974, there was still no relapse; she was working at a factory and her health was very good. In March 1978, eight years had passed since she had been treated and still there was no relapse; she was in good health and could work the entire day without problems. After she had recovered, she gave birth to a son, who was also in good health and was by now in elementary school.

CASE THREE

WIND STRIKE (CEREBRAL ARTERIAL THROMBOSIS)
中风(脑动脉血栓形成)

The patient was a 65-year-old male farmer who was an in-patient at the Héběi Provincial Hospital. His initial examination date was May 10, 1978.

CHIEF COMPLAINT

Hemiplegia on the right side, with a sluggish tongue and difficult speech (aphasia) for the last four days.

INQUIRY EXAMINATION

The patient had had a feeling of numbness four days ago in the upper and lower limbs on the right side, along with discomfort when moving, but he still had some range of motion in his limbs at that time. However, changes occurred in his speech and voice, and he demonstrated difficult sluggish speech. The next day all these symptoms worsened, and he was admitted to the hospital. He had an examination there, and the diagnosis was cerebral arterial thrombosis. At the hospital he received an intravenous (IV) infusion, but he did not improve. The hemiplegia had gradually worsened, so he requested a Chinese medical consultation.

At the initial examination, the patient remained conscious and could respond to questions. He had the following symptoms: dizziness, somnolence, inability to talk and move, and difficult sluggish speech. When he really made an effort, he could hear clearly. His right arm was completely paralyzed; he could lift the right leg from the bed only with great effort, but could not bend it or move it around. The lower half of the right side of his face was weak and limp, his mouth deviated to the left, the right corner of his mouth drooped, and he drooled. He was constipated and already several days had passed without his having a bowel movement.

INSPECTION EXAMINATION

His development was normal and his nutrition was average. His mouth and face were deviated, his mental state was cloudy, and he was drowsy. His tongue fur was white, thick, and slightly yellow; the right side of his body was paralyzed.

LISTENING AND SMELLING EXAMINATION

His speech was difficult and sluggish, but his voice was not low, and breathing was normal.

Palpation examination

The pulses were stringlike, slippery, and forceful. Abdominal examination revealed no abnormalities. The upper and lower limbs on the right side of his body were paralyzed as already mentioned.

Pattern identification

I knew from the patient's age, dizzy head, somnolence, thick white tongue fur, deviated face and mouth, difficult sluggish speech, hemiplegia, and a stringlike, slippery pulse that this was liver wind stirring internally, wind-phlegm harassing the upper body and clouding the clear orifices, phlegm obstructing the network vessels, and the loss of smooth movement of qì and blood. Wind is a yáng evil; wind-phlegm obstruction creates depression, which transforms into heat. Consequently, in this case heat was binding yáng brightness (yáng míng), so the tongue fur became yellow and the bowels did not move. After correlating the four examinations, I diagnosed wind strike disease and channel strike pattern (the disease was already shifting into a bowel strike pattern).

Treatment method

Dispel wind and transform phlegm while clearing heat and quickening the network vessels.

Prescription

I gave the patient two packets of the following prescription:

sāng zhī (桑枝 mulberry twig, Mori Ramulus) 30 g

fáng fēng (防风 saposhnikovia, Saposhnikoviae Radix) 6 g

dǎn xīng (胆星 bile arisaema, Arisaema cum Bile) 9 g

bàn xià (半夏 pinellia, Pinelliae Rhizoma) 9 g

huà jú hóng (化橘红 Huazhou pomelo rind, Citri Grandis Exocarpium Rubrum) 12 g

fú líng (茯苓 poria, Poria) 9 g

zhǐ shí (枳实 unripe bitter orange, Aurantii Fructus Immaturus) 9 g

qiāng huó (羌活 notopterygium, Notopterygii Rhizoma et Radix) 6 g

guā lóu (栝楼 trichosanthes, Trichosanthis Fructus) 30 g

shēng dà huáng (生大黄 raw rhubarb, Rhei Radix et Rhizoma Crudi) 3 g

hóng huā (红花 carthamus, Carthami Flos) 9 g

piàn jiāng huáng (片姜黄 sliced turmeric, Curcumae Longae Rhizoma Sectum) 9 g

Formula explanation

The prescription was modified from two formulas: dí tán tāng (Phlegm-Flushing Decoction) and sān huà tāng (Three Transformations Decoction). As chief medicinals, *qiāng huó* (notopterygium) and *dǎn xīng* (bile arisaema) dispel wind and transform phlegm.

As support medicinals, *bàn xià* (pinellia) and *jú hóng* (red tangerine peel) transform phlegm and rectify qì; *fáng fēng* (saposhnikovia) and *sāng zhī* (mulberry twig) dispel wind and quicken the network vessels; and *fú líng* (poria) percolates dampness and dispels phlegm.

As assistant medicinals, *guā lóu* (trichosanthes), *zhǐ shí* (unripe bitter orange), and *dà huáng* (rhubarb) transform phlegm and downbear qì, clear and transform yáng brightness, and free the intestines and drain heat; *hóng huā* (carthamus) quickens blood and frees the network vessels.

As the courier medicinal, *piàn jiāng huáng* (sliced turmeric) quickens blood and frees the channels, and simultaneously brings the medicinals to the shoulder and arm.

This prescription dispels wind and transforms phlegm, frees the intestines and drains heat, and dispels phlegm and quickens the network vessels.

FOLLOWUP TREATMENT

Second visit on May 12: After two packets, the bowels were uninhibited. The patient was able to move his right arm and lift it from the bed; his right leg moved without restraint; it was stronger, but could only bear slight weight. However, his dizziness was still present. The tongue body was dark with white fur; the pulse was still stringlike and slippery.

I gave the patient three packets of the same prescription with only minor modifications as follows:

dǎn xīng (胆星 bile arisaema, Arisaema cum Bile) 9 g

qiāng huó (羌活 notopterygium, Notopterygii Rhizoma et Radix) 6 g

bàn xià (半夏 pinellia, Pinelliae Rhizoma) 9 g

huà jú hóng (化橘红 Huazhou pomelo rind, Citri Grandis Exocarpium Rubrum) 12 g

fú líng (茯苓 poria, Poria) 9 g

sāng zhī (桑枝 mulberry twig, Mori Ramulus) 30 g

guā lóu (栝楼 trichosanthes, Trichosanthis Fructus) 30 g

zhǐ shí (枳实 unripe bitter orange, Aurantii Fructus Immaturus) 9 g

shēng dà huáng (生大黄 raw rhubarb, Rhei Radix et Rhizoma Crudi) 3 g

hóng huā (红花 carthamus, Carthami Flos) 9 g

táo rén (桃仁 peach kernel, Persicae Semen) 9 g

piàn jiāng huáng (片姜黄 sliced turmeric, Curcumae Longae Rhizoma Sectum) 9 g

bái jiāng cán (白僵蚕 silkworm, Bombyx Batryticatus) 6 g

<u>Third visit on May 15</u>: His spirit-mind was clear, and his speech had greatly improved. He could bend and lift his right arm, which certainly showed improvement since his last visit. He could also bend, flex, lift, and bear his own weight on his right leg, and he was capable of any kind of leg movement, as if he were nearly normal. However, his stools were still dry and bound. His dizziness was gone. There were stasis macules on the tongue, and the fur had changed to thin white. The right pulse was stringlike and slippery and the left slightly stringlike, and the right pulse was larger than the left. I gave the patient one packet of the above-mentioned prescription, but removed *bái jiāng cán* (silkworm) and changed the dosage of *dà huáng* (rhubarb) to 9 grams. I added:

yuán míng fěn (元明粉 refined mirabilite, Natrii Sulfus Exsiccatus) 15 g

The dosage of *yuán míng fěn* (refined mirabilite) was to be divided in two and taken drenched. I instructed the patient to take the first half after decocting the first dose. If a bowel movement occurred, then he did not need to take the second half after decocting the second dose.

<u>Fourth visit on May 16</u>: The bowels moved after taking just one packet, and his appetite increased. I removed *yuán míng fěn* (refined mirabilite) and *táo rén* (peach kernel) from the prescription and gave two more packets to the patient. When these proved effective, I gave him three more.

<u>Fifth visit on May 22</u>: Since the limbs on the right side of his body could move freely as normal, the patient left his bed and was walking. His facial paralysis was completely gone. His speech was clear; he had recovered and appeared normal. His bowels moved twice a day. The tongue fur was normal and the pulse slightly stringlike. He had essentially recovered from his illness, and I gave him three more packets of the following prescription to consolidate the therapeutic effect:

qiāng huó (羌活 notopterygium, Notopterygii Rhizoma et Radix) 6 g
dǎn xīng (胆星 bile arisaema, Arisaema cum Bile) 9 g
bàn xià (半夏 pinellia, Pinelliae Rhizoma) 9 g
fú líng (茯苓 poria, Poria) 12 g
guā lóu (栝楼 trichosanthes, Trichosanthis Fructus) 30 g
shēng dà huáng (生大黄 raw rhubarb, Rhei Radix et Rhizoma Crudi) 6 g
hóng huā (红花 carthamus, Carthami Flos) 9 g
táo rén (桃仁 peach kernel, Persicae Semen) 9 g
dì lóng (地龙 earthworm, Pheretima) 9 g
chì sháo yào (赤芍药 red peony, Paeoniae Radix Rubra) 12 g
bái jí lí (白蒺藜 tribulus, Tribuli Fructus) 9 g
sāng zhī (桑枝 mulberry twig, Mori Ramulus) 30 g

On May 24, the patient happily walked out of the hospital and returned home to recuperate.

CASE FOUR
A SERIOUS CASE OF INSOMNIA
严重失眠

The patient was a 36-year-old male thoracic surgeon at a Běijīng hospital. His initial examination date was December 17, 1967.

CHIEF COMPLAINT
Sleepless nights for the last three to four days.

INQUIRY EXAMINATION
The patient's insomnia had been ongoing for several years, and the sleeping pills that he had taken every evening, including a name brand called Miltown, were all ineffective, so he turned to chloral hydrate (also known as knock-out drops). Each dosage of these drops exceeded the last, until his regular dose was many times the recommended amount. He became accustomed to the higher dosages and had constant diarrhea. As a member of the Health Department, he traveled with the Northwest medical team to Gānsù Province, yet still continued to take the chloral hydrate sleeping pills. Six or seven days passed, and due to the heavy demands of his surgical schedule and to his excessively overworked condition, he was tense. As a result, he could not fall asleep at any time during the night, even though he took large doses of sedatives. Before bedtime for the last two to three nights he took a 10% solution of chloral hydrate in 100 ml liquid, but still could not fall asleep. Instead, he had an opposite reaction and was fidgety and agitated and could not be still at all. He was in and out of bed one moment, and then the next would be squatting on the floor for awhile. At times he stood with the door open for casual conversation with colleagues, other times he paced back and forth outside the door. In short, he could neither lie down nor fall asleep. He was dizzy, gave no thought to food, and had diarrhea six or seven times a day. He showed flusteredness, his heart throbbed (sometimes the heart rate reached 140 beats/minute), and he had a vexed and agitated temperament. For these reasons, he had moved from the dormitory to a single-bed hotel room for the last several days.

INSPECTION EXAMINATION
His development and nutrition were normal. His spirit-mind was tense. The tongue fur was white and slightly lacking fluids.

LISTENING AND SMELLING EXAMINATION
His speech was clear and his voice normal.

Palpation examination

An abdominal examination revealed no abnormalities. The pulse was sunken, fine, slippery, and rapid, and the right cubit pulse was weak.

Pattern identification

The liver is the basis of resistance to fatigue. Noting this patient's excessive fatigue and sleeplessness, irritable temperament, and dizziness, I knew that this was effluent liver yáng leading to a yīn and yáng disharmony, with yáng failing to enter yīn. When liver effulgence damaged the spleen, there was no desire for food, and diarrhea occurred. Later heaven was deprived of nourishment, the source of engendering transformation (the spleen) was lacking, the pulse was fine, and the blood was vacuous. Blood could not provide luxuriance to the heart, and when combined with excessive mental work, caused the heart-spirit to fail to keep its composure. As a result there was serious loss of sleep, and symptoms such as flusteredness and throbbing of the heart occurred. The weak right cubit pulse indicated insufficiency of kidney yáng. When kidney yáng vacuity was unable to warm the center burner, center dampness did not transform. This condition not only caused serious diarrhea, but also influenced the heart-kidney interaction and aggravated sleeplessness. After comprehensive observation of the pulse and symptoms, my diagnosis was insomnia caused by effulgent liver yáng, heart-spirit failing to keep its composure, and dual vacuity of the spleen and kidney.

Treatment method

Calm the liver and subdue yáng, nourish the heart and quiet the spirit, and fortify the spleen and harmonize the center.

Prescription

I gave the patient one packet of the following prescription:

shēng shí jué míng (生石决明 raw abalone shell, Haliotidis Concha Cruda) 30 g (pre-decocted)

shēng lóng gǔ (生龙骨 crude dragon bone, Mastodi Ossis Fossilia Cruda) 15 g (pre-decocted)

shēng mǔ lì (生牡蛎 raw oyster shell, Ostreae Concha Cruda) 15 g (pre-decocted)

shēng zhě shí (生赭石 crude hematite, Haematitum Crudum) 25 g (pre-decocted)

chǎo zǎo rén (炒枣仁 stir-fried spiny jujube, Ziziphi Spinosi Semen Frictum) 15 g

zhū yuǎn zhì (朱远志 cinnabar polygala, Polygalae Radix et Cinnabare) 9 g

zhū fú shén (朱茯神 cinnabar root poria, Poria cum Pini Radice et
Cinnabare) 12 g

bái sháo yào (白芍药 white peony, Paeoniae Radix Alba) 9 g

shēng bái zhú (生白朮 raw ovate atractylodes, Atractylodis Ovatae
Rhizoma Crudum) 9 g

qīng bàn xià (清半夏 purified pinellia, Pinelliae Tuber Depuratum) 9 g

běi shú mǐ (北秫米 sorghum, Sorghi Semen) 9 g

tiān má (天麻 gastrodia, Gastrodiae Rhizoma) 6 g

gōu téng (钩藤 uncaria, Uncariae Ramulus cum Uncis) 15 g

zhì gān cǎo (炙甘草 mix-fried licorice, Glycyrrhizae Radix cum Liquido
Fricta) 4 g

FORMULA EXPLANATION

As chief medicinals, *shēng shí jué míng* (raw abalone shell) nourishes liver
yīn and subdues liver yáng, *shēng lóng gǔ* (crude dragon bone) and *shēng mǔ lì*
(raw oyster shell) subdue yáng and quiet the spirit, and *shēng zhě shí* (crude
hematite) calms the liver and quiets the spirit with its heavy settling nature.

As support medicinals, *chǎo zǎo rén* (stir-fried spiny jujube) constrains
the spirit and nourishes the heart; *zhū yuǎn zhì* (cinnabar polygala) promotes
heart-kidney interaction and quiets the spirit; *zhū fú shén* (cinnabar root poria)
nourishes the heart, quiets the spirit, and boosts the spleen; and *bái sháo yào*
(white peony) emolliates the liver and boosts the spleen.

As assistant medicinals, *qīng bàn xià* (purified pinellia) combined with *běi
shú mǐ* (sorghum) harmonize the center, boost the spleen, and quiet the spirit;
shēng bái zhú (raw ovate atractylodes) combined with *zhì gān cǎo* (mix-fried
licorice) fortify the spleen and boost qì.

Gōu téng (uncaria) and *tiān má* (gastrodia) are the couriers; they calm the
liver and subdue wind.

As a whole, this prescription calms the liver and subdues yáng, nourishes
the heart and quiets the spirit, and harmonizes the center and fortifies the
spleen.

FOLLOWUP TREATMENT

Second visit: After taking the prescribed packet, the patient was able to lie
quietly in bed, and according to his wife, he slept for awhile. The previous
evening he had taken the Chinese medicinals and two tablets of Miltown, but
did not take the chloral hydrate. Bowel frequency had increased, approximately ten times a day, his essence-spirit had improved, and his dizziness was
alleviated. The tongue fur had become thinner. I made the following modifications to his prescription and gave him another packet:

shēng shí jué míng (生石决明 raw abalone shell, Haliotidis Concha
    Cruda) 15 g (pre-decocted)

duàn lóng gǔ (煅龙骨 calcined dragon bone, Mastodi Ossis Fossilia
    Calcinata) 15 g (pre-decocted)

duàn mǔ lì (煅牡蛎 calcined oyster shell, Ostreae Concha Calcinata) 15 g
    (pre-decocted)

zhū yuǎn zhì (朱远志 cinnabar polygala, Polygalae Radix et Cinnabare) 9 g

zhū fú shén (朱茯神 cinnabar root poria, Poria cum Pini Radice et
    Cinnabare) 12 g

qīng bàn xià (清半夏 purified pinellia, Pinelliae Tuber Depuratum) 9 g

běi shú mǐ (北秫米 sorghum, Sorghi Semen) 9 g

bái sháo yào (白芍药 white peony, Paeoniae Radix Alba) 9 g

chǎo bái zhú (炒白术 stir-fried white atractylodes, Atractylodis
    Macrocephalae Rhizoma Frictum) 9 g

tiān má (天麻 gastrodia, Gastrodiae Rhizoma) 6 g

gōu téng (钩藤 uncaria, Uncariae Ramulus cum Uncis) 15 g

chǎo zǎo rén (炒枣仁 stir-fried spiny jujube, Ziziphi Spinosi Semen
    Frictum) 12 g

pào jiāng (炮姜 blast-fried ginger, Zingiberis Rhizoma Praeparatum) 3 g

zhì gān cǎo (炙甘草 mix-fried licorice, Glycyrrhizae Radix cum Liquido
    Fricta) 6 g

hē zǐ (诃子 chebule, Chebulae Fructus) 9 g

gé gēn (葛根 pueraria, Puerariae Radix) [roasted] 6 g

Third visit on December 19: The patient could lie down comfortably and
fall asleep for awhile at night. His bowels moved just three times a day, and
his appetite had increased. He had discontinued his Western medications and
sleeping pills, but could fall asleep without them. His body was renewing itself, and he was almost completely back to his previous self. The tongue and
pulse signs were the same as the previous visit, so I gave him two packets of
the modified prescription as follows:

duàn lóng gǔ (煅龙骨 calcined dragon bone, Mastodi Ossis Fossilia
    Calcinata) 15 g (pre-decocted)

duàn mǔ lì (煅牡蛎 calcined oyster shell, Ostreae Concha Calcinata) 15 g
    (pre-decocted)

zhū yuǎn zhì (朱远志 cinnabar polygala, Polygalae Radix et Cinnabare)
    9 g

zhū fú shén (朱茯神 cinnabar root poria, Poria cum Pini Radice et
    Cinnabare) 12 g

chǎo bái zhú (炒白术 stir-fried white atractylodes, Atractylodis
  Macrocephalae Rhizoma Frictum) 9 g

dǎng shēn (党参 codonopsis, Codonopsis Radix) 9 g

bái sháo yào (白芍药 white peony, Paeoniae Radix Alba) 9 g

ròu dòu kòu (肉豆蔻 nutmeg, Myristicae Semen) 9 g

hē zǐ (诃子 chebule, Chebulae Fructus) 9 g

gé gēn (葛根 pueraria, Puerariae Radix) *[roasted]* 6 g

bǔ gǔ zhī (补骨脂 psoralea, Psoraleae Fructus) 9 g

ròu guì (肉桂 cinnamon bark, Cinnamomi Cortex) 2.5 g

zhì gān cǎo (炙甘草 mix-fried licorice, Glycyrrhizae Radix cum Liquido
  Fricta) 5 g

gōu téng (钩藤 uncaria, Uncariae Ramulus cum Uncis) 15 g

<u>Fourth visit on December 21</u>: Since the last visit, the patient could fall
asleep anytime during the day or night. At night, he slept for 2–3 hours at a
time. He had discontinued all the Western medications and sleeping pills and
had voluntarily moved back into the medical team dormitory. His appetite was
good, his bowels moved five times a day, and he was clearheaded and alert.
The tongue fur had been completely transformed; the pulse spirit was tranquil
without any stringlike or rapid manifestation, but slightly slippery and fine.
Again, I modified the prescription as follows and gave him two packets:

duàn lóng gǔ (煅龙骨 calcined dragon bone, Mastodi Ossis Fossilia
  Calcinata) 15 g (pre-decocted)

duàn mǔ lì (煅牡蛎 calcined oyster shell, Ostreae Concha Calcinata) 15 g
  (pre-decocted)

zhū yuǎn zhì (朱远志 cinnabar polygala, Polygalae Radix et Cinnabare)
  9 g

zhū fú shén (朱茯神 cinnabar root poria, Poria cum Pini Radice et
  Cinnabare) 9 g

chǎo zǎo rén (炒枣仁 stir-fried spiny jujube, Ziziphi Spinosi Semen
  Frictum) 12 g

běi shú mǐ (北秫米 sorghum, Sorghi Semen) 9 g

chǎo bái zhú (炒白术 stir-fried white atractylodes, Atractylodis
  Macrocephalae Rhizoma Frictum) 9 g

bái sháo yào (白芍药 white peony, Paeoniae Radix Alba) 15 g

dǎng shēn (党参 codonopsis, Codonopsis Radix) 9 g

bǔ gǔ zhī (补骨脂 psoralea, Psoraleae Fructus) 9 g

wǔ wèi zǐ (五味子 schisandra, Schisandrae Fructus) 3 g

gé gēn (葛根 pueraria, Puerariae Radix) 6 g

hē zǐ (诃子 chebule, Chebulae Fructus) 9 g

pào jiāng (炮姜 blast-fried ginger, Zingiberis Rhizoma Praeparatum) 5 g

zhì gān cǎo (炙甘草 mix-fried licorice, Glycyrrhizae Radix cum Liquido Fricta) 5 g

<u>Fifth visit on December 23</u>: His sleeping was stabilized and his essence-spirit and appetite were very good. He had not taken the Western drugs and sleeping pills for some time, and he could sleep for approximately three hours at a time. At other times he was tranquil enough to lie down and rest. I gave him three more packets of the prescription to consolidate the therapeutic effect. His essence-spirit and appetite remained healthy, and he returned to his normal schedule.

CASE FIVE
INSOMNIA AND SEMINAL EMISSION
失眠、遗精

The patient was a 29-year-old male whose initial examination date was April 2, 1962.

CHIEF COMPLAINT

Insomnia, headache, and seminal emission for the last year.

INQUIRY EXAMINATION

For more than a year, the patient suffered from insomnia and was unable to sleep longer than 1–2 hours a night. Sometimes he remained completely awake throughout the night. He had a headache on the right side of his forehead and during the daytime had occasional dizziness. Usually at night he would lie down, but was unable to fall asleep; if he did sleep, he would experience night sweating, profuse dreaming, and seminal emission. This occurred three to four times a week. Sometimes he had numbness in his hands and feet, and 3–4 times a night he experienced frequent painless urination, and the urine was not yellow in color. Occasionally he had palpitations and nosebleeds, but his stools were normal.

INSPECTION EXAMINATION

His development and nutrition were normal, but his essence-spirit did not appear healthy. The tongue body was slightly red and the fur thin and white.

LISTENING AND SMELLING EXAMINATION

No abnormalities were seen.

PALPATION EXAMINATION

Palpation of the chest, abdomen, and limbs revealed nothing unusual, but the pulse was equally fine on both wrists.

PATTERN IDENTIFICATION

I knew the pattern was yīn vacuity and non-interaction of heart and kidney, because his insomnia had continued for more than a year accompanied by seminal emission, and he had night sweating and a fine pulse. Kidney yīn was insufficient and unable to help the heart, so heart blood was insufficient and unable to help kidney essence below. The heart and kidney were not able to aid each other; thus, symptoms such as insomnia, heart palpitations, seminal emission, and nocturia appeared. Vacuous kidney yīn was also unable to nourish the liver, so liver yáng easily stirred and harassed the upper body. Therefore, there was headache on the right side of the forehead and dizziness. Yīn vacuity engendered internal heat, and internal heat distressed the blood; thus, the nosebleed occurred. Correlation of the four examinations supported my diagnosis of insomnia and seminal emission due to yīn vacuity and yáng effulgence and to non-interaction of heart and kidney.

TREATMENT METHOD

Enrich yīn and boost the kidney, calm the liver and subdue yáng, and quiet the heart-spirit and secure the lower origin.

PRESCRIPTION

I gave the patient three packets of the following prescription, to be decocted in water:

> shēng dì huáng (生地黄 dried rehmannia, Rehmanniae Radix Exsiccata) 12 g
>
> bái sháo yào (白芍药 white peony, Paeoniae Radix Alba) 9 g
>
> shēng shí jué míng (生石决明 raw abalone shell, Haliotidis Concha Cruda) 24 g (pre-decocted)
>
> suān zǎo rén (酸枣仁 spiny jujube, Ziziphi Spinosi Semen) 12 g
>
> shēng mǔ lì (生牡蛎 raw oyster shell, Ostreae Concha Cruda) 15 g (pre-decocted)
>
> xiāng fù (香附 cyperus, Cyperi Rhizoma) 6 g
>
> zhū yuǎn zhì (朱远志 cinnabar polygala, Polygalae Radix et Cinnabare) 6 g
>
> yè jiāo téng (夜交藤 flowery knotweed stem, Polygoni Multiflori Caulis) 12 g
>
> qiàn shí (芡实 euryale, Euryales Semen) 9 g
>
> lián xū (莲须 lotus stamen, Nelumbinis Stamen) 6 g
>
> cí zhū wán (磁朱丸 Loadstone and Cinnabar Pill) 6 g (wrapped in cloth)

FORMULA EXPLANATION

This prescription is based on my empirical formula, yì shén tāng (Spirit-Lifing Decoction), with modifications according to the pattern. As chief medicinals, *shēng dì huáng* (dried rehmannia) supplements the kidney by enriching and nourishing kidney yīn, and *shēng shí jué míng* (raw abalone shell) enriches liver yīn and subdues liver yáng.

As support medicinals, *shēng bái sháo* (raw white peony) supplies nourishment to the blood, emolliates the liver, and boosts the heart; *suān zǎo rén* (spiny jujube) nourishes the liver and supplements blood while boosting the heart and quieting the spirit; *zhū yuǎn zhì* (cinnabar polygala) and *yè jiāo téng* (flowery knotweed stem) promote heart-kidney interaction.

As assistant medicinals, *xiāng fù* (cyperus) soothes liver depression and clears depressed heat; *mǔ lì* (oyster shell) subdues liver yáng and stops night sweating; *qiàn shí* (euryale) secures the kidney and astringes essence; and *lián xū* (lotus stamen) clears the heart and secures essence.

Cí zhū wán (Loadstone and Cinnabar Pill) is the courier and consists of cí shí (磁石 loadstone, Magnetitum) and *zhū shā* (朱砂 cinnabar, Cinnabaris) *Cí shí* (loadstone) settles and restrains lesser yīn (*shào yīn*) fire from floating upward, and *zhū shā* (cinnabar) clears heart heat, settles the heart, and quiets the spirit. Hence *cí zhū wán* (Loadstone and Cinnabar Pill) causes the heart and kidney to help each other, thereby stabilizing the mind and quieting the spirit. The entire formula enriches yīn and subdues yáng, calms the liver and boosts the kidney, and quiets the spirit and secures essence.

FOLLOWUP TREATMENT

Second visit on April 5: The headache was greatly relieved by taking the decoction, and the symptoms of dizziness, bodily fatigue, and numbness in the limbs had all disappeared. However, the insomnia and frequent nocturia were still present. The patient had no desire for fluids even though his lips and throat were dry. The tongue fur was thin and white and the tongue body slightly red. He had a fine pulse. So, from the previous prescription, I removed *xiāng fù* (cyperus) to avoid aromatic dry damage to yīn, and I added nine grams of *zhī mǔ* (anemarrhena) to clear heat from the heart and stomach and enrich the kidney. I also added nine grams of *hé huān huā* (silk tree flower) to strengthen the heart-kidney interaction. I changed the dosage of *yè jiāo téng* (flowery knotweed stem) and *suān zǎo rén* (spiny jujube) to fifteen grams and eighteen grams respectively. I divided the dosage of *suān zǎo rén* equally between the fresh medicinal and the prepared to strengthen the effect of harmonizing both yīn and yáng and quieting the spirit. I gave the patient four packets.

Third visit on April 9: Good results were evident after taking the decoction, because the patient could now sleep for more than three hours at a time, and dreaming was less frequent. Both the headaches and the night sweating had stopped. There had been no recurrence of seminal emission during the last week. However, he still occasionally had some dizziness and was easily fatigued. Since there was improvement in all the symptoms, I knew that the medicinals were appropriate for the pathocondition. Therefore, the effect was good, and I did not change the prescription, but kept the original method in mind and prescribed the following:

> *shēng dì huáng* (生地黄 dried rehmannia, Rehmanniae Radix Exsiccata) 9 g
>
> *shēng shí jué míng* (生石决明 raw abalone shell, Haliotidis Concha Cruda) 30 g (pre-decocted)
>
> *bái sháo yào* (白芍药 white peony, Paeoniae Radix Alba) 9 g
>
> *suān zǎo rén* (酸枣仁 spiny jujube, Ziziphi Spinosi Semen) 18 g (equally divided between fresh and cooked)
>
> *zhū yuǎn zhì* (朱远志 cinnabar polygala, Polygalae Radix et Cinnabare) 6 g
>
> *yè jiāo téng* (夜交藤 flowery knotweed stem, Polygoni Multiflori Caulis) 15 g
>
> *hé huān huā* (合欢花 silk tree flower, Albizziae Flos) 9 g
>
> *shēng mǔ lì* (生牡蛎 raw oyster shell, Ostreae Concha Cruda) 18 g (pre-decocted)
>
> *zhī mǔ* (知母 anemarrhena, Anemarrhenae Rhizoma) 9 g
>
> *cí zhū wán* (磁朱丸 Loadstone and Cinnabar Pill) 6 g (wrapped in cloth)

All the symptoms disappeared after three packets of this prescription. I continued with this method using slight modifications and treating him three more times until he had indeed fully recovered and resumed his normal work.

EMPIRICAL KNOWLEDGE

Concerning the diagnosis of *jiē nüè* (malaria)

The disease we call "malaria" is referred to in the *Huáng Dì Nèi Jīng* ("The Yellow Emperor's Inner Canon"). In the *Sù Wèn* ("Plain Questions"), it states, "All malaria is engendered by wind." It also states, "If the patient suffers damage by summerheat during the summer, then malaria occurs in the autumn."

The understanding and explanation of malaria by later generations of physicians was for all practical purposes identical. Generally speaking, they held three common theories:

1. The term "malaria" is a general term for all malaria-like diseases.

2. The onset of malaria-like signs recurs every two days or on a regular basis.

3. The term "malaria" also refers to enduring malaria or old malaria.

The *Dān Xī Xīn Fǎ* ("Dān Xī's Heart-Approach") states, "There is malaria, and there is old malaria." The *Yī Xué Gāng Mù* ("Compendium of Medicine") explains, "The patient who suffers from enduring malaria also suffers from malaria." I believe that the patient in Case 1 followed the above-mentioned third theory because his residence was in the southern region of the country, and he had ample opportunity to be affected by the hot summer weather. As the *Huáng Dì Nèi Jīng* ("The Yellow Emperor's Inner Canon") says:

> "The patient who suffers from malaria first experiences cold and afterwards heat; why does this happen? When damage by great heat happens in summer, there is great sweating and the interstices open; then summer qì meets chilly water-cold, which is stored in the interstices and within the skin. Consequently, in the following autumn when the patient suffers damage by wind, disease occurs."

At the initial onset of disease, the treatment may not be timely enough, the treatment method may not be correctly chosen, or the right qì may be insufficient; for whatever reason, the disease evil is not resolved, and it remains hidden half-exterior and half-interior in the lesser yáng (*shào yáng*). Thus, when a struggle occurs between right and evil, disease is manifest; when right and evil separate from each other, disease stops; this process repeats itself continuously. Physicians of the past said that "when heat is predominant over cold, then in the hot summer weather, wind and cold are also less frequent." The patient in Case 1 had a fever more frequently than he had feelings of cold, to the extent that he had the fever every 2–3 days and then it resolved, so I knew this condition was due to exuberant depressed heat. Whenever this patient used antipyretic medicines, he could not reduce the fever; on the contrary, if he left the fever untreated, it would resolve itself after a period of time. This is exactly how the *Huáng Dì Nèi Jīng* ("The Yellow Emperor's Inner Canon") explains it thus:

> "When the patient experiences the cold manifestation of this disease, hot soup and fire cannot warm him; during warm manifestation, ice water cannot cool him. At these times even a skilled physician cannot stop the course of the disease. You should allow the disease to weaken on its own accord before attempting an acupuncture treatment."

Furthermore, the previously mentioned theories of enduring malaria and old malaria by Dān Xī and Lóu Yīng coincide with the patient in Case 1, who had already suffered his disease for over two years. Certainly the illness could be called "enduring and old." Therefore, my diagnosis was malaria due to disharmony of the lesser yáng (*shào yáng*) and enduring exuberance of depressed heat.

The physicians of ancient China were bound by historical circumstances, and thus they did not recognize malarial parasites as we know them today. What we call malaria today was described by physicians in the past as alternating cold and heat occurring at fixed periods of time, first cold and then heat, predominant cold with less frequent heat, predominant heat with less frequent cold, or even sometimes first heat and later cold. They also recognized the conditions of heat without cold and cold without heat. From a modern perspective, many of these conditions are not recognized as part of the medical diagnosis of malaria, which instead emphasizes a positive diagnostic test for malarial parasites or plasmodium. However, these descriptions of old play a larger role when diagnostic tests are negative for malarial parasites. Although physicians in ancient times could not recognize malaria with the precision that the modern world provides, their understanding of this disease deserves attention because until modern times we relied on the theories of our predecessors concerning malaria, and used their methods of pattern identification to treat this disease and obtain satisfactory results. Moreover, acumoxa treatments have proven effective to prevent the occurrence of malaria-like symptoms, and this approach certainly merits more study.

Concerning the use of the harmonization method

Physicians of the past believed that malarial symptoms were directly related to the lesser yáng (*shào yáng*). To treat malaria they used *chái hú* (bupleurum) as the chief medicinal in formulas that harmonize the lesser yáng. The "harmonization" method is one of the eight methods of disease treatment. However, to use only the harmonization method to treat malarial symptoms would mean fixating on just one treatment principle. If you do not formulate the harmonization method to specific circumstances by modifying, changing, and flexibly applying the treatment according to the specific requirements of the patient and his condition, then you can never obtain ideal results.

An example here is the patient in Case 1, who, prior to my examination, had taken more than 200 packets of Chinese medicinals. Some of these prescriptions had indeed used the harmonization method. Yet all these formulas were ineffective, and thus there was some doubt as to whether any of them were modified and flexibly applied according to the pattern. At the time of this patient's initial visit he was 63 years old, his illness had already been active for more than two years, his pulse was fine, and his complexion was without luster; all these signs indicated right vacuity. However, upon further analysis, and according to his account, every time the illness recurred, there was more heat than cold. The high fever abated after 2–3 days, but his body temperature reached approximately 40°C. He had a sensation of fullness in the right rib-side, yellow tongue fur, and a stringlike pulse. These symptoms indicated repletion evil. In this particular case, a comprehensive understanding of the relative strength of evil and right was necessary, and the tendency toward exuberance of evil qì determined the true nature of this disease. Even though there was, in fact, vacuity within repletion, the repletion pattern was foremost, and I decided to treat him using *xiǎo chái hú tāng* (Minor Bupleurum Decoction) with modifications. The use of *xiǎo chái hú tāng* to harmonize is a general treatment method; thus it was necessary to consider the specific characteristics of this patient's symptoms, namely, that the occurrence of heat was greater than the occurrence of cold. I chose to combine the formulas *bái hǔ jiā guì zhī tāng* (White Tiger Decoction Plus Cinnamon Twig) and *xiǎo chái hú tāng* (Minor Bupleurum Decoction). *Bái hǔ jiā guì zhī tāng* (White Tiger Decoction Plus Cinnamon Twig) treats malarial symptoms characterized by heat that is greater than cold or heat without cold. I paid particular attention to the general approach to treatment of malarial symptoms and closely integrated the specific characteristics of the disease in this patient.

At the time of the second visit, since the medicinals had proven effective for the disease, I added *cháng shān* (dichroa), *bīng láng* (areca), and *cǎo guǒ* (tsaoko) to strengthen the phlegm-eliminating, dampness-transforming, malaria-treating, and evil-outthrusting effect. Then I followed the changes in the condition of the disease and in the transformation of the exuberance and depletion of evil and right. By the time of the sixth visit, I saw that evil qì had gradually abated. When this happened, right vacuity was in a transitional phase, so I changed the dosage of *dǎng shēn* (codonopsis) to 30 g and added *hé shǒu wū* (flowery knotweed). Basically, I took the essence of the treatment of malaria from *hé rén yǐn* (Flowery Knotweed and Ginseng Beverage) and used it in this prescription to strengthen support for right qì. The medicinals in *hé rén yǐn* (Flowery Knotweed and Ginseng Beverage) are listed below. This formula treats enduring malaria with constitutional vacuity:

hé shǒu wū (何首乌 flowery knotweed, Polygoni Multiflori Radix)

rén shēn (人参 ginseng, Ginseng Radix)

dāng guī (当归 Chinese angelica, Angelicae Sinensis Radix)

chén pí (陈皮 tangerine peel, Citri Reticulatae Pericarpium)

shēng jiāng (生姜 fresh ginger, Zingiberis Rhizoma Recens)

The combined use of *hòu pò* (officinal magnolia bark), *xìng rén* (apricot kernel), and *zǐ wǎn* (aster) was directed at treating the patient's symptom of cough, since these medicinals in this case treated the tip. When a symptom existed, I added a medicinal to the formula; when a symptom was alleviated, I subtracted it. These particular medicinals were not the most important in the formula. After the eighth visit, the evil qì had abated, the symptoms were gone, the tongue fur had transformed, and the pulse was moderate; the disease condition had been quite altered. At this time I decreased the dosage of *chái hú* (bupleurum) and *huáng qín* (scutellaria) and removed *shēng shí gāo* (raw gypsum). I also altered my treatment to emphasize support for right qì and used the method of combining *xiǎo chái hú tāng* (Minor Bupleurum Decoction) and *hé rén yǐn* (Flowery Knotweed and Ginseng Beverage) with modifications according to the pattern. In the pill prescription, I not only increased the dosage of *dǎng shēn* (codonopsis) and *hé shǒu wū* (flowery knotweed), but I also added *bái zhú* (white atractylodes), which combines with *dǎng shēn* (codonopsis) and *fú líng* (poria) to strengthen and fortify the center burner.

This combination comes from the experience of past physicians and refers to "primarily supplementing the spleen as the treatment method for malarial symptoms." Because the lesser yáng and the liver stand in exterior-interior relationship, the lesser yáng is associated with enduring depression and influences the spleen and stomach. Furthermore, the spleen and stomach are the root of later heaven, and I have noticed that in later stages of disease, the method of spleen supplementation supports the weak against the strong and harmonizes the liver and spleen. When spleen movement is healthy and vigorous, then the body will be also.

In summary, when using the harmonization method, you must flexibly consider the special circumstances of the patient's condition, the transitions in the course of disease, and the presence of exuberance and depletion of evil and right. It is exactly as the famous Qīng dynasty physician, Chéng Zhōng-Líng, said:

> "There is the method of clearing and harmonizing, the method of warming and harmonizing, the method of dispersing and harmonizing, of supplementing and harmonizing, of drying and harmonizing, and of moisturizing and harmonizing. There is also the method of simultaneous treatment of the exterior and harmonization, and of simultaneous attack and harmonization. This is the meaning of harmonization, and the methods are infinite in their variations."

Concerning the liver-calming wind-extinguishing method

The liver-calming wind-extinguishing method is primarily used in the treatment of liver wind stirring internally. The patient who suffers from liver wind stirring internally not only presents with symptoms such as dizziness and tremors, but also with symptoms such as sudden clouding, deviation of mouth and eyes, convulsions of the four limbs, grinding of the teeth, and up-turned eyes. As the *Huáng Dì Nèi Jīng* ("The Yellow Emperor's Inner Canon") says:

> "All fulminant rigidity is ascribed to wind.... All wind with shaking and dizzy vision is ascribed to the liver.... When wind prevails, there is stirring."

The liver-calming wind-extinguishing method is commonly used to treat liver wind stirring internally. However, this is just one treatment principle and should be taken into account along with the specific circumstances and condition of the patient. By doing so, you will select medicinals for the prescription with flexible application and modification and thereby obtain ideal treatment results.

In Case 2, even though the patient was diagnosed with liver wind stirring internally, I did not merely apply a "liver-calming wind-extinguishing formula" using medicinals such as *shēng shí jué míng* (raw abalone shell), *shēng dài zhě shí* (crude hematite), *bái sháo yào* (white peony), *xiāng fù* (cyperus), *huáng qín* (scutellaria), *bái jí lí* (tribulus), *gōu téng* (uncaria), *quán xiē* (scorpion), and *wú gōng* (centipede). Instead, I comprehensively observed her other symptoms such as slippery pulse, white tongue fur, inhibited tongue body, and greatly diminished memory. With these symptoms in mind, I took into consideration the fact that liver disease most easily harms the spleen (this is traditionally called wood overwhelming earth), and that when the spleen is invaded, center dampness cannot transform, but rather gathers to form phlegm. Then wind evil and phlegm harass the upper body and exacerbate the condition of the patient, causing dizziness and collapse. Furthermore, clouding of the clear orifices may occur with symptoms of spiritlessness, loss of alertness, forgetfulness, and confusion. Phlegm obstructs the tongue root and causes inhibited speech and sluggish tongue aphasia.

Since I knew that the symptoms of slippery pulse, white tongue fur, and indistinct speech were caused by wind-phlegm harassing the upper body, I selected *dí tán tāng* (Phlegm-Flushing Decoction) and modified it according to the pattern. Moreover, since heat signs were not prevalent, I removed *huáng qín* (scutellaria) from *píng gān xī fēng tāng* (Calm the Liver and Extinguish Wind Decoction). However, I used this formula as the chief of both formulas since the symptom of wind-stirred convulsions was obviously critical. Thus, I selected only *bàn xià* (pinellia), *jú hóng* (red tangerine peel), and *dǎn xīng* (bile arisaema) from *dí tán tāng* (Phlegm-Flushing Decoction) to assist the damp-dispelling and phlegm-transforming effect. Because her forgetfulness and inability to sleep day or night were serious, I substituted *zhū yuǎn zhì* (cinnabar polygala) for *shí chāng pú* (acorus) in *dí tán tāng* (Phlegm-Flushing Decoction). This substitution not only preserved the phlegm-transforming orifice-opening principle of *dí tán tāng*, but also strengthened the spirit-quieting mind-stabilizing effect of this formula. I also took into consideration the constant convulsions of limbs and body and added *sāng zhī* (mulberry twig) to extinguish wind, free and penetrate the four limbs, and soothe the inhibited channels and network vessels.

At the second visit, wind had been gradually extinguished, but the forgetfulness and insomnia remained, so I added *shí chāng pú* (acorus) at that time to open the orifices and arouse the brain, and *zhū shā* (cinnabar) and *hǔ pò* (amber) to settle the heart and quiet the spirit. The tongue fur became thin and white at the third visit, and the pulse changed to slightly slippery. Since the patient had essentially recovered from all the symptoms, I removed *dǎn xīng* (bile arisaema) to prevent an excessive drying effect since this medicinal was not suitable for long-term use. I added *tiān zhú huáng* (bamboo sugar), which profoundly influences the elimination of phlegm from the heart channel, and *fú líng* (poria), which transforms phlegm and fortifies the spleen to eliminate the source of phlegm formation. I increased the dosage of *dài zhě shí* (hematite) to settle the liver and quiet the spirit; while it settles the liver, it indirectly assists the spleen, which in turn fortifies and moves the center burner. Thus, the entire body is restored to health. By the time of this visit there was no longer any need for *zhū shā* (cinnabar) or *hǔ pò* (amber), and since *zhū shā* is not suitable for long-term use, I removed both medicinals from his prescription.

We can see by the treatment process and outcome of this case that determination of treatment method according to pattern identification must be carefully combined with the specific circumstances of the patient and the disease. Only by doing so can you modify the formula and flexibly apply it to achieve satisfactory results.

Concerning the integration of treatment principles and treatment method

Strictly speaking, treatment principles and treatment method are different from each other; however, they bear a close relationship to each other, and even though they are distinguished from each other, they are nevertheless related. Treatment principles primarily refer to the general rules guiding the treatment of disease. The *Huáng Dì Nèi Jīng* ("The Yellow Emperor's Inner Canon") gives the following as examples:

"To treat disease, seek its root."

"Keep to the pathomechanisms; each belongs to a category. If something exists, seek why; if something does not exist, question it. First determine the five overcomings, then course, regulate, and harmonize qì and blood."

"To treat disease above, mildly supplement; to treat disease below, urgently drain. In acute conditions, use richly flavored qì medicinals, and in mild conditions, use weakly flavored qì medicinals; each has its appropriate use."

"For cold signs, use a warming principle; for heat, use a cooling one. Mild conditions are treated by counteraction; severe conditions are treated by coaction. Hardness is treated by whittling; intrusion is treated by eliminating; taxation is treated by warming; binding is treated by dissipating. Counteraction is straight treatment; coaction is paradoxical treatment. Treat heat with cold; treat cold with heat; treat the stopped by unstopping; treat the unstopped by stopping. For all cold disease and for heat, treat yīn; for all heat disease and cold, treat yáng. When disease is in the skin, sweat and effuse it; when it is fierce or stubborn, suppress and astringe it. When disease is mild, raise it; when disease is severe, reduce it; when qì and blood are debilitated, strengthen them; when the form is insufficient, warm with qì; when the essence is insufficient, supplement with flavor; when disease is in the upper burner, lead it up and out; in the lower burner, guide and draw it down."

These principles apply to the tip and the root and to the mild and the urgent.

Treatment method refers to a particular method of treatment such as the liver-settling yáng-subduing method, the liver-calming wind-extinguishing method, the spleen-fortifying stomach-harmonizing method, the acrid-warming exterior-resolving method, the lesser yáng-harmonizing method, the heat-clearing toxin-resolving method, the blood-quickening phlegm-transforming method, the urgent precipitation to rescue yīn method, and the qì-supplementing blood-nourishing method. By combining these we say that the treatment method is the specific realization of the treatment principles. Treatment method and treatment principles are distinctly different and yet share a close relationship.

We discussed above the respective meanings of treatment principles and treatment methods, but in the context of "principles, methods, formulas, and medicinals," the term "method" includes both treatment principles and methods. The "method" of "principles, methods, formulas, and medicinals" is to resolve the issue of "determining treatment." Thus, establishing methods means careful combination of treatment principles and treatment methods together with their practical application. In this way, health is restored.

Concerning the treatment principle in Case 1, we could say that I used the principle of "eliminating that which intrudes." When an evil guest intrudes in the lesser yáng, you must eliminate it. However, as far as the particular method of "eliminating" is concerned, I used a treatment method to harmonize the lesser yáng and outthrust evil to the exterior. As far as the flexible application of the treatment method is concerned, the characteristic of much heat and less cold and the principle of "treating heat with cold" were combined with the use of *bái hǔ jiā guì zhī tāng* (White Tiger Decoction Plus Cinnamon Twig) to clear heat and outthrust the exterior, thereby assisting the outthrusting of evil to the exterior.

The principle in Case 2 was "when disease is fierce or stubborn, suppress and astringe it." I used heavy-settling medicinals that subdue and absorb, such as *shēng dài zhě shí* (crude hematite), *shēng shí jué míng* (raw abalone shell), and *zhū shā* (cinnabar). This patient had constant limb and body convulsions, and the principles associated with this symptom include "the liver governs wind; wind is a yáng evil; wind by nature moves; and wind is swift and changeable." For this one particular symptom I formulated a liver-calming wind-extinguishing treatment method; in conjunction with this, and according to the pattern identification, I also used the phlegm-transforming orifice-opening method. When the application follows the pattern, satisfactory results are achieved.

The importance of freeing the stool when treating channel strike and bowel strike patterns during wind strike disease

Wind strike disease as defined in Chinese medicine is associated with the Western medical conditions of cerebral thrombosis, cerebral hemorrhage, cerebrovascular spasm, cerebral embolism, and facial paralysis. Chinese medicine clinically categorizes wind strike disease as either network vessel strike, channel strike, bowel strike, or visceral strike. The network strike pattern is the most mild of these and primarily presents as mouth and eye deviation. Visceral strike pattern is the most serious and presents with symptoms such as deep coma, mouth deviation, drooling, paralysis of limbs and body, and involuntary discharge of urine and stool. Physicians of the past called this the half-dead, half-alive pattern, and it is easy to see how extremely critical this condition is.

The remaining two patterns, channel strike and bowel strike, lie between the other two in their degree of severity. The chief characteristic of channel strike is hemiplegia sometimes with inhibited speech, but this pattern is without the aspect of spirit-mind obstruction. The bowel strike pattern is also marked by hemiplegia and aphasia or inhibited speech, but it is especially characterized to some extent by spirit-mind obstruction. Furthermore, these various patterns sometimes transform; for instance, channel strike can change into bowel strike, bowel strike can become visceral strike, bowel strike can transform into channel strike, or visceral strike can transform into bowel strike. Other patterns are distinguished within bowel strike and visceral strike such as block patterns and desertion patterns, and these, in turn, may also transform. However, I will not go into further detail on this topic, but rather encourage the reader to research additional sources.

Here I would like to discuss my experience concerning some particulars of the treatment of channel strike and bowel strike. The Ming dynasty physician, Sūn Wén-Yuán (Sūn Yī-Kuí) agreed with Liú Hé-Jiān (Liú Wán-Sù) when he said in the *Dān Tái Yù Àn* ("Cinnabar Platform and the Jade Table"):

> "Visceral strike mostly concerns stagnation of the nine orifices of the body, so there are symptoms of difficult or slow speech, loss of speech, nasal congestion, deafness, dim eyesight, and blocked bowels. Bowel strike mostly concerns the four limbs; thus, there are symptoms of hemiplegia or paralysis of the limbs."

From my own experience in clinical practice, I know that the symptom of constipation is seen not only in the visceral strike pattern, but also frequently accompanies the bowel strike pattern. For this reason, you should "use the method of freeing the six bowels." If wind strike affects the bowels, then there is stoppage of qì and blood and obstruction of bowel qì; therefore, the obstructed stool does not descend. After many years of clinical observation, I have concluded that in patients with bowel strike patterns, there is also a spirit-mind obstruction to some extent, and more often than not, a resemblance to yáng brightness (*yáng míng*) bowel repletion pattern. There will be symptoms such as incoherent speech, inappropriate movements of hands and feet, manic raving and nonsensical speech, failure to recognize others, vexation and agitation, constipation, late afternoon tidal heat and worsening of symptoms, thick yellow tongue fur, and a surging, slippery, stringlike, or large pulse.

This complies with the record of Hàn dynasty physician Zhāng Zhòng-Jǐng, who stated, "In yáng brightness disease, there is also stomach domain (stomach and intestine) repletion." The stomach is the sea of the six bowels; therefore, the treatment method for bowel strike pattern is often combined with the treatment for yáng brightness bowel repletion pattern. Thus, the Yuán dynasty physician Liú Hé-Jiān formulated *sān huà tāng* (Three Transformations Decoction) to free the intestines and drain heat, to quicken stasis and dispel wind, and to cause bowel qì to transform and engender the new. He used the following medicinals in the formula:

hòu pò (厚朴 officinal magnolia bark, Magnoliae Officinalis Cortex)

zhǐ shí (枳实 unripe bitter orange, Aurantii Fructus Immaturus)

dà huáng (大黄 rhubarb, Rhei Radix et Rhizoma)

qiāng huó (羌活 notopterygium, Notopterygii Rhizoma et Radix)

The "three transformations" define the principle of freeing the intestines and draining heat, and quickening stasis and dispelling wind to enable the triple burner to regain its ability to conduct and transform. The idea that the bowel strike pattern "is mostly concerned with the four limbs" explains the close relationship between the four limbs and bowel qì. On the other hand, the limb and body paralysis in the channel strike pattern also shows relevance to bowel qì. Therefore, channel strike pattern frequently includes the symptom of constipation with movement of the bowels only every few days.

The patient in Case 3 is an example of wind strike disease where channel strike has tended to transform into a bowel strike pattern. He was constipated and several days passed without a bowel movement. Thus, I combined *dí tán tāng* (Phlegm-Flushing Decoction) and *sān huà tāng* (Three Transformations Decoction) and modified them according to the pattern; once the stools were kept unobstructed, the remaining symptoms were quite quickly resolved.

Recently at my hospital, I treated a certain physician who had suffered from cerebral thrombosis. The Chinese medical pattern identification was wind strike disease of the channel strike pattern; however, at the early stage of treatment I paid no attention to treating the dry and scant stool, and consequently recovery for his left-sided paralysis was not ideal. Later, to transform phlegm and dispel wind and to quicken blood and free the network vessels, I added the following medicinals to his prescription:

dà huáng (大黄 rhubarb, Rhei Radix et Rhizoma) 6 g

qiāng huó (羌活 notopterygium, Notopterygii Rhizoma et Radix) 6 g

guā lóu (栝楼 trichosanthes, Trichosanthis Fructus) 30 g

bīng láng (槟榔 areca, Arecae Semen) 10 g

These medicinals freed the intestine and moistened the stool, regulated and smoothed bowel qì, and caused stools to move once a day. After this, the patient could move his limbs around and recovery was greatly accelerated. His physical strength went quickly from level III to level IV. When he had taken the medicinals for 3–4 weeks, he could stand by supporting himself with a hand on the bed railing and, with the help of his wife, walk about ten steps. Upon further inquiry, I learned that although the patient had one bowel movement a day, it was not much in amount and was ungratifying. I increased the dosage of *dà huáng* (rhubarb) to 8–10 grams, and after that the bowel movements still occurred once a day but were greater in amount and were gratifying. From then on, his appetite greatly increased, the tongue fur changed from thick and slimy to thin and not slimy, the physical strength of his limbs and his ability to exercise greatly improved, and he could manage a short walk with some support. Many years later, I definitely pay more attention to this point in clinic, and because of this clinical experience, I obtain more satisfactory results.

When the stool is unobstructed and bowel qì is free and normalized, the center burner can regain its function of conducting, moving, and transforming, and the source of qì and blood engenderment and transformation is sufficient. Qì and blood move smoothly in the channels and network vessels, static blood is removed and new blood is engendered, phlegm turbidity is transformed, and clear qì penetrates. Thus, the patient receives a satisfactory result. This is the reason why I believe that in the treatment of channel strike and bowel strike patterns in wind strike disease, it is important to maintain the smooth function of the stool. By doing this, patients will undergo a quick rate of recovery, especially in the use of their limbs and body. However I do not want to overemphasize the need to "free the stool," or to cause the stool to move several times a day, or for this method to turn into the method of offensive precipitation. Although they may appear to have a repletion pattern, patients suffering from wind strike disease generally have a pattern of right qì vacuity. You should discontinue medication when the disease is largely eliminated, and avoid excessive use of the attacking method, particularly when treating an elderly patient. Just as the *Zá Bìng Guǎng Yāo* ("Broad Essentials of Miscellaneous Diseases") said concerning "wind strike," as derived from the *Yī Jīng Huì Jiě* ("Resolving Medical Classics"):

> "In the treatment of wind strike, do not indiscriminately use *dà jǐ* (euphorbia/knoxia), *yuán huā* (genkwa) and *gān suì* (kansui), for these medicinals drain the large intestine and damage yīn and blood to the extent that there is no remedy. When it is necessary to precipitate phlegm, but excretion is obstructed, then it is especially appropriate to use qì-normalizing intestine-lubricating medicinals to mildly disinhibit. In the treatment of

toxic heat and phlegm-fire with signs of replete qì and a replete pulse, you may also use the clearing and disinhibiting method."

I was once connected to another case of an elderly woman who suffered from wind strike disease with channel strike pattern. The previous doctor had already used the draining and precipitating method, and each day the stools drained several times. This situation had been on-going for several days, there was no improvement in the disease condition, and the patient was fatigued and sluggish in movement. I advised the physician to change to the wind-dispelling, phlegm-transforming and blood-quickening, network-freeing treatment method, assisted by the center-regulating and qì-boosting method. Afterwards, all the patient's symptoms gradually improved. Thus, you can see that excessive use of the draining method can have a negative effect by damaging right qì, and thereby rendering an unsuccessful recovery. You certainly should pay attention to this point.

Concerning sleeplessness

In Chinese medical theory, yīn and yáng and the qì and blood of the human body circulate unceasingly day and night. At night yáng enters yīn, and when yīn and yáng are harmonious, a person can lie down and sleep. Just as the Míng dynasty physician Zhāng Jǐng-Yuè said:

> "The heart stores the spirit and is the residence of yáng qì; defense governs qì and is in charge of the transformation of yáng qì. Whenever defense qì enters yīn, there is tranquility. When yīn is tranquil, there is sleep; then right qì and yáng qì have a place to return; thus the spirit is quiet and there is sleep."

> "Whenever the heart is harassed, the spirit stirs and is not tranquil, and there is no sleep. Thus when you desire to sleep, you must nourish yáng within yīn and remove stirring from tranquility; by doing this, you achieve the goal."

Because the patient in Case 4 was excessively fatigued and had much tension in the workplace, he was sleepless throughout the night. The diagnosis, after correlating the pulse and the pathocondition together with the four examinations, was liver yáng effulgence, heart blood vacuity, and yáng unable to enter yīn, with the spirit failing to keep to its abode. I used *shēng shí jué míng* (raw abalone shell), *shēng bái sháo* (raw white peony), *shēng mǔ lì* (raw oyster shell), and *shēng lóng gǔ* (crude dragon bone) to nourish liver yīn and subdue liver yáng. This is the meaning of "nourishing yáng within yīn." Furthermore, I used *shēng zhě shí* (crude hematite) to greatly settle and calm the liver, and I combined it with *suān zǎo rén* (spiny jujube) to nourish liver blood as well as to nourish the heart and quiet the spirit. *Shēng zhě shí* (crude hematite) is also able to nourish blood; these two medicinals, *suān zǎo rén* (spiny jujube) and *shēng zhě shí* (crude hematite), are interconnected to nourish the blood and heart and to greatly settle and quiet the spirit. This treatment approach is the essence of what is meant by "the removal of stirring from tranquility." To subdue and constrain yáng efflugence so it can enter yīn, you must succeed in nourishing yīn-blood vacuity so it will accept yáng with yīn. When yáng enters yīn, there is tranquility, and the spirit obtains blood and nourishment and is quiet; when the spirit is quiet, there is sleep. Based on this theory, pattern identification to determine treatment obtained very good results.

The patient in Case 5 also suffered from sleeplessness, but he presented with symptoms of night sweating, frequent nocturia, and a serious case of seminal emission occurring 3–4 times a week. The pathomechanism was primarily yīn vacuity internal heat and non-interaction of heart and kidney. His case was somewhat different in terms of its treatment principle and treatment method. The former patient (Case 4) was excessively fatigued, yáng did not enter yīn, and the spirit failed to keep to its abode; therefore, I treated him by calming the liver and subduing yáng, nourishing the heart and quieting the spirit, and fortifying the spleen and harmonizing the center. The latter patient (Case 5) I treated by enriching yīn and boosting the kidney, calming the liver and subduing yáng, quieting the heart-spirit, and securing the lower origin. This approach also obtained very good results. From these examples it is evident that when determining treatment methods and principles, by all means avoid inflexibility and rigidity. You must instead change, adapt, and flexibly apply the methods and principles to obtain ideal results.

Chapter Four

Flexible application of prescriptions and medicinals is important in treatment based on pattern identification.

Principles, methods, formulas, and medicinals are the concrete embodiment of the process of using pattern identification to determine treatment. Of these four aspects, formulas and medicinals occupy a large proportion of the process, and it is extremely important to use them flexibly when identifying patterns to determine treatment. Therefore, after you have identified patterns and established the method, you must select formulas and medicinals to create a specific prescription that meets the patient's circumstances based on variations according to presenting patterns. Thus, this process is an important step in obtaining excellent results. Here are five case histories based on my experience that discuss several points concerning the flexible application of formulas and medicinals.

Case Studies

Case One
Swelling in both rib-sides
两肋肿块

The patient was a 61-year-old female whose initial examination date was December 9, 1961.

Chief complaint

A large swelling, sometimes painful, that was located transversely on both rib-sides for the last ten years.

INQUIRY EXAMINATION

The swelling was situated transversely from the lower edge of each breast to her back. The posterior section was higher and thicker than the anterior section which was lower and thinner. Its shape resembled an inverted cow horn. Ordinarily, the swelling was slightly soft and quite small, and she did not notice it when lying down. Yet, whenever her emotions were upset or she was fatigued, the swelling became distended, painful, hard, and enlarged, even to the extent of being brick-like, and then she could not lie down on either side. She had visited hospitals in Běijīng in the past and had received many diagnoses and treatments including a biopsy, but there had been no definitive diagnosis, and the treatments had yielded no results. In the last several days, the swelling had become painful; when she bent over forward or stooped over, the pain worsened. Urine and stools were normal. Sometimes she was aware of throbbing of the heart, and she also had a medical history of hypertension.

INSPECTION EXAMINATION

Her development was normal and nutrition very good and she was slightly overweight. Acute pain and suffering showed in her complexion, yet her essence-spirit was still good. The tongue body and fur were normal. The enlarged swelling that started below each breast was without any changes in skin color (see the palpation examination section below).

LISTENING AND SMELLING EXAMINATION

There were no abnormalities.

PALPATION EXAMINATION

Examination of the head, neck, abdomen, and four limbs revealed no abnormalities. There was a swelling that was symmetrical on both sides at the chest and rib-sides, under both breasts and aligned with the sixth and seventh ribs. The swelling was slightly higher as it extended posterior, and slightly thicker in size as it reached up behind the armpit. Toward the anterior portion of the body, the swelling was lower and thinner and ended at the lateral border of the sternum. The swelling itself was thick and easily defined by palpation, and it was hard as a brick. The exterior portion was uneven in appearance, immobile, and painful under pressure. The pulses of both wrists were sunken and slippery.

PATTERN IDENTIFICATION

Because the swelling appeared on both rib-sides, I knew the disease belonged to the liver channel, and because the lump became distended and painful when her emotions were upset, I knew the disease was caused by binding depression of liver qì. Since the pulse was sunken and slippery, and the patient was overweight, I knew that congealing phlegm was also present. Enduring disease had entered the blood. Qì, phlegm, and blood were binding together and not dissipating; they had accumulated over a long period of time to form a hard lump. Phlegm and blood have form; therefore, the swelling had increased in size due to prolonged non-dissipation. Since liver qì was sometimes depressed and other times outthrusting, the painful distention was intermittent, and the swelling itself changed in size depending on the depression and outthrusting of liver qì. Correlation of the four examinations supported my diagnosis of liver qì depression with congealing of phlegm and blood.

TREATMENT METHOD

Course the liver and move qì while dispersing and dissipating binding phlegm, assisted by quickening the network vessels and quieting the spirit.

PRESCRIPTION

I prescribed two formulas with modifications: *chái hú shū gān sǎn* (Bupleurum Liver-Coursing Powder) and *xiāo luǒ wán* (Scrofula-Dispersing Pill). I gave the patient three packets of the following prescription to be decocted in water:

chái hú (柴胡 bupleurum, Bupleuri Radix) 5 g

zhì xiāng fù (制香附 processed cyperus, Cyperi Rhizoma Praeparatum) 10 g

chǎo zhǐ qiào (ké) (炒枳壳 stir-fried bitter orange, Aurantii Fructus Frictus) 10 g

shēng shí jué míng (生石决明 raw abalone shell, Haliotidis Concha Cruda) 19 g (pre-decocted)

shēng mǔ lì (生牡蛎 raw oyster shell, Ostreae Concha Cruda) 12 g (pre-decocted)

zhè bèi mǔ (浙贝母 Zhejiang fritillaria, Fritillariae Thunbergii Bulbus) 12 g

xuán shēn (玄参 scrophularia, Scrophulariae Radix) 10 g

huà jú hóng (化橘红 Huazhou pomelo rind, Citri Grandis Exocarpium Rubrum) 6 g

bái jiè zǐ (白芥子 white mustard, Sinapis Albae Semen) 5 g

fú líng (茯苓 poria, Poria) 10 g

zhū yuǎn zhì (朱远志 cinnabar polygala, Polygalae Radix et Cinnabare) 6 g

lù lù tōng (路路通 liquidambar fruit, Liquidambaris Fructus) 2 pieces

FORMULA EXPLANATION

As chief medicinals, *xiāng fù* (cyperus) moves qì and dissipates binds, and *chái hú* (bupleurum) courses the liver and resolves depression.

As support medicinals, *zhǐ ké* (bitter orange) loosens the chest and disinhibits the diaphragm; *shēng shí jué míng* (raw abalone shell) enriches liver yīn and subdues liver yáng; *shēng mǔ lì* (raw oyster shell) subdues yáng, softens hardness, and dissipates binds. *Zhè bèi mǔ* (Zhejiang fritillaria) dissipates depression and disperses phlegm. *Xuán shēn* (scrophularia) downbears fire and resolves toxin while dispersing lumps. *Mǔ lì* (oyster shell), *zhè bèi mǔ* (Zhejiang fritillaria), and *xuán shēn* (scrophularia) are the medicinals in *xiāo luǒ wán* (Scrofula-Dispersing Pill).

As assistant medicinals, *jú hóng* (red tangerine peel) transforms phlegm; *fú líng* (poria) dispels dampness; *bái jiè zǐ* (white mustard) dispels phlegm between the skin and the inner membrane and disperses and dissipates phlegm nodes and lumps. *Yuǎn zhì* (polygala) opens the heart and sweeps phlegm and quiets the spirit and stabilizes the mind.

The courier medicinal, *lù lù tōng* (liquidambar fruit), frees the channels and quickens the network vessels.

This entire formula courses the liver and resolves depression, moves qì and disperses phlegm, quickens the network vessels and dissipates binds, and quiets the spirit and stabilizes the mind.

FOLLOWUP TREATMENT

Second visit on December 12: After the patient had taken three packets of the prescription, the distended pain was slightly alleviated, but the size and hardness of the swelling remained the same. Considering the enduring nature of the diseased lump, I appropriately increased the dosage of blood-quickening stasis-dispelling medicinals in the original prescription, and I added *bái jīn wán* (Alum and Curcuma Pill) [*bái fán* (alum) and *yù jīn* (curcuma)] to strengthen the depression-resolving phlegm-dispersing effect. I gave the patient three more packets of the following:

xiāng fù (香附 cyperus, Cyperi Rhizoma) 10 g
zhǐ qiào (*ké*) (枳壳 bitter orange, Aurantii Fructus) 10 g
yù jīn (郁金 curcuma, Curcumae Radix) 6 g
shēng shí jué míng (生石决明 raw abalone shell, Haliotidis Concha Cruda) 25 g (pre-decocted)
shēng mǔ lì (生牡蛎 raw oyster shell, Ostreae Concha Cruda) 19 g (pre-decocted)
zhè bèi mǔ (浙贝母 Zhejiang fritillaria, Fritillariae Thunbergii Bulbus) 12 g
xuán shēn (玄参 scrophularia, Scrophulariae Radix) 10 g
bái jiè zǐ (白芥子 white mustard, Sinapis Albae Semen) 6 g
dān shēn (丹参 salvia, Salviae Miltiorrhizae Radix) 12 g

zhì shān jiǎ (炙山甲 mix-fried pangolin scales, Manis Squama cum Liquido Fricta) 5 g

shí chāng pú (石菖蒲 acorus, Acori Tatarinowii Rhizoma) 5 g

yuǎn zhì (远志 polygala, Polygalae Radix) 6 g

I prescribed 15 grams of *bái jīn wán* (Alum and Curcuma Pill), to be taken twice a day at a dose of 1.5 grams each time.

Third visit on December 20: By now, the patient had taken eight packets of medicinals, and the swelling was greatly reduced. There was no distended pain and no pain when she bent over. There was only a slight sensation of pain when she stretched her arms, but no other symptoms remained. The pulse was slippery, yet harmonious and moderate. I advised her to continue with the *bái jīn wán* (Alum and Curcuma Pill) at the same dosage as before, and I decided to give her the same prescription as before with only slight modifications. I added 10 grams of *niú xī* (achyranthes) and increased the amount of *dān shēn* (salvia) to 15 grams.

Fourth visit on December 27: The patient had finished another seven packets of medicinals. At this time, the swelling on both sides had basically disappeared, their shape was no longer visible upon inspection, and palpation examination revealed that the skin and muscles were only slightly stiff at the location where the swelling had been. She moved her arms and body with no feelings of discomfort. She could freely move from side to side when lying down, and she slept well. The tongue fur was thick and slimy and the pulse sunken and slippery. I modified the prescription again to continue with the recovery and gave her six more packets of the following:

xiāng fù (香附 cyperus, Cyperi Rhizoma) 10 g

zhè bèi mǔ (浙贝母 Zhejiang fritillaria, Fritillariae Thunbergii Bulbus) 12 g

shēng shí jué míng (生石决明 raw abalone shell, Haliotidis Concha Cruda) 15 g (pre-decocted)

shēng mǔ lì (生牡蛎 raw oyster shell, Ostreae Concha Cruda) 19 g (pre-decocted)

xuán shēn (玄参 scrophularia, Scrophulariae Radix) 10 g

bái jiè zǐ (白芥子 white mustard, Sinapis Albae Semen) 5 g

tiān zhú huáng (天竹黄 bamboo sugar, Bambusae Concretio Silicea) 6 g

zhì shān jiǎ (炙山甲 mix-fried pangolin scales, Manis Squama cum Liquido Fricta) 6 g

shēng dì huáng (生地黄 dried rehmannia, Rehmanniae Radix Exsiccata) 9 g

xià kū cǎo (夏枯草 prunella, Prunellae Spica) 6 g

hǎi zǎo (海藻 sargassum, Sargassum) 9 g

niú xī (牛膝 achyranthes, Achyranthis Bidentatae Radix) 6 g

<u>Follow-up visit on June 24, 1962</u>: The patient said that the swelling on both rib-sides had completely disappeared, and she had not suffered a relapse up to this time. I saw her on subsequent follow-up visits in 1963 and 1964, and there still was no recurrence of disease.

CASE TWO

LIVER-KIDNEY QÌ STAGNATION, DAMP AMASSMENT IN THE URINARY BLADDER (URINARY CALCULI)

肝肾气滞，湿蓄膀胱（泌尿系结石）

The patient, a 42-year-old male, was an army commander from Běijīng whose initial examination date was September 12, 1978.

CHIEF COMPLAINT

Lesser-abdominal pain and hematuria for the last two months.

INQUIRY EXAMINATION

For two months the patient had suffered pain in the right side of the lesser abdomen, often accompanied by hematuria. Normally, the red blood cells were detected using a microscope, but when the illness was critical, blood in the urine was easily visible. At one time he had had a detailed examination done at the Chinese People's Liberation Army Hospital, but a pyelographic test had revealed no organic pathology. The usual x-rays had been done, but they also had revealed no evidence of urinary calculi. Since the hematuria had been undiagnosed, he left the hospital. Some time later, after talking with someone, he became suspicious that cancer pathology may have been present, so he requested Chinese medical examination and treatment.

At the time of the initial examination, the patient felt pain, sometimes mild and sometimes severe, on the right side of the lesser abdomen, and he felt a slight discomfort in the lumbus and smaller abdomen. He also experienced discomfort but not pain in the urethra when he urinated. The urine was red in color, but the stools were still regular.

INSPECTION EXAMINATION

Physically his development was very good, and his nutrition was good, but he had an anxious expression on his face. The tongue fur was thin and white and completely covered the tongue.

LISTENING AND SMELLING EXAMINATION

There were no abnormalities.

PALPATION EXAMINATION

His head, neck, chest, and four limbs were normal. His abdomen, liver, and spleen were not enlarged. The muscles on the right side of the lower abdomen were stiff, and not as soft and supple as on the left, but there was no pain upon pressure and no swelling. The lumbus showed no pain when tapped. All pulses were stringlike, slippery, and slightly fine.

PATTERN IDENTIFICATION

The lesser abdomen and the smaller abdomen are the domain of the liver, kidney, and urinary bladder channels. When qì and blood in the liver and kidney channels is stagnant or moves counterflow, the channel becomes obstructed, intermittent pain occurs in the lesser abdomen, there is discomfort in the smaller abdomen, and the muscles become unyielding and stiff. The kidney and urinary bladder stand in interior-exterior relationship; the kidney governs water-damp and qì transformation. In this case, liver and kidney qì became stagnant, and the waterways lost their ability to disinhibit; dampness amassed in the urinary bladder, and enduring damp depression gradually transformed into heat. Thus, the urine became red in color, and there was discomfort in the urethra. White, thin tongue fur that spread evenly over the tongue and a slippery pulse indicated damp evil. Since all six pulses were stringlike, I knew that the pain was associated with the liver channel. After correlating the four examinations, I diagnosed stagnation of liver-kidney qì and damp amassment in the urinary bladder.

TREATMENT METHOD

Regulate the liver and relax tension, move qì and disinhibit dampness, assisted by boosting the kidney and stopping the bleeding.

PRESCRIPTION

I modified two formulas for this prescription, *sháo yào gān cǎo tāng* (Peony and Licorice Decoction) and *tiān tái wū yào sǎn* (Tiantai Lindera Powder). I gave the patient six packets of the following prescription, to be decocted in water:

bái sháo yào (白芍药 white peony, Paeoniae Radix Alba) 15 g

zhì gān cǎo (炙甘草 mix-fried licorice, Glycyrrhizae Radix cum Liquido Fricta) 6 g

wū yào (乌药 lindera, Linderae Radix) 12 g

chǎo chuān liàn zǐ (炒川楝子 stir-fried toosendan, Toosendan Fructus Frictus) 12 g

chǎo xiǎo huí xiāng (炒小茴香 stir-fried fennel, Foeniculi Fructus
    Frictus) 5 g

chǎo jú hé (炒橘核 stir-fried tangerine pip, Citri Reticulatae Semen
    Frictum) 9 g

fú líng (茯苓 poria, Poria) 12 g

zé xiè (泽泻 alisma, Alismatis Rhizoma) 10 g

jīn qián cǎo (金钱草 moneywort, Lysimachiae Herba) 15 g

huáng bǎi tàn (黄柏炭 charred phellodendron, Phellodendri Cortex
    Carbonisatus) 12 g

xiǎo jì tàn (小蓟炭 charred cephalanoplos, Cephalanoploris Herba seu
    Radix Carbonisata) 21 g

xù duàn tàn (续断炭 charred dipsacus, Dipsaci Radix Carbonisata) 21 g

FORMULA EXPLANATION

As chief medicinals, *bái sháo yào* (white peony) nourishes blood and emolliates the liver while soothing the sinews and relaxing tension. *Wū yào* (lindera) normalizes counterflow qì.

As support medicinals, *gān cǎo* (licorice), from *sháo yào gān cǎo tāng*
(Peony and Licorice Decoction), relaxes tension and relieves pain. *Chuān liàn
zǐ* (toosendan) and *xiǎo huí xiāng* (fennel) are combined with *wū yào* (lindera)
and *jú hé* (tangerine pip) to treat liver-kidney qì counterflow with intermittent
pain in the umbilicus and abdomen.

As assistant medicinals, *fú líng* (poria), *zé xiè* (alisma), and *jīn qián cǎo*
(moneywort) disinhibit dampness; *huáng bǎi* (phellodendron) consolidates the
kidney and clears heat; *xù duàn* (dipsacus) strengthens the kidney and invigorates the lumbus. A few medicinals were prepared by char-frying; these provided a blood-stanching effect.

Because *xiǎo jì* (field thistle) is an important medicinal to treat blood in
the urine, it was the courier medicinal.

FOLLOWUP TREATMENT

<u>Second visit on September 19</u>: All the subjective symptoms were
alleviated after the patient took the medicinals. He had his urine retested and
found that the red blood cell count was now only 30–40 in the microscopic
field of vision, which clearly indicated an improvement. However, he now felt
a pain in the abdomen as if qì were piercing or attacking in a downward direction. The tongue fur was white and thin; the pulse was the same as before. I
modified the original prescription and gave him six packets of the following,
to be decocted in water:

bái sháo yào (白芍药 white peony, Paeoniae Radix Alba) 15 g

zhì gān cǎo (炙甘草 mix-fried licorice, Glycyrrhizae Radix cum Liquido Fricta) 6 g

wū yào (乌药 lindera, Linderae Radix) 9 g

chǎo chuān liàn zǐ (炒川楝子 stir-fried toosendan, Toosendan Fructus Frictus) 12 g

chǎo xiǎo huí xiāng (炒小茴香 stir-fried fennel, Foeniculi Fructus Frictus) 5 g

chǎo jú hé (炒橘核 stir-fried tangerine pip, Citri Reticulatae Semen Frictum) 9 g

hǎi jīn shā (海金沙 lygodium spore, Lygodii Spora) 12 g

jī nèi jīn (鸡内金 gizzard lining, Galli Gigeriae Endothelium Corneum) 9 g

jīn qián cǎo (金钱草 moneywort, Lysimachiae Herba) 15 g

xiǎo jì tàn (小蓟炭 charred cephalanoplos, Cephalanoploris Herba seu Radix Carbonisata) 21 g

xù duàn tàn (续断炭 charred dipsacus, Dipsaci Radix Carbonisata) 15 g

huáng bǎi tàn (黄柏炭 charred phellodendron, Phellodendri Cortex Carbonisatus) 9 g

<u>Third visit on September 26</u>: The patient had taken 12 packets of the Chinese medicinals, and all the subjective symptoms had essentially disappeared. The muscles in the lower abdomen on the right side were soft and supple. Although the urine was still sometimes red in color, the diagnostic tests showed overall improvement. Now when the patient urinated, he felt scurrying, piercing pain in the lesser abdomen as if qì were descending, but he did not find any calculi in the urine. The tongue fur was thin and white, and the pulse was the same as before. I modified the prescription again; this time I removed the qì-rectifying tension-relaxing medicinals and increased the dosage of kidney-boosting, stasis-breaking, orifice-lubricating, and strangury-freeing medicinals. The patient received six packets of this prescription, to be decocted in water:

xù duàn tàn (续断炭 charred dipsacus, Dipsaci Radix Carbonisata) 30 g

shēng dì huáng (生地黄 dried rehmannia, Rehmanniae Radix Exsiccata) 15 g

dōng kuí zǐ (冬葵子 mallow seed, Malvae Semen) 10 g

qū mài (瞿麦 dianthus, Dianthi Herba) 12 g

zé xiè (泽泻 alisma, Alismatis Rhizoma) 10 g

fú líng (茯苓 poria, Poria) 12 g

jīn qián cǎo (金钱草 moneywort, Lysimachiae Herba) 15 g

xuán shēn (玄参 scrophularia, Scrophulariae Radix) 12 g

huáng qín (黄芩 scutellaria, Scutellariae Radix) 9 g

huáng bǎi tàn (黄柏炭 charred phellodendron, Phellodendri Cortex
  Carbonisatus) 15 g

xiǎo jì tàn (小蓟炭 charred cephalanoplos, Cephalanoploris Herba seu
  Radix Carbonisata) 25 g

On October 21, I received the following letter from the patient:

> "I finished the six packets of medicinals on October 2. During
> the time that I was taking these last six packets, some changes
> occurred. First, the abdominal pain was more frequent, some-
> times every other day. Second, each time the pain occurred, it
> grew worse. The pain that previously lasted a half hour now
> lasted up to 4–5 hours. During these times I drank many cups
> of boiled water as you advised, taking a little at a time. On Oc-
> tober 15, my urethra discharged a stone the size of a jujube pit.
> I was extremely happy about this. For four days afterwards, I
> continued to urinate without observing any blood."

In November, the patient personally sent me the urinary calculus which
was the size of a red date pit and was yellowish-brown in color. He told me he
had long ago gone back to work.

<u>Fourth visit, early December</u>: The patient said he was back at work and
carrying out his flight assignments. On a later follow-up visit in March of
1979, his health was still continuously good, and he was back to flying.

CASE THREE
VOMITING AND CONSTIPATION (TRAUMATIC BONE FRACTURE SEQUELAE)
呕吐便秘(外伤骨折后遗症)

The patient was a 40-year-old female, a farm worker in the mountains in
the northern province of Hēilóngjiāng.

CHIEF COMPLAINT

Stomach distention, abdominal pain, and vomiting for over six months.

INQUIRY EXAMINATION

While the patient was at work in August 1971, she had been buried in
gravel after a landslide occurred on the mountaintop. Her co-workers immediately dug her out from the rubble and took her to the hospital where she was
examined. The diagnosis was cervical nerve damage, compression fracture of
two thoracic vertebrae, and multiple rib fractures. Four broken ribs had
pierced the right lung and caused hemato-pneumothorax. She received emer-

gency medical treatment, and after two months, she regained movement in the upper body, with the exception of her right arm, which was still numb and painful. She was nauseous and she vomited several times a day; she sometimes vomited in the evening, and her abdomen was distended and painful. She experienced painful voidings of scant reddish urine. She continued to receive treatment until the end of that year, when she could stand and walk with assistance. However, the nausea, stomach distention, and abdominal pain gradually worsened. She came to Běijīng for treatment for several months in 1972, but had no clear results. In March 1973, she consulted with doctors at the Hēilóngjiāng Provincial Hospital and received a diagnosis of bone fracture sequelae. The second, third, fourth, and fifth rib group was broken and the intestinal tract was mildly narrowed and had adhesions and blockage. With the possibility of colon cancer present, she was referred to Běijīng for treatment. She went to several hospitals in Běijīng for diagnosis and treatment, but everyone agreed that the diagnosis was bone fracture sequelae. Following many recommendations to Chinese medical treatment, she arrived at my hospital.

At my clinic, she presented with the following symptoms: stomach duct distention, abdominal pain, lumbar pain, nausea, vomiting seven or eight times a day, and vomiting at night. Before vomiting, she belched, yawned, had runny teary eyes, and shivered. The smaller abdomen was distended like a drum, and abdominal pain was severe. The stools moved once every 5–7 days, were dry, bound, and ball-like, and the bowel movements extremely difficult. She had a ravenous appetite and ate six to seven meals a day, but was never satisfied after eating. The right side of her body was numb, especially the right arm, which was also sometimes painful. She perspired on the left side of the body, but not on the right, and she was forgetful and slept only about three hours a night.

INSPECTION EXAMINATION

Her complexion was blue-green, dark, and without luster. She was thin, weighing only about 45 kilograms, and could not walk without assistance. There were stasis macules on her tongue, her lips were relatively dark, and her tongue fur was thick and quite yellow.

LISTENING AND SMELLING EXAMINATION

The sound of her voice was low and her breathing was fine and timid.

PALPATION EXAMINATION

The abdomen was distended and painful, and resisted pressure; tapping revealed a drum-like sound, and the lower abdomen was quite distended. The pulse was stringlike, slippery, and relatively fine.

PATTERN IDENTIFICATION

This was post-traumatic illness. The tongue had stasis macules and the lips were dark blue-green, so I knew that static blood was involved. There was blood stasis in the chest and abdomen, and qì and blood had lost their ascending and descending regularity. Center burner qì had moved counterflow, so there was frequent vomiting. Turbid yīn did not descend so the stools were dry, bound, and difficult. Blood did not nourish the heart, so there was forgetfulness and insomnia. The essence-blood was not able to reach the face, thus, the complexion was dark blue-green and without luster. Qì and blood of the channels and network vessels had lost their smooth flow; thus, half the body was numb and without sweating. The fine pulse was the chief indicator of blood vacuity, and the stringlike pulse the chief indicator of pain. The correlation of the four examinations supported the diagnosis of abdominal pain and vomiting caused by blood stasis.

TREATMENT METHOD

Quicken stasis, downbear counterflow, moisten the intestines, and free the bowels.

PRESCRIPTION

I gave the patient 3–6 packets of the following prescription, to be decocted in water:

chái hú (柴胡 bupleurum, Bupleuri Radix) 15 g

dāng guī (当归 Chinese angelica, Angelicae Sinensis Radix) 12 g

hóng huā (红花 carthamus, Carthami Flos) 9 g

táo rén (桃仁 peach kernel, Persicae Semen) 9 g (smashed into pieces)

chì sháo yào (赤芍药 red peony, Paeoniae Radix Rubra) 12 g

zhì shān jiǎ (炙山甲 mix-fried pangolin scales, Manis Squama cum Liquido Fricta) 6 g

shēng zhě shí (生赭石 crude hematite, Haematitum Crudum) 45 g (pre-decocted)

bàn xià (半夏 pinellia, Pinelliae Rhizoma) 9 g

guā lóu (栝楼 trichosanthes, Trichosanthis Fructus) 45 g

liú jì nú (刘寄奴 anomalous artemisia, Artemisiae Anomalae Herba) 12 g

zhēn zhū mǔ (珍珠母 mother-of-pearl, Concha Margaritifera) 30 g (pre-decocted)

shēng dà huáng (生大黄 raw rhubarb, Rhei Radix et Rhizoma Crudi) 9 g

shēng gān cǎo (生甘草 raw licorice, Glycyrrhizae Radix Cruda) 6 g

máng xiāo (芒硝 mirabilite, Natrii Sulfas) 6 g (divided in half and taken drenched)

In addition, I prescribed 20 pills of *dà huáng zhè chóng wán* (Rhubarb and Ground Beetle Pill); one pill twice a day, to be taken with warm boiled water.

FORMULA EXPLANATION

This prescription was a modification of *fù yuán huó xuè tāng* (Origin-Restorative Blood-Quickening Decoction). The liver governs the storage of blood; thus, static blood often remains in the chest and rib-side. This patient had suffered rib-side bone fractures, so, as chief medicinals, I prescribed *chái hú* (bupleurum) since it enters the liver channel, and *dāng guī* (Chinese angelica) since it quickens the blood and nourishes the liver.

As support medicinals, *hóng huā* (carthamus), *táo rén* (peach kernel), *liú jì nú* (anomalous artemisia), *chì sháo yào* (red peony), and *zhì shān jiǎ* (mix-fried pangolin scales) quicken static blood and free the channels.

As assistant medicinals, *shēng zhě shí* (crude hematite) downbears counterflow and harmonizes the center, while *bàn xià* (pinellia) harmonizes the stomach and stops vomiting. *Quán guā lóu* (whole trichosanthes) downbears qì and moistens the intestines. *Zhēn zhū mǔ* (mother-of-pearl) nourishes the heart and quiets the spirit. *Gān cǎo* (licorice) relaxes tension and harmonizes the center. *Shēng dà huáng* (raw rhubarb) breaks vanquished blood, dispels stasis, and engenders the new. When *dà huáng* is used with *gān cǎo* (licorice), the formula is called *dà huáng gān cǎo tāng* (Rhubarb and Licorice Decoction), and it is used to stop vomiting.

As the courier medicinal, *máng xiāo* (mirabilite) moistens dryness and frees the bowels.

Since this was a case of enduring illness, I also prescribed *dà huáng zhè chóng wán* (Rhubarb and Ground Beetle Pill) to disperse and eliminate dry blood and to dispel stasis and engender the new [blood].

FOLLOWUP TREATMENT

<u>Second visit on June 2</u>: All symptoms had been alleviated to some extent after the patient took twelve packets of the prescription, and bowel movements occurred once every day. Abdominal distention was alleviated and vomiting reduced, but when the patient did not take the Chinese medicinals, the stool did not move. The tongue fur became thin and the pulse slippery. I modified the prescription as follows and gave her 3–6 packets to continue the therapeutic effect. I changed the dosage of the following medicinals:

chái hú (柴胡 bupleurum, Bupleuri Radix 12 g

zhì shān jiǎ (炙山甲 mix-fried pangolin scales, Manis Squama cum Liquido Fricta) 5 g

máng xiāo (芒硝 mirabilite, Natrii Sulfa)) 5 g

chì sháo yào (赤芍药 red peony, Paeoniae Radix Rubra) 15 g

And I added:

chén pí (陈皮 tangerine peel, Citri Reticulatae Pericarpium) 6 g

Third visit on June 19: All symptoms were alleviated, and her essence-spirit had improved. I modified the prescription as follows and gave her 6–12 packets. I changed the dosage of the following:

guā lóu (栝楼 trichosanthes, Trichosanthis Fructus) 30 g

zhì shān jiǎ (炙山甲 mix-fried pangolin scales, Manis Squama cum Liquido Fricta) 6 g

chén pí (陈皮 tangerine peel, Citri Reticulatae Pericarpium) 7.5 g

And I added:

piàn jiāng huáng (片姜黄 sliced turmeric, Curcumae Longae Rhizoma Sectum) 9 g

guì zhī (桂枝 cinnamon twig, Cinnamomi Ramulus) 3 g

Fourth visit on June 30: The patient was now having successful bowel movements every 1–2 days, the vomiting was reduced, and the abdominal distention and pain was relieved. Yet, in the last few days the urine was scant yellow, and she felt as if she were catching a cold. The tongue fur and pulse had not changed. Consequently, I gave her 3–6 packets of the following prescription:

chái hú (柴胡 bupleurum, Bupleuri Radix) 9 g

hóng huā (红花 carthamus, Carthami Flos) 9 g

táo rén (桃仁 peach kernel, Persicae Semen) 9 g

sū mù (苏木 sappan, Sappan Lignum) 9 g

liú jì nú (刘寄奴 anomalous artemisia, Artemisiae Anomalae Herba) 12 g

chì sháo yào (赤芍药 red peony, Paeoniae Radix Rubra) 15 g

piàn jiāng huáng (片姜黄 sliced turmeric, Curcumae Longae Rhizoma Sectum) 9 g

xiāng fù (香附 cyperus, Cyperi Rhizoma) 9 g

zǐ sū yè (紫苏叶 perilla leaf, Perillae Folium) 9 g

jīng jiè (荆芥 schizonepeta, Schizonepetae Herba) 6 g

shēng dà huáng (生大黄 raw rhubarb, Rhei Radix et Rhizoma Crudi) 3 g

chén pí (陈皮 tangerine peel, Citri Reticulatae Pericarpium) 9 g

zhū líng (猪苓 polyporus, Polyporus) 12 g

fú líng (茯苓 poria, Poria) 12 g

mù tōng (木通 trifoliate akebia, Akebiae Trifoliatae Caulis) 5 g

huáng bǎi (黄柏 phellodendron, Phellodendri Cortex) 9 g

zé xiè (泽泻 alisma, Alismatis Rhizoma) 9 g

guì zhī (桂枝 cinnamon twig, Cinnamomi Ramulus) 3 g

<u>Fifth visit on July 6</u>: The abdominal distention was greatly relieved, and since starting the prescription, the patient had no recurrence of the drum-like condition of the abdomen. Now she vomited only once every week, and sometimes not at all. The pre-vomiting symptoms of belching, yawning, and tearing of the eyes had all disappeared. The feelings of ravenous hunger had been greatly reduced. Slight damp-moist sweating occurred on the right side of the body, and she could sleep 8–9 hours a night. The urine was no longer yellow in color and was normal in amount. As a patient in the hospital, she was free to walk around. However, she still had a feeling of anxiety in the heart, and when she did not take the decoction, she did not have bowel movements. When there were no bowel movements, then the vomiting and abdominal distention recurred. Thus, every day I gave her one packet of the prescription. There was still pain in the lumbus and occasional dizziness. The tongue fur had transformed, and the pulse was slightly slippery. So, I gave the patient 12 packets of the following:

chái hú (柴胡 bupleurum, Bupleuri Radix) 9 g

xiāng fù (香附 cyperus, Cyperi Rhizoma) 9 g

hóng huā (红花 carthamus, Carthami Flos) 9 g

táo rén (桃仁 peach kernel, Persicae Semen) 9 g

chì sháo yào (赤芍药 red peony, Paeoniae Radix Rubra) 15 g

sāng jì shēng (桑寄生 mistletoe, Loranthi seu Visci Ramus) 25 g

xù duàn (续断 dipsacus, Dipsaci Radix) 12 g

shēng dà huáng (生大黄 raw rhubarb, Rhei Radix et Rhizoma Crudi) 6 g

guā lóu (栝楼 trichosanthes, Trichosanthis Fructus) 30 g

shēng zhě shí (生赭石 crude hematite, Haematitum Crudum) 30 g (pre-decocted)

zhēn zhū mǔ (珍珠母 mother-of-pearl, Concha Margaritifera) 30 g (pre-decocted)

gōu téng (钩藤 uncaria, Uncariae Ramulus cum Uncis) 12 g

piàn jiāng huáng (片姜黄 sliced turmeric, Curcumae Longae Rhizoma Sectum) 6 g

huáng qín (黄芩 scutellaria, Scutellariae Radix) 9 g

bàn xià (半夏 pinellia, Pinelliae Rhizoma) 9 g

dǎng shēn (党参 codonopsis, Codonopsis Radix) 9 g

<u>Sixth visit on July 19</u>: The emotions had stabilized and the symptoms had gradually abated. Nevertheless, in recent days, the tongue fur had become slightly thick, the pulse slippery, and sleeping was disturbed. At this time, I made some changes to the prescription. I removed *zhě shí* (hematite), *dǎng shēn* (codonopsis), *huáng qín* (scutellaria), *gōu téng* (uncaria), and *guā lóu* (trichosanthes). Then I added the following:

shēng lóng gǔ (生龙骨 crude dragon bone, Mastodi Ossis Fossilia Cruda)
   30 g (pre-decocted)

shēng mǔ lì (生牡蛎 raw oyster shell, Ostreae Concha Cruda) 30 g (pre-decocted)

dāng guī (当归 Chinese angelica, Angelicae Sinensis Radix) 9 g

shēng pú huáng (生蒲黄 raw typha pollen, Typhae Pollen Crudum) 9 g

jīng jiè (荆芥 schizonepeta, Schizonepetae Herba) 9 g

huò xiāng (藿香 patchouli, Pogostemonis Herba) 9 g

zhū líng (猪苓 polyporus, Polyporus) 12 g

fú líng (茯苓 poria, Poria) 12 g

I gave the patient 6–18 packets.

<u>Seventh visit on August 9</u>: Her complexion was moist and lustrous, her lips and tongue were no longer blue-green in color, her body weight had increased from 45 to 59 kg, and she could now shop on her own at the local department store. Sometimes she had a dull pain in the lower abdomen and yellow vaginal discharge with malign odor. The tongue fur was normal and the pulse relaxed. I knew the yellow vaginal discharge and malign odor was caused by lower burner blood stasis transforming into heat and damp-heat amassment and stagnation. Therefore, to the original formula described above, I added some medicinals to disperse and transform damp-heat. I gave the patient 6–10 packets of the following to continue the therapeutic effect:

chái hú (柴胡 bupleurum, Bupleuri Radix) 9 g

dāng guī (当归 Chinese angelica, Angelicae Sinensis Radix) 12 g

hóng huā (红花 carthamus, Carthami Flos) 9 g

táo rén ní (桃仁泥 crushed peach kernel, Persicae Semen Tusum) 5 g

qīng bàn xià (清半夏 purified pinellia, Pinelliae Tuber Depuratum) 9 g

chì sháo yào (赤芍药 red peony, Paeoniae Radix Rubra) 12 g

bái sháo yào (白芍药 white peony, Paeoniae Radix Alba) 12 g

guā lóu (栝楼 trichosanthes, Trichosanthis Fructus) 30 g

shēng dà huáng (生大黄 raw rhubarb, Rhei Radix et Rhizoma Crudi) 9 g

dǎng shēn (党参 codonopsis, Codonopsis Radix) 9 g

bái zhú (白术 white atractylodes, Atractylodis Macrocephalae Rhizoma)
   6 g

fú líng (茯苓 poria, Poria) 12 g

zhì shān jiǎ (炙山甲 mix-fried pangolin scales, Manis Squama cum
   Liquido Fricta) 6 g

xù duàn (续断 dipsacus, Dipsaci Radix) 12 g

wú zhū yú (吴茱萸 evodia, Evodiae Fructus) 5 g

huáng lián (黄连 coptis, Coptidis Rhizoma) 5 g

pèi lán (佩兰 eupatorium, Eupatorii Herba) 9 g

wū yào (乌药 lindera, Linderae Radix) 9 g

<u>Eighth visit on August 30</u>: Her pain in the lower abdomen and lumbus was greatly relieved, her body weight had increased, her physical strength and essence-spirit had all improved, and she could now stroll around by herself in the marketplace. The yellow vaginal discharge had lessened. However, in the last two days, her urine was yellow in color and she felt a sagging pain; also recently, due to the common cold, she had vomited once. The tongue fur was slightly yellow and the pulse slippery. To continue the effect, I prescribed the following, six to twelve packets:

hóng huā (红花 carthamus, Carthami Flos) 9 g

táo rén ní (桃仁泥 crushed peach kernel, Persicae Semen Tusum) 9 g

qīng bàn xià (清半夏 purified pinellia, Pinelliae Tuber Depuratum) 9 g

chì sháo yào (赤芍药 red peony, Paeoniae Radix Rubra) 15 g

shēng dà huáng (生大黄 raw rhubarb, Rhei Radix et Rhizoma Crudi) 9 g

huáng bǎi (黄柏 phellodendron, Phellodendri Cortex) 12 g

huáng qín (黄芩 scutellaria, Scutellariae Radix) 12 g

wú zhū yú (吴茱萸 evodia, Evodiae Fructus) [stir-fried] 6 g

zhū líng (猪苓 polyporus, Polyporus) 15 g

fú líng (茯苓 poria, Poria) 15 g

biǎn xù (萹蓄 knotgrass, Polygoni Avicularis Herba) 9 g

shēng yǐ mǐ (生苡米 raw coix seed, Coicis Semen Crudum) 15 g

shú yǐ mǐ (熟苡米 cooked coix, Coicis Semen Conquitum) 15 g

shēng zhě shí (生赭石 crude hematite, Haematitum Crudum) 30 g (pre-decocted)

xuán fù huā (旋覆花 inula flower, Inulae Flos) 9 g (wrapped in cloth)

xù duàn (续断 dipsacus, Dipsaci Radix) 12 g

zé xiè (泽泻 alisma, Alismatis Rhizoma) 12 g

After this, I made changes to the prescription following the symptoms and the seasons and modified according to the pattern, and the patient continued to take the decoction until October 4. By that time, all her symptoms had been eliminated and her appetite increased, as did her weight and her strength. So with ten packets of the prescription to treat the vaginal discharge, she returned to her home town. On a follow-up visit in October of 1974, I learned she had completely recovered and had been working again for nearly a year.

CASE FOUR

POST-MISCARRIAGE PLACENTAL RETENTION (PARTIAL PLACENTAL RETENTION)

小产后胞衣不下(部分胎盘组织留滞)

The patient was a 40-year-old female from the mountainous region of Gānsù Province whose initial examination was a house call on October 27, 1967.

CHIEF COMPLAINT

Post-miscarriage retention of the placenta and unceasing uterine bleeding for more than eight days.

INQUIRY EXAMINATION

The patient was almost four months pregnant when she miscarried on October 19. The placenta did not completely discharge and the uterus continued to bleed without stopping. Her local physician had given her daily injections of glucose and *xiān hè cǎo* (agrimony) with other blood-stanching medicinals, but these remedies were ineffective. Because of the remote mountain location and the lack of a facility to do dilatation and curettage, the patient first wanted to seek diagnosis and treatment from a Chinese medical physician. She was flustered and dizzy, and her entire body was without strength. There was continuous vaginal bleeding sometimes with blood clots and dull pain in the lower abdomen. She had a poor appetite, but urine and stools were still normal.

INSPECTION EXAMINATION

She looked pale, her lips and tongue were pale, her essence-spirit was listless, and she was completely bed-ridden.

LISTENING AND SMELLING EXAMINATION

Her breathing was thin and her voice low.

PALPATION EXAMINATION

The smaller abdomen was relatively painful when lightly pressed; I did not dare to press firmly or to palpate for swellings or lumps. The liver and spleen were not enlarged. The pulse was sunken, rapid, and forceless.

PATTERN IDENTIFICATION

This was a case of incomplete miscarriage and partial placental retention within the uterus with unstoppable bleeding. Chinese medicine calls this post-miscarriage retention of the placenta. I knew that this was due to excessive blood loss and dual vacuity of qì and blood since she looked pale, her lips and tongue were pale, her breathing was thin, her voice was low, and her pulse was sunken and forceless. Moreover, there was also dull pain in the lower abdomen that resisted pressure, and sometimes blood clots were present; thus, there was still static blood in the thoroughfare (*chōng*) and controlling (*rèn*) vessels, as well as the remainder of the undelivered placenta. Therefore, this was a pattern of repletion within vacuity. If I just used a blood-stanching prescription, I feared that the placenta and the static blood would stagnate even more and be difficult to descend, and furthermore, that the condition would remain as it was, namely, that the bleeding would not stop. On the other had, if I used a blood-stasis-eliminating prescription to offensively precipitate the placenta, then I feared that such action would cause a great loss of blood. Considering both of these issues and knowing that her condition was critical, I advised her local physician and her family to immediately take the patient from her remote mountain residence to the closest public health clinic and to decoct the Chinese medicinals and take them as quickly as possible.

TREATMENT METHOD

Supplement both qì and blood, assisted by dispelling stasis and stanching bleeding.

PRESCRIPTION

I gave her one prescription packet, to be urgently decocted as follows:

dāng guī (当归 Chinese angelica, Angelicae Sinensis Radix) 12 g

chuān xiōng (川芎 chuanxiong, Chuanxiong Rhizoma) 6 g

pào jiāng tàn (炮姜炭 blast-fried ginger, Zingiberis Rhizoma Praeparatum) 3 g

táo rén (桃仁 peach kernel, Persicae Semen) 6 g

yì mǔ cǎo (益母草 leonurus, Leonuri Herba) 15 g

zhì huáng qí (炙黄芪 mix-fried astragalus, Astragali Radix cum Liquido Fricta) 15 g

dān shēn (丹参 salvia, Salviae Miltiorrhizae Radix) 12 g

bǎi zǐ rén (柏子仁 arborvitae seed, Platycladi Semen) 9 g

ài yè tàn (艾叶炭 charred mugwort, Artemisiae Argyi Folium Carbonisatum) 9 g

ē jiāo (阿胶 ass hide glue, Asini Corii Colla) 9 g (melted)

zōng tàn (棕炭 charred trachycarpus, Trachycarpi Petiolus Carbonisatus) 9 g

dù zhòng tàn (杜仲炭 charred eucommia, Eucommiae Cortex Carbonisatus) 9 g

I instructed her family to give her 3–5 more packets if the first packet of medicinals was effective, and to send her to the public health clinic if the first packet was not effective.

FORMULA EXPLANATION

This prescription is a combined and modified version of *dāng guī bǔ xuè tāng* (Chinese Angelica Blood-Supplementing Decoction) and *shēng huà tāng* (Engendering Transformation Decoction). The chief medicinals are *dāng guī* (Chinese angelica) and *huáng qí* (astragalus), which combine to achieve dual supplementation of blood and qì. *Dāng guī* (Chinese angelica) supplements blood, and *huáng qí* (astragalus) supplements qì.

As support medicinals, *chuān xiōng* (chuanxiong) and *táo rén* (peach kernel) quicken the blood and dispel stasis; *dān shēn* (salvia) engenders new blood and eliminates stasis and stagnation, and combined with *yì mǔ cǎo* (leonurus), expels stasis and engenders the new, and stanches bleeding. *Ē jiāo* (ass hide glue) enriches and supplements yīn-blood while stanching bleeding.

As an assistant medicinal, *yì mǔ cǎo* (leonurus) quickens static blood in the thoroughfare (*chōng*) and controlling (*rèn*) vessels and stanches bleeding, and combined with *dān shēn* (salvia) and *dāng guī* (Chinese angelica), engenders new blood, quickens static blood, and stanches uterine bleeding. *Ài yè tàn* (charred mugwort) and *zōng tàn* (charred trachycarpus) astringe blood to stanch bleeding and prevent the medicinals that dispel static blood and remove placental stagnation from resulting in massive hemorrhage. Since these two medicinals only possess blood-astringing and stanching action and lack the ability to quicken blood, it is inappropriate to use them here in large doses. *Dù zhòng* (eucommia) boosts the kidney and secures the thoroughfare (*chōng*) and controlling (*rèn*) vessels, and *bǎi zǐ rén* (arborvitae seed) nourishes heart blood and quiets the heart spirit.

As the courier medicinal, *pào jiāng tàn* (blast-fried ginger) warms and assists yáng in the thoroughfare (*chōng*) and controlling (*rèn*) vessels, and warms the uterus and stanches bleeding.

When all these medicinals are used together, they supplement qì and blood, secure the thoroughfare (*chōng*) and controlling (*rèn*) vessels, warm the uterus, dispel stasis, and engender the new and stanch bleeding.

FOLLOWUP TREATMENT

<u>Second examination on November 6</u>: In the afternoon on the day after the last examination, the patient passed the placenta approximately one half hour after taking the decoction. It was about the size of the palm of her hand, purplish-red in color, and one side of it had already turned black. The precipitation of the placenta was followed by profuse bleeding. She was dizzy, so no time was wasted in preparing and taking the second decoction, and within an hour, she felt her heart spirit stabilize and the uterine bleeding decrease. After this, she took one packet of medicinals every day for four days and the bleeding completely stopped. She discontinued the medicinals then for four days

while recovering and the bleeding did not recur. She still felt dizzy and flustered, and had a fear of cold in her lumbus. Her essence-spirit had already improved, her speech was almost normal, but her lips and tongue were still pale, and all six pulses were weak. She felt that she was catching a cold the day before, but today she had already recovered. On the basis of her condition, I prescribed first a decoction to boost qì and resolve the exterior, and then a decoction to take later to supplement both qì and blood, assisted by warming the kidney.

FIRST FOLLOWUP PRESCRIPTION

I gave the patient one packet; when finished, she should take the second prescription:

zhì huáng qí (炙黄芪 mix-fried astragalus, Astragali Radix cum Liquido
   Fricta) 15 g

dāng guī (当归 Chinese angelica, Angelicae Sinensis Radix) 9 g

jīng jiè (荆芥 schizonepeta, Schizonepetae Herba) 6 g

fáng fēng (防风 saposhnikovia, Saposhnikoviae Radix) 9 g

dǎng shēn (党参 codonopsis, Codonopsis Radix) 9 g

zǐ sū yè (紫苏叶 perilla leaf, Perillae Folium) 9 g

guì zhī (桂枝 cinnamon twig, Cinnamomi Ramulus) 3 g

gān cǎo (甘草 licorice, Glycyrrhizae Radix) 3 g

shēng jiāng (生姜 fresh ginger, Zingiberis Rhizoma Recens) 2 slices

SECOND FOLLOWUP PRESCRIPTION

I gave the patient ten packets of the following:

zhì huáng qí (炙黄芪 mix-fried astragalus, Astragali Radix cum Liquido
   Fricta) 21 g

dāng guī (当归 Chinese angelica, Angelicae Sinensis Radix) 9 g

shú dì huáng (熟地黄 cooked rehmannia, Rehmanniae Radix Praeparata)
   15 g (stir-fried with shā rén (砂仁 amomum, Amomi Fructus))

dǎng shēn (党参 codonopsis, Codonopsis Radix) 15 g

bái zhú (白术 white atractylodes, Atractylodis Macrocephalae Rhizoma)
   9 g

fú líng (茯苓 poria, Poria) 9 g

chuān xiōng (川芎 chuanxiong, Chuanxiong Rhizoma) 2.4 g

pào jiāng tàn (炮姜炭 blast-fried ginger, Zingiberis Rhizoma
   Praeparatum) 6 g

chén pí (陈皮 tangerine peel, Citri Reticulatae Pericarpium) 6 g

ròu guì (肉桂 cinnamon bark, Cinnamomi Cortex) 3 g

chǎo dù zhòng (炒杜仲 stir-fried eucommia, Eucommiae Cortex Frictus)
   9 g

zhì gān cǎo (炙甘草 mix-fried licorice, Glycyrrhizae Radix cum Liquido
   Fricta) 6 g

<u>Third examination on November 21</u>: The patient had recovered. There was no recurrence of bleeding; her essence-spirit and her physical strength had greatly improved. She was able to walk to work, cook meals, and tend to household chores. At that time I advised her to take several more packets of the prescription given to her on November 6 to promote her recovery.

CASE FIVE
HAIR LOSS
脱发

The patient was a 30-year-old female, an outpatient at Héběi Provincial Hospital, whose initial examination date was May 27, 1972.

CHIEF COMPLAINT

Hair loss was her chief complaint.

INQUIRY EXAMINATION

The patient had been losing her hair for almost one year. In the previous year, she began to lose her black hair completely from the top of her head and was left with a few strands of white hair in its place. She had given birth to three children in the past, she had a scanty menstruation, her menstrual cycle was irregular, and on many occasions she had delayed menstruation.

INSPECTION EXAMINATION

Her development was normal. She was completely bald on top of her head and usually wore a head scarf. The tongue fur was thin and white.

LISTENING AND SMELLING EXAMINATION

No abnormalities were noted.

PALPATION EXAMINATION

All six pulses were fine (thin).

PATTERN IDENTIFICATION

"The hair is the surplus of blood"; "the kidney governs the bones and engenders marrow; its bloom is in the hair of the head." This patient had delivered three children over several years, and her essence-blood was damaged. The liver and kidney were insufficient; thus, the amount of the menses was scant and menstruation was delayed. The hair did not receive nourishment from blood, and therefore fell out. "Wind is swift and changeable"; the head hair had fallen out very quickly, indicating a pattern of blood vacuity stirring wind.

TREATMENT METHOD

Boost the liver and kidney, supplement essence-blood, assisted by dispelling wind.

PRESCRIPTION

I gave her three packets of the following prescription to be decocted in water, and I advised her to get the repeat prescriptions herself if these proved to be ineffective:

hé shǒu wū (何首乌 flowery knotweed, Polygoni Multiflori Radix) 30 g

dāng guī (当归 Chinese angelica, Angelicae Sinensis Radix) 9 g

shú dì huáng (熟地黄 cooked rehmannia, Rehmanniae Radix Praeparata) 10 g

gǒu qǐ zǐ (枸杞子 lycium, Lycii Fructus) 15 g

tù sī zǐ (菟丝子 cuscuta, Cuscutae Semen) 15 g

chuān xiōng (川芎 chuanxiong, Chuanxiong Rhizoma) 7.5 g

tiān mén dōng (天门冬 asparagus, Asparagi Radix) 9 g

mài mén dōng (麦门冬 ophiopogon, Ophiopogonis Radix) 9 g

bái sháo yào (白芍药 white peony, Paeoniae Radix Alba) 7.5 g

gōu téng (钩藤 uncaria, Uncariae Ramulus cum Uncis) 9 g

fáng fēng (防风 saposhnikovia, Saposhnikoviae Radix) 9 g

FORMULA EXPLANATION

The chief medicinal is *hé shǒu wū* (flowery knotweed); it supplements the liver and kidney, nourishes essence-blood, and blackens the hair and beard.

As support medicinals, *dāng guī* (Chinese angelica) and *shú dì huáng* (cooked rehmannia) supplement blood, and *gǒu qǐ zǐ* (lycium) and *tù sī zǐ* (cuscuta) engender essence.

As assistant medicinals, *tiān mén dōng* (asparagus) and *mài mén dōng* (ophiopogon) boost yīn; *bái sháo yào* (white peony) nourishes blood; and *chuān xiōng* (chuanxiong) quickens blood and prevents stagnation from rich sticky medicinals such as *hé shǒu wū* (flowery knotweed), *shú dì huáng* (cooked rehmannia), *tiān mén dōng* (asparagus), and *mài mén dōng* (ophiopogon).

As courier medicinals, *gōu téng* (uncaria) dispels wind and *fáng fēng* (saposhnikovia) guides the medicinals upward and outward.

Furthermore, I prescribed these medicinals as an external wash:

> *màn jīng zǐ* (蔓荆子 vitex, Viticis Fructus) 9 g
>
> *bò hé* (薄荷 mint, Menthae Herba) 6 g (add at end)
>
> *fáng fēng* (防风 saposhnikovia, Saposhnikoviae Radix) 9 g
>
> *shēng ài yè* (生艾叶 raw mugwort, Artemisiae Argyi Folium Crudum)
> 9 g
>
> *sāng yè* (桑叶 mulberry leaf, Mori Folium) [raw] 9 g
>
> *jú huā* (菊花 chrysanthemum, Chrysanthemi Flos) 9 g
>
> *gǎo běn* (藁本 Chinese lovage, Ligustici Rhizoma) 9 g
>
> *cè bǎi yè* (侧柏叶 arborvitae leaf, Platycladi Cacumen) 9 g
>
> *jīng jiè* (荆芥 schizonepeta, Schizonepetae Herba) 9 g
>
> *huò xiāng* (藿香 patchouli, Pogostemonis Herba) 9 g

I advised the patient to decoct one packet each day and use the decoction as a hair wash 3–4 times a day. After every wash, it was important for her to avoid exposure to wind.

Followup Treatment

Second visit on June 6: The patient saw no changes after taking six packets of medicinals. The tongue and pulse were the same as before. I gave her three more packets, but removed *tiān mén dōng* (asparagus) and *mài mén dōng* (ophiopogon) and added the following:

> *hēi zhī má* (黑脂麻 black sesame, Sesami Semen Nigrum) 30 g
>
> *bǔ gǔ zhī* (补骨脂 psoralea, Psoraleae Fructus) 9 g
>
> *cè bǎi yè* (侧柏叶 arborvitae leaf, Platycladi Cacumen) 9 g

I also gave her the same prescription for the hair wash, but this time with added *sāng shèn* (mulberry) 30 g.

Third visit on June 10: The bald place at the top of her head was beginning to show a few black roots. However, in the last few days, her appetite had decreased, so I added 30 grams of *jiāo sān xiān* (scorch-fried three immortals) and 9 grams of *chén pí* (tangerine peel) to the above-mentioned oral decoction to aid digestion. I advised her to take one packet every other day and gave her three packets. I also gave her the same hair wash prescription as the previous visit. In addition to these, I prepared for her a prescription in pill form to take simultaneously; the pill prescription contained the following medicinals:

> *hé shǒu wū* (何首乌 flowery knotweed, Polygoni Multiflori Radix) 60 g
>
> *hēi zhī má* (黑脂麻 black sesame, Sesami Semen Nigrum) 60 g
>
> *dāng guī* (当归 Chinese angelica, Angelicae Sinensis Radix) 90 g

> *shēng dì huáng* (生地黄 dried rehmannia, Rehmanniae Radix Exsiccata)
>   30 g
> *shú dì huáng* (熟地黄 cooked rehmannia, Rehmanniae Radix Praeparata)
>   30 g
> *bái sháo yào* (白芍药 white peony, Paeoniae Radix Alba) 30 g
> *chuān xiōng* (川芎 chuanxiong, Chuanxiong Rhizoma) 30 g
> *nǚ zhēn zǐ* (女贞子 ligustrum, Ligustri Lucidi Fructus) 30 g
> *tù sī zǐ* (菟丝子 cuscuta, Cuscutae Semen) 30 g
> *wǔ wèi zǐ* (五味子 schisandra, Schisandrae Fructus) 20 g
> *bǔ gǔ zhī* (补骨脂 psoralea, Psoraleae Fructus) 30 g
> *shān yào* (山药 dioscorea, Dioscoreae Rhizoma) 30 g
> *jú huā* (菊花 chrysanthemum, Chrysanthemi Flos) 30 g

These medicinals were ground into a fine powder and mixed with refined honey to form pills weighing nine grams. The dosage was one pill twice a day, early in the morning and in the evening, to be taken with boiled water.

Fourth visit on June 29: She finished the oral decoction and then took the pill prescription. After she had taken the pills for eight days, she noticed a gradual outgrowth of several tufts of black hair on top of her head. Toward the front there was one section of black hair, and towards the back of the head, two sections, each section measuring about 2–3 centimeters in length. Her appetite had improved and her essence-spirit was good. I advised her to combine two ingredients to continue the therapy after finishing the pill prescription. I told her to decoct *shēng ài yè* (raw mugwort) and *sāng yè* (mulberry leaf) in appropriate amounts and use it often as a hair wash.

EMPIRICAL KNOWLEDGE

When using the formulas of past physicians, be flexible with modifications and make changes according to the pattern.

In China, skilled physicians of the past, because of their long history in medical practice, have provided us with many effective formulas. However, we have an obligation to further investigate these formulas to develop greater proficiency. When we use the formulas of past physicians in clinic today, we must pay careful attention to remain flexible and adaptive according to the special circumstances of each patient. As the Míng dynasty physician Lǐ Chān said concerning the modification of formulas:

"Whether the pattern is one of external contraction or of internal damage, you must add, subtract, and combine medicinals from other formulas, thereby creating a tailored formula to meet the needs of the patient. Thousands of formulas, countless circumstances, and individual medicinals must be considered in this way. If you understand this concept, then you know that your prescription has a solid framework. This is precisely what Dōng-Yuán (Lǐ Gǎo) called being effective at using formulas, neither keeping rigidly to the formula, nor straying far from its essence."

Chén Shí-Gōng maintained that "skilled use of formulas lies not in the number of formulas, but rather in the skillful manipulation of formulas to produce the desired effects." During the Qīng dynasty, some people maintained that when the number of formulas were few, they were most valuable for their modifications. So, it is clear that when selecting and using the prescriptions of physicians of the past, you should never copy them mechanically or apply them indiscriminately.

When the condition of the patient surely fits the source formula that governs the treatment, you can simply use the source formula with dosage modifications, taking into account such circumstances as the person, season, or place. Such a process clearly alters the source formula in a different way. Thus, the formulas that you can copy mechanically ingredient by ingredient are very few indeed, and the vast majority of formulas definitely require flexible modifications and changes according to the pattern.

For instance, the patient in Case 1 had a hard swelling due to liver depression and qì stagnation with congealing qì and phlegm. This was a case of chronic disease entering the blood and causing the mutual binding of qì, blood, and phlegm. Following the treatment method of coursing the liver and moving qì while dispersing phlegm and dissipating binds, I selected *chái hú shū gān sǎn* (Bupleurum Liver-Coursing Powder). In this formula, *chái hú* (bupleurum), *xiāng fù* (cyperus), and *zhǐ ké* (bitter orange) move qì and course the liver. I then selected *shēng shí jué míng* (raw abalone shell) because it enriches liver yīn and subdues liver yáng while regulating the liver and moving qì. To strengthen the qì-moving function, I increased the dosage of *xiāng fù* (cyperus) and *zhǐ ké* (bitter orange) as compared to their dosage in the source formula. Since I feared that the yáng-ascending function of *chái hú* (bupleurum) would have an unfavorable effect on the patient's hypertension, I later substituted *yù jīn* (curcuma) for *chái hú*. To enhance the phlegm-transforming function, I substituted *huà jú hóng* (Huazhou pomelo rind) for *chén pí* (tangerine peel) in the source formula. Thus, I used four of the seven ingredients from the source formula.

To disperse phlegm and dissipate binds effectively, I added acrid-flavored *bái jiè zǐ* (white mustard); this medicinal frees and dissipates, moves qì and sweeps phlegm, and disperses phlegm binding between the skin and inner membranes. To disperse and eliminate the swelling, besides choosing qì-moving phlegm-dispersing medicinals, I also selected *xiāo luǒ wán* (Scrofula-Dispersing Pill), which consists of *mǔ lì* (oyster shell), *bèi mǔ* (fritillaria), and *xuán shēn* (scrophularia). This formula resolves depression and emolliates the liver, softens hardness and dissipates binds, and disperses phlegm nodes, so I used it to strengthen the lump-dispersing and eliminating effect. Because this was a condition of enduring disease entering the blood with binding of qì, phlegm, and blood, I was not able to hastily disperse and dissipate, so I did not use blood-quickening stasis-dissipating medicinals. I did, however, at the time of the second visit, add *dān shēn* (salvia) and *zhì shān jiǎ* (mix-fried pangolin scales) to the prescription. These two medicinals quicken blood and dissipate stasis, and transform concretions and disperse accumulations. Considering that the disease had endured for over ten years, the treatment required medicinals that were not only focused but also long-lasting. Therefore, in addition to the decoction, I added *bái jīn wán* (Alum and Curcuma Pill). This pill formula consists of *bái fán* (alum), which dispels dampness and disperses phlegm, and *yù jīn* (curcuma), which resolves depression, courses the liver, and simultaneously quickens blood.

The prescription for this case was flexibly modified according to the pattern and consisted of three source formulas; namely, *chái hú shū gān sǎn* (Bupleurum Liver-Coursing Powder), *xiāo luǒ wán* (Scrofula-Dispersing Pill), and *bái jīn wán* (Alum and Curcuma Pill). The dosages of the medicinals were monitored and changed to reflect any differences in the patient and the pattern.

In Case 2, I used a treatment method of regulating the liver and relaxing tension, and moving qì and disinhibiting dampness, assisted by boosting the kidney and stanching the bleeding. According to the requirements of the treatment method, and considering that the patient had presented with pain in the right side of the lesser abdomen at the time of the initial and second visits, I selected *sháo yào gān cǎo tāng* (Peony and Licorice Decoction) to emolliate the liver and relax tension and to treat the abdominal pain. I used *wū yào* (lindera), *huí xiāng* (fennel), *chuān liàn zǐ* (toosendan), *jú hé* (tangerine pip), and *bīng láng* (areca) from *tiān tái wū yào sǎn* (Tiantai Lindera Powder), and I added *fú líng* (poria), *zé xiè* (alisma), and *jīn qián cǎo* (moneywort) to move qì and disinhibit dampness. *Xù duàn* (dipsacus) and *huáng bǎi* (phellodendron) boosted the kidney, and as charcoaled medicinals, stanched bleeding, so the tip and the root were treated at the same time.

By the time of the third examination, the patient was already free of lesser-abdominal pain, so I removed *bái sháo yào* (white peony) and *gān cǎo* (licorice) from the prescription. Then, given the fact that the patient presented with scurrying pain which ran in a downward direction whenever he urinated, I considered the possibility that damp depression had transformed into heat and, by scorching dampness, a stone had formed, producing sand-stone strangury disease. Therefore, I modified the prescription and added *dōng kuí zǐ* (mallow seed) and *qū mài* (dianthus) to lubricate the orifice, disinhibit dampness, and treat strangury. I combined these with *zé xiè* (alisma), *fú líng* (poria), and *jīn qián cǎo* (moneywort) to enhance the orifice-lubricating, dampness-disinhibiting, and sand-stone–expelling effect. However, there was still an aspect of right vacuity present, given the fact that the disease had endured for more than two months and the pulse was fine. Thus, I increased the dosage of the medicinals that supplement the kidney and boost yīn; namely, I changed the dosage of *xù duàn tàn* (charred dipsacus) to 30 grams and added *shēng dì huáng* (dried rehmannia) and *xuán shēn* (scrophularia). This action produced a satisfactory effect to heighten the patient's physical resistance to disease, in other words, this action "supported right to expel evil" and prevented excessive damage to yīn.

For Case 3, I selected *fù yuán huó xuè tāng* (Origin-Restorative Blood-Quickening Decoction) with modifications according to the pattern, and combined it with *dà huáng gān cǎo tāng* (Rhubarb and Licorice Decoction) and *dà huáng zhè chóng wán* (Rhubarb and Ground Beetle Pill). I obtained results by changing the formulas according to the differences in the course of the disease and according to the transformations in the condition of the patient. When treating the patient in Case 4, I used the same concept by prescribing *dāng guī bǔ xuè tāng* (Chinese Angelica Blood-Supplementing Decoction) together with *shēng huà tāng* (Engendering Transformation Decoction), modifying the prescription according to the pattern. Thus, the treatment was effective.

Have confidence to compose a new prescription according to the pattern requirements.

Even if you practice in clinic always modifying according to pattern changes and requirements of the treatment method, and comply with the formulas of past physicians, you will still find that formulas sometimes do not satisfy the requirements. You may also find that formulas used in the past do not always achieve ideal results today. When this happens, you must choose suitable medicinals and attempt a self-composed, new prescription in accordance with the condition of the patient and the requirements of the treatment method. You should follow the rules of formula composition and medicinal compatibility, that is, which medicinals are suitable and which should be avoided, and draw from both ancient and modern experience.

A good example here is the new prescription composed for the patient in the second case at the time of the third visit. The patient had taken a treatment of more than ten packets of medicinals by that time, and the condition of the pattern had changed: the pain on the right side of the lesser abdomen was relieved, the discomfort in the lumbus and smaller abdomen had disappeared, and the bloody urine had clearly improved. Now, when the patient urinated, he felt a scurrying pain moving in a downward direction, so the disease had become sand-stone strangury, despite the fact that not long before tests at the hospital had failed to detect urinary stones. Therefore, given the symptoms on one hand and the fine pulse on the other, I knew right qì was insufficient, so I increased the dosage of *xù duàn* (dipsacus) to strengthen kidney qì, and I added *shēng dì huáng* (dried rehmannia) and *xuán shēn* (scrophularia) to supplement the kidney and nourish yīn and to enhance the formula's capability of supporting right and dispelling evil. Furthermore, I chose *dōng kuí zǐ* (mallow seed) to lubricate the orifice and disinhibit dampness, *qū mài* (dianthus) to quicken blood and disinhibit dampness to treat strangury, and *huáng qín* (scutellaria) to clear heat. These medicinals were coordinated with *jīn qián cǎo* (moneywort), *fú líng* (poria), and *zé xiè* (alisma) to disinhibit dampness and expel stones.

The entire composition of this prescription served to supplement the kidney and boost yīn, assisted by disinhibiting dampness and expelling the stone. The reasoning behind this prescription was clear: It made no difference if the patient actually had a urinary stone or not; by taking the medicinals, the stone would be expelled if it existed. If it did not exist, the patient would still benefit from supplementing the kidney and disinhibiting dampness. There was also benefit in supporting right and dispelling evil and in hastening the period of recovery. Yet, as expected, the patient passed a stone after taking the medicinals, blood in the urine stopped, and he made a complete recovery.

This newly-composed prescription was based on the fundamental theories and experience of past physicians and combined with modern reports on the action of *jīn qián cǎo* (moneywort) to expel stones. In clinic, I often use this prescription modified according to the pattern to treat urinary calculi, and I achieve ideal results. Here are some of the useful modifications to this prescription: When blood in the urine is not severe, do not use char-fried *xù duàn* (dipsacus), *huáng bǎi* (phellodendron), or *xiǎo jì* (field thistle). When there is proof that a stone exists, and the patient has not been able to expel it for a long period of time, add *niú xī* (achyranthes), *zé lán* (lycopus), *jī nèi jīn* (gizzard lining), and *zhì shān jiǎ* (mix-fried pangolin scales); the dosage of *dōng kuí zǐ* (mallow seed) can be 10–20 g; the dosage of *jīn qián cǎo* (moneywort) can be

20–40 g. If there are no symptoms of yīn vacuity, remove *xuán shēn* (scrophularia) and substitute *shēng dì huáng* (dried rehmannia) for *shú dì huáng* (cooked rehmannia) or prescribe *shēng dì huáng* (dried rehmannia) and *shú dì huáng* (cooked rehmannia) in equal amounts. My experience in treating urinary stones has been to emphasize kidney-supplementing medicinals; my advice is that the composition of the prescription should not just contain dampness-disinhibiting and strangury-freeing medicinals.

I composed the prescription in Case 5 according to the specific condition of the patient, that is, her condition of excessive childbearing and insufficient essence-blood. Not only did I use *hé shŏu wū* (flowery knotweed) as the chief medicinal to nourish essence-blood, but I also combined it with medicinals such as *tù sī zĭ* (cuscuta), *dāng guī* (Chinese angelica), *bái sháo yào* (white peony), and *gŏu qĭ zĭ* (lycium) to enrich essence-blood. Assisted by dispelling wind, the prescription proved efficacious. The external hair wash formula for this particular patient had certainly produced results. I had carefully combined the dosage with the condition of the patient, and by doing so, very quickly obtained an ideal result. In summary, do not be afraid to carefully compose a new prescription.

The method of prescription modification

Physicians of the past accumulated abundant experience in the practice of formula modification, and they have provided us with this knowledge to study and use. Here I will discuss the method by which physicians of the past handled formula modifications, and combined with my own experience, offer below several formula methods for your reference.

1. "Add" refers to adding one or more medicinals to a source formula; "add" also refers to the action of increasing the dosage of one or more medicinals that are already in the formula.

2. "Remove" refers to removing one or more medicinals from a source formula or to reducing the dosage of one or more medicinals.

3. "Trim," as trimming a garment, refers to trimming out the portions of a source formula that are not required for the relevant patterns and symptoms.

4. "Picking" refers to picking or retaining the chief medicinals from the source formula or picking certain highly efficacious medicinals in combination in one formula and placing these in other formulas.

5. "Stringing" refers to taking the essential portion of two or three, sometimes three or four prescriptions and weaving them together to create one formula, simultaneously considering the primary and secondary roles for each

formula. For example, to create my self-composed formula, *má xìng èr sān tāng* (Ephedra and Apricot Kernel Two-Three Decoction), I selected *má huáng* (ephedra) and *xìng rén* (apricot kernel) from *má huáng tāng* (Ephedra Decoction) and combined them with *èr chén tāng* (Two Matured Ingredients Decoction) and *sān zǐ yǎng qīn tāng* (Three-Seed Filial Devotion Decoction). In most situations, I remove *bái jiè zǐ* (white mustard) and *gān cǎo* (licorice).

6. "Combine" refers to combining two or more than two formulas into one formula. Whenever I treat enduring stomach duct pain that is difficult to resolve, I use my own formula "*sān hé tāng* (Triple Combination Decoction)," which is a combination of three other formulas: *liáng fù wán* (Lesser Galangal and Cyperus Pill), *bǎi hé tāng* (Lily Bulb Decoction), and *dān shēn yǐn* (Salvia Beverage). When the location of the pain is fixed, or if the stools are sometimes black and the pain is severe, I combine *sān hé tāng* (Triple Combination Decoction) with *shī xiào sǎn* (Sudden Smile Powder), which is also known as *sì hé tāng* (Quadruple Combination Decoction).

7. "Integration" refers to both a method and a requirement. The methods mentioned above—adding, removing, trimming, picking, stringing, and combining—are sometimes used alone and sometimes used in conjunction with each other. Above all, it is important to remain flexible and to avoid rigidity. After you select a formula and add or remove medicinals, the next step is to appropriately trim, pick, string together, or combine them; afterwards you will still need to pay attention to the "transformation" of the formula. This means that besides reconfirming the appropriateness of the formula in relation to the symptoms, the treatment method, the patient, the place, and the time, you must also carefully analyze each medicinal's suitability in the composition in terms of compatibility, proportional medicinal strength, dosage, cooking methods, and medicinal preparations. For instance, you should ask whether the medicinal should be pre-decocted, added later, roasted, wrapped, ground, or stir-fried. You must also consider each medicinal with respect to the symptoms and the treatment method and confirm that they bear an organic relationship with each other, which succeeds in bringing out the greatest therapeutic efficacy and at the same time minimizes shortcomings. When this process is successful, the new prescription conforms better to the treatment requirements than the source formula.

Physicians in the past understood this integrative process and developed formulas that were highly effective; these individuals were acclaimed as the superb masters of medicinals and formulas. Some very effective new prescriptions emerged from this process of "integration." This process is not just the "mixing together" of an assortment of individual medicinals. "Integration" is, instead, the process in which the composition, compatibility, and modifications of the medicinals proficiently corresponds to the symptoms and treatment method.

In summary, the formulas of past physicians and your own new formulas are both valuable. However, both approaches are intimately related to the condition of the patient and based on the requirements of the treatment method, together with modifications following the pattern and flexible application depending on the person, the time, and the place. By following this principle, you can obtain outstanding results.

The importance of assimilating the strong points of classical formulas, post-antique formulas, and empirical formulas

"Classical formulas" generally refer to medicinal formulas from one of the medical classics, such as *Huáng Dì Nèi Jīng* ("The Yellow Emperor's Inner Canon"), *Shāng Hán Lùn* ("On Cold Damage"), and *Jīn Guì Yào Lüè* ("Essential Prescriptions of the Golden Coffer"). These formulas have many merits; for example, they contain relatively few medicinals, their composition is concise, and they reflect profound principles. Within these formulas there are clear distinctions between the four medicinal roles (i.e. chief, support, assistant, and courier), and the seven formula types (i.e. large, small, moderate, urgent, odd, even, and compound). Furthermore, the compilers of these books worked out the medicinal processing, cooking, and administration methods, as well as the dosages and formula modifications. The formula is united as one with the method, and the treated patterns are explicit.

Certain classical formulas treat specific diseases, and certain methods use specific formulas; if the condition of the patient changes, then the formula changes. In some cases, the medicinals in formulas may be the same, but the dosages are different; thus, formulas with different guiding principles are formed, the treatment follows a different pattern, and the formula name changes. Because of these features, classical formulas are still extensively used in the modern clinic. In my treatment of Case 3 in this chapter, I selected the formula *dà huáng gān cǎo tāng* (Rhubarb and Licorice Decoction) from the *Jīn Guì Yào Lüè* ("Essential Prescriptions of the Golden Coffer") to treat constipation and vomiting immediately after eating caused by accumulation and stagnation that had transformed into heat. I selected *sháo yào gān cǎo tāng* (Peony and Licorice Decoction) from the *Shāng Hán Lùn* ("On Cold Damage") for the patient in Case 2 to nourish blood and relax tension and to treat the fixed abdominal pain. I further prescribed for this patient *dà huáng zhè chóng wán* (Rhubarb and Ground Beetle Pill), as it appears in the *Jīn Guì Yào Lüè* ("Essential Prescriptions of the Golden Coffer") to dispel stasis and engender new blood.

Post-antique formulas were later developments founded on classical formulas. The elements of post-antique formulas reflect the composition of classical formulas, such as the role of medicinals (chief, support, assistant, and courier), the aim of the formula structure, the assessment of medicinal dosage, the nature of medicinal relationships (need, empowerment, fear, and clashing), and appropriate use of medicinal preparation, cooking, and administration techniques. All these factors reflect the profound developments of Chinese medical theory, and physicians who wish to effectively prescribe post-antique formulas must be knowledgeable of this. Post-antique formulas developed from the principles and spirit of classical formulas in terms of formula composition, pattern treatment, and formula transformation. Furthermore, they supplement areas in the classical formulary that are insufficient. For example, although there are simply too many of these formulas to mention here, the following well-known post-antique formulas are still in common usage and produce reliable, effective results:

- *Fáng fēng tōng shèng sǎn* (Saposhnikovia Sage-Inspired Powder) created by Liú Hé-Jiān

- *Bǔ zhōng yì qì tāng* (Center-Supplementing Qì-Boosting Decoction) created by Lǐ Dōng-Yuán

- *Liáng gé sǎn* (Diaphragm-Cooling Powder), *zǐ xuě dān* (Purple Snow Elixir), and *zhì bǎo dān* (Supreme Jewel Elixir) from the *Tài Píng Huì Mín Hé Jì Jú Fāng* ("Tài-Píng Imperial Grace Pharmacy Formulas")

- *Sān zǐ yǎng qīn tāng* (Three-Seed Filial Devotion Decoction) from the text *Hán Shì Yī Tōng* ("Han's Clear View of Medicine")

- *Ān gōng niú huáng wán* (Peaceful Palace Bovine Bezoar Pill), *yín qiào sǎn* (Lonicera and Forsythia Powder), and *zēng yè chéng qì tāng* (Humor-Increasing Qì-Infusing Decoction) from the *Wēn Bìng Tiáo Biàn* ("Systematized Identification of Warm Diseases")

- *Gé xià zhú yū tāng* (Infradiaphragmatic Stasis-Expelling Decoction) and *bǔ yáng huán wǔ tāng* (Yáng-Supplementing Five-Returning Decoction) from the *Yī Lín Gǎi Cuò* ("Correction of Errors in Medical Classics")

For the cases in this chapter, I selected several post-antique formulas. Among them were *chái hú shū gān sǎn* (Bupleurum Liver-Coursing Powder) and *xiāo luǒ wán* (Scrofula-Dispersing Pill) for the patient in Case 1; *tiān tái wū yào sǎn* (Tiantai Lindera Powder) in Case 2; and *fù yuán huó xuè tāng* (Origin-Restorative Blood-Quickening Decoction) for Case 3. For the patient in Case 4, I selected post-antique formulas *dāng guī bǔ xuè tāng* (Chinese Angelica Blood-Supplementing Decoction) and *shēng huà tāng* (Engendering Transformation Decoction). Everyone should learn and use the principles of composition, concepts, pattern treatment, and medicinal compatibility of these post-antique formulas and modify them according to the pattern. These comments are simply based on my experience.

Empirical formulas are those formulas that are defined through folklore and in "formula books," or they may be secret or experiential formulas from physicians. Some may concern certain medicinal herbs or even home remedies and folk prescriptions. These are exceptionally effective formulas, and there is a great deal of knowledge that is passed by word of mouth from teachers to disciples and from parents to children. These prescriptions have many merits; they are simple, convenient, effective, and inexpensive, and they are also concise and appropriate in their compatibility. By studying these formulas, we can often find new ways of thinking about medicinals and thereby strengthen our knowledge base. I assimilated the empirically-known medicinal *jīn qián cǎo* (moneywort) into the prescription for the patient in Case 2 to treat stone strangury, and I used *liú jì nú* (anomalous artemisia) to empirically treat blood and qì distention and fullness for the patient in Case 3. Finally, in Case 5, I assimilated *hé shǒu wū* (flowery knotweed) into the prescription; this medicinal is empirically known to blacken the hair and beard.

When using these types of formulas, it is essential to remain free of bias. Some practitioners like supplementing medicinals and prescribe supplementing formulas for all their patients. Some like attacking medicinals and prescribe attacking formulas for their patients. Some practitioners frequently write prescriptions for cold and cool medicinals because that is their bias; others write prescriptions for only warm and hot medicinals because that is their preference. The physicians who use classical formulas ridicule those who use post-antique formulas as traitors to classical orthodoxy. Those physicians preferring post-antique formulas say that physicians who use only classical formulas are trapped in the past and are inflexibly conservative. These biased points of view do not benefit our intellectual progress or our development of Chinese herbal medicine. I believe that the clinical application of medicine should meet the needs of the patient. When it is appropriate to supplement, then supplement; when appropriate to drain, drain; when heating is appropriate, use heat; and when cooling is suitable, cool. When a classical formula is appropriate, then select a classical formula. When a post-antique formula is suitable for the treatment, use it. When an empirical formula is useful, by all means use it. In fact, all three of these formula types can be combined and modified and can be integrated and organically applied.

In summary, be flexible and avoid prejudice. Use and flexibly assimilate these three formula types to improve treatment efficacy. Recall the statement by Míng dynasty physician Lǐ Shān in the *Yī Xué Rù Mén* ("The Gateway to Medicine"), recording the words of Lǐ Dōng-Yuán:

> "The physician who effectively uses formulas neither keeps
> rigidly to the formula, nor strays far from its essence."

CHAPTER FIVE

When treating diseases diagnosed by Western medicine, use pattern identification as a basis for determining treatment.

It is essential for the Chinese medical physician to use the principles of Chinese medical theory to diagnose the illness of the patient, even when a Western biomedical diagnosis has already been provided. In my experience, you must pay attention to the theories and methods of pattern identification to determine treatment and thereby distinguish the disease and the patterns through Chinese medical principles. Follow the rules of pattern identification, choose the formula and the medicinals, organize the prescription, and formulate the treatment step-by-step. Be certain to take into account the specific circumstances and condition of the patient, and also consider the knowledge of modern medical science and modern scientific research. By deliberating over all these factors you can integrate them into a holistic model, and thus formulate a treatment that is goal-oriented. Continued practice of this model will obtain good therapeutic effectiveness. Here are five case studies from my clinical experience with brief discussions to illustrate these points.

CASE STUDIES

CASE ONE
HYPERACTIVE TONGUE WIND (PEDIATRIC CHOREA)
弄舌风(小舞蹈病)

The patient, a 10-year-old male student at the village school, was an outpatient at the Héběi Provincial Hospital, first examined May 21, 1972.

CHIEF COMPLAINT

Protrusion of the tongue, constant eye blinking, flailing of the arms and legs, and fidgetiness for more than three months.

INQUIRY EXAMINATION

The patient was angered by a fellow student six months ago. On the following day, the patient presented with flailing limbs that moved involuntarily. He visited a Western medical physician who diagnosed him with pediatric chorea and administered injections such as sulfuric acid and magnesium. The patient seemed to recover. Then on the Chinese New Year, after being frightened by the sound of firecrackers, the patient had a relapse. He went to the hospital again for the same type of injections and for a variety of other treatments, but this time there were no results at all. At the time of the initial examination in my clinic, the patient presented with symptoms of unceasing protrusion of the tongue and eye blinking, flailing involuntary movement of both arms, and random involuntary movement of both legs. Urine and stools were still normal.

INSPECTION EXAMINATION

His development and nutrition appeared normal. The tongue tip was continuously protruding, and his eyes were constantly blinking. His head was shaking, his arms and legs were flailing involuntarily, and he was fidgety. All these symptoms would not stop for even a moment. The tongue fur was thin and white and the tongue body slightly red.

LISTENING AND SMELLING EXAMINATION

His speech was clear and distinct; his voice was normal.

PALPATION EXAMINATION

His head, neck, chest, abdomen, and four limbs were without any other abnormalities. Since the arm movement was constant and involuntary, it was difficult to conduct a detailed pulse examination; however, the pulse was stringlike.

At that time I had fellow classmates in clinical practice that were allopathic physicians trained in Chinese medicine, and we jointly conferred on this case. We found a reference to pediatric chorea in a basic Western medical text that cited an article on the treatment of chorea in Chinese medicine with a certain Chinese medicinal prescription. Here is the prescription exactly as it was given in the text:

> *ài yè* (艾叶 mugwort, Artemisiae Argyi Folium) 3 g
> *fáng jǐ* (防己 fangji, Stephaniae Tetrandrae Radix) 1.5 g
> *guì zhī* (桂枝 cinnamon twig, Cinnamomi Ramulus) 3 g
> *qín jiāo* (秦艽 large gentian, Gentianae Macrophyllae Radix) 1.5 g

fáng fēng (防风 saposhnikovia, Saposhnikoviae Radix) 3 g

nǚ zhēn zǐ (女贞子 ligustrum, Ligustri Lucidi Fructus) 1.5 g

shí chāng pú (石菖蒲 acorus, Acori Tatarinowii Rhizoma) 3 g

huā jiāo (花椒 zanthoxylum, Zanthoxyli Pericarpium) 1.5 g

mèng huā (梦花 edgeworthia, Edgeworthiae Flos) 3 g

jú hé (橘核 tangerine pip, Citri Reticulatae Semen) 3 g

gān jiāng (干姜 dried ginger, Zingiberis Rhizoma) 0.9 g

It was my understanding at the time that this prescription was empirically based and expressly for the treatment of pediatric chorea, so I made no modifications and advised his family to administer 3–6 packets of the prescription.

FOLLOWUP TREATMENT

<u>Second visit on May 29:</u> After taking the six packets of medicinals, the patient still experienced no alleviation of the symptoms. My colleagues and I still diagnosed the disease as chorea, but also decided to conduct Chinese medical pattern identification to determine treatment.

PATTERN IDENTIFICATION

I knew that the liver and heart channels were involved since the illness arose after the patient had been angered and frightened, and since the tongue tip protruded continuously. The liver governs wind; the tongue is associated with the heart. This patient's pulse was stringlike and the tongue body was relatively red; these signs and symptoms revealed that liver depression had formed heat and engendered wind, and heart fire resulted from liver heat burning the upper body. Wind and fire are both yáng evils and by nature govern movement. Since wind was moving, the eyes were blinking and hyperactive, and there was flailing of the limbs. Since heart heat was present, the tongue tip protruded and was unceasingly active. After correlating the four examinations, I diagnosed hyperactive tongue wind disease caused by movement of wind in the liver channel and exuberant heat in the heart channel.

TREATMENT METHOD

Settle the liver and subdue yáng while extinguishing wind and clearing the heart.

PRESCRIPTION

I prescribed six packets of the following, to be decocted in water:

shēng dài zhě shí (生代赭石 crude hematite, Haematitum Crudum) 21 g (pre-decocted)

shēng mǔ lì (生牡蛎 raw oyster shell, Ostreae Concha Cruda) 24 g (pre-decocted)

tiān zhú huáng (天竹黄 bamboo sugar, Bambusae Concretio Silicea) 6 g *bái jí lí* (白蒺藜 tribulus, Tribuli Fructus) 9 g

gōu téng (钩藤 uncaria, Uncariae Ramulus cum Uncis) 15 g

quán xiē (全蝎 scorpion, Scorpio) 9 g

fáng fēng (防风 saposhnikovia, Saposhnikoviae Radix) 9 g

dāng guī wěi (当归尾 tangkuei tail, Angelicae Sinensis Radicis
     Extremitas) 9 g

bái sháo yào (白芍药 white peony, Paeoniae Radix Alba) 12 g

sāng zhī (桑枝 mulberry twig, Mori Ramulus) 30 g

I also prescribed 12 pills of *niú huáng zhèn jīng wán* (Bovine Bezoar Fright-Settling Pill), one pill twice a day, taken after the decoction.

FORMULA EXPLANATION

As chief medicinals, *shēng dài zhě shí* (crude hematite) and *shēng mǔ lì* (raw oyster shell) settle the liver and subdue yáng.

As support medicinals, *tiān zhú huáng* (bamboo sugar) clears heart heat, and *bái jí lí* (tribulus) and *gōu téng* (uncaria) calm the liver and extinguish wind.

As assistant medicinals, *quán xiē* (scorpion) combined with *fáng fēng* (saposhnikovia) enhance the wind-extinguishing action of the formula, and *dāng guī wěi* (tangkuei tail) and *bái sháo yào* (white peony) nourish blood and emolliate the liver.

As the courier medicinal, *sāng zhī* (mulberry twig) not only treats wind, but also frees and penetrates the four limbs, and when combined with *dāng guī wěi* (tangkuei tail), moves blood to automatically extinguish wind.

I additionally prescribed *niú huáng zhèn jīng wán* (Bovine Bezoar Fright-Settling Pill) to clear heart heat and extinguish liver wind while settling fright and quieting the spirit.

<u>Third visit on June 6:</u> The patient basically recovered after six packets of the above-mentioned prescription. The limbs were no longer flailing about and he could sit quietly while the physician diagnosed the pulse. Occasionally the tongue protruded and the eyes blinked, but these symptoms were not obvious unless close attention was paid. The tongue diagnosis bordered on normal; the pulse tended to be stringlike. Using the above-mentioned prescription, I changed the dosage for *shēng dài zhě shí* (crude hematite) and *shēng mǔ lì* (raw oyster shell) to 30 g each and gave the patient three more packets. I advised the family that several more packets were necessary for an effective outcome.

<u>Fourth visit on June 30:</u> I found that the patient had fully recovered, and there had been no relapse.

CASE TWO

CHEST IMPEDIMENT (ACUTE MYOCARDITIS)

胸痹(急性心肌炎)

The patient was a 37-year-old female, a factory worker from Běijīng, whose initial examination date was July 7, 1978.

CHIEF COMPLAINT

Flusteredness, heart palpitations, and occasional chest and back pain for more than three months.

INQUIRY EXAMINATION

Earlier that year on March 16, the patient had a pregnancy in the isthmic portion of the right uterine tube that had caused rupture of the uterine tube, resulting in hemorrhagic shock. She had been rushed to a Běijīng hospital to undergo emergency surgery in the gynecology and obstetrics department. At that time she had lost 2,200 ml of blood, but was given a transfusion of only 1,800 ml. She seemed to be in good condition after the surgery. On March 20, however, she felt flustered and nauseous and sought a consultation with an intern. Several times she received an electrocardiogram test, and the diagnosis was acute myocarditis. She then received injections of compounded *dān shēn* (salvia), ATP (adenosine triphosphate), vitamin C, and orally administered propranolol and persantin. After taking these medications, she received 80 packets of Chinese medicinal prescriptions that were given to her with some modifications. Several medicinals included in these prescriptions were as follows:

huáng qí (黄芪 astragalus, Astragali Radix)

dǎng shēn (党参 codonopsis, Codonopsis Radix)

bái zhú (白术 white atractylodes, Atractylodis Macrocephalae Rhizoma)

dāng guī (当归 Chinese angelica, Angelicae Sinensis Radix)

shēng dì huáng (生地黄 dried rehmannia, Rehmanniae Radix Exsiccata)

mài mén dōng (麦门冬 ophiopogon, Ophiopogonis Radix)

dān shēn (丹参 salvia, Salviae Miltiorrhizae Radix)

shān yào (山药 dioscorea, Dioscoreae Rhizoma)

lián ròu (莲肉 lotus seed, Nelumbinis Semen)

hé huān pí (合欢皮 silk tree bark, Albizziae Cortex)

yuǎn zhì (远志 polygala, Polygalae Radix)

suān zǎo rén (酸枣仁 spiny jujube, Ziziphi Spinosi Semen)

chén pí (陈皮 tangerine peel, Citri Reticulatae Pericarpium)

bàn xià (半夏 pinellia, Pinelliae Rhizoma)
fú líng (茯苓 poria, Poria)
gān cǎo (甘草 licorice, Glycyrrhizae Radix)

Yet after all the medications and the Chinese medicinals, the electrocardiogram results remained abnormal. On April 14, the results were as follows: sinus tachycardia 103 beats/minute, P–R intervals 0.16 second, Q–T intervals 0.37 second. Each lead of the QRS waves was normal. ST: V3 depression 0.1mV. T: I, II, III, aVF, V3–V6 inverted; V3 was most distinct and profound 0.1mV; aVL and V1 both low and flat; aVR vertical.

On June 24: sinus tachycardia; ST: II, III, aVF, V3–V6 mildly depressed. T: V3 inverted; II, III, aVF, V6 low and flat <1/10 R.

On July 7, the patient came to my outpatient clinic at the hospital. At the time of her initial examination, her chief complaint was the feeling of chest oppression, flusteredness, shortness of breath when walking, and occasional aching pain in the chest and back which was relatively severe on the left side. She was nauseous and her appetite was poor. She experienced no adequate sleep, her menses were profuse, her spirit-essence was devitalized, and her lumbus was aching, limp, and lacking strength. Urine and stool remained normal.

INSPECTION EXAMINATION

Her development was normal and nutrition average; her mind was clear, but her spirit was fatigued. Her tongue fur was white.

LISTENING AND SMELLING EXAMINATION

Her speech was clear and distinct, but her voice was not loud and clear. There was some shortness of breath whenever she moved.

PALPATION EXAMINATION

On the left hand the inch pulse was weak and the bar and cubit pulses were sunken and fine. On the right hand the inch and cubit pulses were sunken and fine and the bar pulse was sunken, slippery, and fine. There were no other remarkable signs and symptoms.

PATTERN IDENTIFICATION

The heart governs blood, and illness in this patient had arisen due to a great amount of blood loss. When combined with the evidence of the weak left inch pulse, I knew that the pattern was insufficiency of heart blood. The heart resides in the center of the chest and governs yáng qì in the chest. Yīn and yáng are rooted in each other, so when heart blood was insufficient, chest yáng was devitalized, and the patient presented with symptoms such as chest oppression, flusteredness, and a sunken, weak inch pulse. When chest yáng was devitalized, the flow of qì and blood was irregular and unsmooth in the blood vessels, so sometimes there was aching in the chest and back. When blood could not nourish the heart, the heart-spirit became disquieted and sleep was not peaceful.

The spleen and stomach are the source of blood production and nourishment for the vessels. In this case, there was insufficient heart blood depriving vessel qì of nourishment; both these events influenced center burner stomach qì. Therefore the patient had symptoms of nausea with a desire to vomit, poor appetite, white tongue fur, and a sunken, slippery bar pulse on the right hand. The loss of blood was excessive during the pregnancy and injured the lower origin. The kidney governs the lower origin, so whenever the lower origin is damaged, there is also injury to the thoroughfare (*chōng*) and controlling (*rèn*) vessels. Consequently, menstruation was profuse, the lumbus was aching and weak, and the essence-spirit was devitalized. After correlating all four examinations, I decided that the diagnosis was chest impediment disease with insufficient heart blood and devitalized chest yáng.

TREATMENT METHOD

Reinforce yáng and open impediment while nourishing blood and quieting the heart, assisted by boosting the kidney and spleen.

PRESCRIPTION

The patient received six packets of modified *guā lóu xiè bái bái jiǔ tāng* (Trichosanthes, Chinese Chive, and White Liquor Decoction) and *sì wù tāng* (Four Agents Decoction), to be decocted in water:

quán guā lóu (全栝楼 whole trichosanthes, Trichosanthis Fructus Integer) 30 g

xiè bái (薤白 Chinese chive, Allii Macrostemonis Bulbus) 10 g

dāng guī (当归 Chinese angelica, Angelicae Sinensis Radix) 10 g

bái sháo yào (白芍药 white peony, Paeoniae Radix Alba) 12 g

shēng dì huáng (生地黄 dried rehmannia, Rehmanniae Radix Exsiccata) 9 g

shú dì huáng (熟地黄 cooked rehmannia, Rehmanniae Radix Praeparata) 9 g

hóng huā (红花 carthamus, Carthami Flos) 5 g

shēng mǔ lì (生牡蛎 raw oyster shell, Ostreae Concha Cruda) 30 g (predecocted)

bái zhú (白术 white atractylodes, Atractylodis Macrocephalae Rhizoma) 9 g

fú líng (茯苓 poria, Poria) 12 g

sāng jì shēng (桑寄生 mistletoe, Loranthi seu Visci Ramus) 30 g

chǎo xù duàn (炒续断 stir-fried dipsacus, Dipsaci Radix Fricta) 21 g

FORMULA EXPLANATION

As chief medicinals, *guā lóu* (trichosanthes) loosens the chest and dissipates binds while transforming phlegm and downbearing turbidity; acrid *xiè bái* (Chinese chive) frees the heart and chest, reinforces yáng, and opens impediment.

As support medicinals, *dāng guī* (Chinese angelica), *bái sháo yào* (white peony), *shēng dì huáng* (dried rehmannia), and *shú dì huáng* (cooked rehmannia) all nourish the blood to provide luxuriance to the heart.

As assistant medicinals, *bái zhú* (white atractylodes) and *fú líng* (poria) transform dampness, regulate the center, and boost the spleen; *sāng jì shēng* (mistletoe) and *xù duàn* (dipsacus) boost the kidney and secure the thoroughfare (*chōng*) and controlling (*rèn*) vessels; and *shēng mǔ lì* (raw oyster shell) subdues and quiets the heart-spirit.

The small dosage of *hóng huā* (carthamus), which acts as the courier medicinal, dispels stasis and engenders the new while guiding blood-nourishing medicinals to the heart.

When used together, all the medicinals reinforce yáng and open impediment, nourish blood and quiet the heart, boost the kidney and calm the spirit, and simultaneously regulate the center and boost the spleen.

FOLLOWUP TREATMENT

<u>Second visit on July 14:</u> After taking the medicinals, the patient noticed an improvement in sleeping and appetite. However, the chest oppression, flusteredness, chest and back pain, and aching lumbus did not improve at all. The tongue fur had become thin and white; the pulse was primarily sunken and slippery, and the fine manifestation had already changed for the better. According to my analysis of pulse and disease symptoms, I knew the goal of blood-nourishing, heart-calming, and center-regulating had been reached, but the prescription was still not effective for reinforcing yáng and opening impediment. Therefore, I changed to another formula, *guā lóu xiè bái bàn xià tāng* (Trichosanthes, Chinese Chive, and Pinellia Decoction) with added *guì zhī* (cinnamon twig), plus modifications according to the pattern, to reinforce yáng and open impediment, while still supporting the kidney-boosting, center-regulating, and spirit-quieting effect. The patient received six packets of the following prescription:

quán guā lóu (全栝楼 whole trichosanthes, Trichosanthis Fructus Integer) 30 g

xiè bái (薤白 Chinese chive, Allii Macrostemonis Bulbus) 10 g

bàn xià (半夏 pinellia, Pinelliae Rhizoma) 9 g

guì zhī (桂枝 cinnamon twig, Cinnamomi Ramulus) 9 g

zǐ sū gěng (紫苏梗 perilla stem, Perillae Caulis) 9 g

dān shēn (丹参 salvia, Salviae Miltiorrhizae Radix) 12 g

yuǎn zhì (远志 polygala, Polygalae Radix) 9 g

zhēn zhū mǔ (珍珠母 mother-of-pearl, Concha Margaritifera) 30 g (pre-decocted)

sāng jì shēng (桑寄生 mistletoe, Loranthi seu Visci Ramus) 30 g

xù duàn (续断 dipsacus, Dipsaci Radix) 15 g

dǎng shēn (党参 codonopsis, Codonopsis Radix) 9 g

bái zhú (白术 white atractylodes, Atractylodis Macrocephalae Rhizoma) 6 g

fú líng (茯苓 poria, Poria) 12 g

Third visit on July 21: The chest oppression and pain had been alleviated. Her sleep had improved even further, and the lumbar pain had also lessened. Yet the back pain, shortness of breath, and irritability remained. The tongue fur was thin and slightly yellow; the pulse was slightly slippery, but without the fine manifestation. I made the following modifications to the previous prescription and gave the patient six more packets. I reduced the dosage of *guì zhī* (cinnamon twig) to 6 g and increased the dosage of *dān shēn* (salvia) to 15 g; I removed *bái zhú* (white atractylodes), *xù duàn* (dipsacus), and *zǐ sū gěng* (perilla stem) and added:

xiāng fù (香附 cyperus, Cyperi Rhizoma) 9 g

bīng láng (槟榔 areca, Arecae Semen) 9 g

Fourth visit on July 27: The chest pains had not recurred during this last week, and the patient had almost regained her physical strength as before, but she still sometimes experienced shortness of breath and flusteredness. The tongue fur was still slightly yellow at the root; the pulse was sunken and slippery. Two days prior to this examination the patient underwent another electrocardiogram examination, her first since the emergency visit to the hospital some weeks ago. The results showed an improvement since that time: sinus tachycardia; ST: II and V5 had a slight decline. T: V5 low and flat <1/10 R. On the basis of this information, I made the following modifications to the above-mentioned prescription and gave the patient six more packets: I reduced the dosage of *guā lóu* (trichosanthes) to 25 g and increased the dosage of *guì zhī* (cinnamon twig) to 9 g. I removed *dān shēn* (salvia) and *xiāng fù* (cyperus) and added:

chì sháo yào (赤芍药 red peony, Paeoniae Radix Rubra) 9 g

bái sháo yào (白芍药 white peony, Paeoniae Radix Alba) 9 g

lián ròu (莲肉 lotus seed, Nelumbinis Semen) 9 g

Fifth visit on August 7: There had been no recurrence of chest pain, and her essence-spirit had improved, but the chest oppression still remained. The other symptoms were no longer pronounced. The tongue fur was slightly yellow and the pulse manifestation slightly slippery. So, again I modified the above-mentioned prescription as follows: I increased the dosage of *guā lóu* (trichosanthes) to 30 g and reduced the dosage of *sāng jì shēng* (mistletoe) to 21 g. I removed *lián ròu* (lotus seed) and *dǎng shēn* (codonopsis) and added:

> *dān shēn* (丹参 salvia, Salviae Miltiorrhizae Radix) 15 g
>
> *zǐ sū gěng* (紫苏梗 perilla stem, Perillae Caulis) 9 g

I gave the patient 6–10 packets.

Sixth visit on August 17, seventh visit on August 29, and eighth visit on September 12: At each visit, the patient received additional packets of the above-mentioned prescription with minor modifications. The symptoms seemed to gradually disappear at each visit; the chest pain did not recur, and her essence-spirit and physical strength continued to improve. The patient was already back to work for the last month with no sign of a relapse. I advised her to continue with the prescription packets for another 2–3 weeks, each week taking 3–4 packets to strengthen the therapeutic effect. On September 5, the patient returned to the hospital for another electrocardiogram examination. The results were: T: V3 and V5 readings were low and flat <1/10 R. The remaining indicators were normal.

In November of the same year, I happened to see an account of this patient's case at the hospital where she had originally received the emergency surgery. Here are two items extracted from the relevant electrocardiogram reports concerning the daily record of pathology:

1. Dated August 9, 1978: "…[patient] referred to Dōng Zhí Mén hospital of the Academy of Traditional Chinese Medicine, where she has been receiving Chinese medicinals for more than a month. Results very good. Consent to continue treatment there for another three months."

2. Dated August 23, 1978: "…at present the symptoms have taken a turn for the better…the results of the electrocardiogram have definitely improved; no organic murmur of the heart upon auscultation."

Follow-up visit, February 1979: I learned that the patient had long ago discontinued the Chinese medicinal prescription. She had already returned to work, and the illness had not recurred. She did receive a follow-up electrocardiogram, and the results were normal.

Follow-up visit, December 1979: The patient appeared in very good health; she had worked continuously at her job without leave. In October and December, she had returned for follow-up electrocardiogram examinations, and both times had received normal results.

CASE THREE
JAUNDICE (ACUTE INFECTIOUS HEPATITIS)
黄疸（黄疸型急性传染性肝炎）

The patient was a 17-year-old female who was diagnosed with acute infectious hepatitis at Hénán Province People's Hospital. Her initial examination date was November 27, 1969.

CHIEF COMPLAINT
Jaundiced body and yellow urine for more than a month.

INQUIRY EXAMINATION
One month earlier, her entire body had become jaundiced, and her urine turned yellow. She was unable to eat and had a poor appetite, her entire body was weak, and her limbs were aching and heavy. On November 5, she was admitted to the infectious hepatitis division of the local hospital. At that time, an examination revealed that the sclera of her eyes and the skin of her entire body had turned yellow in color. There was no evidence of spider nevi, and the heart and lungs were normal and the abdomen level and flat. The liver was enlarged by 1.5–2 centimeters, but was soft upon palpation. The spleen was normal. The liver function laboratory tests revealed thymol flocculation test (TFT) 6 units; cerebral flocculation test (CCFT) (++); and glutamic-pyruvate transaminase (GPT) 930 units. The diagnosis was acute jaundice due to infectious hepatitis. Three days later on November 8, the icteric (jaundice) index was 50 units and glutamic-pyruvate transaminase (GPT) measured 1,660 units. The patient had received treatment for three weeks, yet all the symptoms remained the same without improvement. Consequently, on November 27, she requested a consultation and diagnosis from a Chinese medical physician. At the time of the initial examination, she presented with a feeling of oppression in the chest and abdomen, phlegm that was difficult to expectorate, no pleasure in eating, and scant yellow urine.

INSPECTION EXAMINATION
Her body was the color of a tangerine, and her eyes were the color of an apricot. The jaundice was bright and distinct, and the tongue fur was white.

LISTENING AND SMELLING EXAMINATION
No abnormalities were seen.

PALPATION EXAMINATION
The abdomen and the four limbs appeared normal. The pulse was slippery.

PATTERN IDENTIFICATION
The patient complained of stifling oppression in the chest and stomach duct. She had a torpid stomach and reduced food intake, urine was scant and

yellow in color, her pulse was slippery, and her tongue fur was white. The jaundice was bright and distinct. From these signs and symptoms, I knew there was exuberant dampness in the center burner causing spleen-stomach stagnation and liver-stomach disharmony. Free coursing had been inhibited, and depressed dampness had formed heat. Damp-heat was depressed and steaming, and gallbladder heat caused humor spillage, so consequently the jaundice appeared. By correlating the four examinations, I concluded that the diagnosis was damp-heat jaundice (yáng jaundice).

TREATMENT METHOD

Disinhibit dampness and clear heat while regulating and harmonizing the liver and stomach.

PRESCRIPTION

The patient received six packets of the following prescription, to be decocted in water:

> *yīn chén hāo* (茵陈蒿 virgate wormwood, Artemisiae Scopariae Herba) 45 g
> *shēng zhī zǐ* (生栀子 raw gardenia, Gardeniae Fructus Crudus) 9 g
> *huáng qín* (黄芩 scutellaria, Scutellariae Radix) 12 g
> *huáng bǎi* (黄柏 phellodendron, Phellodendri Cortex) 12 g
> *zhū líng* (猪苓 polyporus, Polyporus) 12 g
> *chē qián zǐ* (车前子 plantago seed, Plantaginis Semen) 12 g (wrapped in cloth)
> *chái hú* (柴胡 bupleurum, Bupleuri Radix) 9 g
> *xiāng fù* (香附 cyperus, Cyperi Rhizoma) 9 g
> *jiāo shén qū* (焦神曲 scorch-fried medicated leaven, Massa Medicata Fermentata Usta) 12 g
> *jiāo bīng láng* (焦槟榔 scorch-fried areca, Arecae Semen Ustum) 9 g
> *shēng dà huáng* (生大黄 raw rhubarb, Rhei Radix et Rhizoma Crudi) 1 g

FORMULA EXPLANATION

As chief medicinals, *yīn chén hāo* (virgate wormwood) disinhibits dampness and abates jaundice, and *shān zhī zǐ* (gardenia) clears heat and dispels dampness. When these two medicinals are combined with *shēng dà huáng* (raw rhubarb), they form *yīn chén hāo tāng* (Virgate Wormwood Decoction).

As support medicinals, *huáng bǎi* (phellodendron) and *huáng qín* (scutellaria) clear heat, and *zhū líng* (polyporus) and *chē qián zǐ* (plantago seed) disinhibit dampness.

As assistant medicinals, *chái hú* (bupleurum) and *xiāng fù* (cyperus) regulate the liver, and *bīng láng* (areca) and *shén qū* (medicated leaven) harmonize the stomach.

As the courier medicinal, *shēng dà huáng* (raw rhubarb) guides heat downward, clears heat, and resolves toxins.

FOLLOWUP TREATMENT

<u>Second visit on December 2</u>: The jaundice had abated; the icteric (jaundice) index was 15 units. For the last few days, the patient had suffered aching pain and distention in the lower abdomen, yellow urine, and no pleasure in eating. The tongue fur was white and the pulse was slippery. I modified the previous prescription as follows and gave the patient three more packets:

> *yīn chén hāo* (茵陈蒿 virgate wormwood, Artemisiae Scopariae Herba) 30 g
>
> *shēng zhī zǐ* (生栀子 raw gardenia, Gardeniae Fructus Crudus) 9 g
>
> *huáng bǎi* (黄柏 phellodendron, Phellodendri Cortex) 9 g
>
> *shēng dà huáng* (生大黄 raw rhubarb, Rhei Radix et Rhizoma Crudi) 6 g
>
> *xiāng fù* (香附 cyperus, Cyperi Rhizoma) 9 g
>
> *zhū líng* (猪苓 polyporus, Polyporus) 12 g
>
> *fú líng* (茯苓 poria, Poria) 12 g
>
> *mù xiāng* (木香 costusroot, Aucklandiae Radix) 9 g
>
> *bái sháo yào* (白芍药 white peony, Paeoniae Radix Alba) 12 g
>
> *jiāo bīng láng* (焦槟榔 scorch-fried areca, Arecae Semen Ustum) 9 g
>
> *wū yào* (乌药 lindera, Linderae Radix) 9 g
>
> *yán hú suǒ* (延胡索 corydalis, Corydalis Rhizoma) 9 g
>
> *chén pí* (陈皮 tangerine peel, Citri Reticulatae Pericarpium) 9 g

<u>Third visit on December 5</u>: The jaundice was no longer visible. The urine remained scant yellow, and the patient still felt oppression and distention throughout her entire body. The tongue fur was white and the pulse was slippery. Considering the pulse and the symptoms, this was still a condition of exuberant dampness. I modified the prescription to strengthen the damp-disinhibiting effect and gave the patient six packets, to be decocted in water:

> *yīn chén hāo* (茵陈蒿 virgate wormwood, Artemisiae Scopariae Herba) 30 g
>
> *shēng zhī zǐ* (生栀子 raw gardenia, Gardeniae Fructus Crudus) 9 g
>
> *huáng qín* (黄芩 scutellaria, Scutellariae Radix) 12 g
>
> *huáng bǎi* (黄柏 phellodendron, Phellodendri Cortex) 12 g
>
> *zhū líng* (猪苓 polyporus, Polyporus) 12 g
>
> *zé xiè* (泽泻 alisma, Alismatis Rhizoma) 9 g
>
> *chē qián zǐ* (车前子 plantago seed, Plantaginis Semen) 12 g (wrapped in cloth)
>
> *zǐ sū gěng* (紫苏梗 perilla stem, Perillae Caulis) 6 g
>
> *shēng dà huáng* (生大黄 raw rhubarb, Rhei Radix et Rhizoma Crudi) 5 g
>
> *yán hú suǒ* (延胡索 corydalis, Corydalis Rhizoma) 9 g

Fourth visit on December 10: The tongue and pulse signs were the same as before, but the jaundice had completely abated. However, the patient had a feeling that a lump of roasted meat was in her throat; this could not be swallowed or coughed up, and some puffy swelling was still present in the lower limbs. Now it was appropriate to add qì-regulating, depression-resolving, and phlegm-transforming medicinals to the prescription. I changed the dosage of *zǐ sū gěng* (perilla stem) to 10 grams and *shēng dà huáng* (raw rhubarb) to 3 grams and added the following to the above-mentioned prescription:

> *xiāng fù* (香附 cyperus, Cyperi Rhizoma) 12 g
> *chái hú* (柴胡 bupleurum, Bupleuri Radix) 9 g

The patient received three more packets of this prescription.

Fifth visit on December 13: Her menses arrived with abdominal pain; the color of the menses was dark purple and contained many clots. I removed *huáng qín* (scutellaria), *huáng bǎi* (phellodendron), *zé xiè* (alisma), and *zǐ sū gěng* (perilla stem) from the prescription. I added the following and gave the patient three packets:

> *dāng guī* (当归 Chinese angelica, Angelicae Sinensis Radix) 9 g
> *ài yè* (艾叶 mugwort, Artemisiae Argyi Folium) 9 g
> *táo rén ní* (桃仁泥 crushed peach kernel, Persicae Semen Tusum) 9 g

I made only minor modifications to the prescription after December 5th. On December 15th, the patient's liver functions were retested. The icteric (jaundice) index was 4 units; thymol turbidity test (TTT) 2 units; cerebral flocculation test (CCFT) (±); and glutamic-pyruvate transaminase (GPT) 115 units. On December 20th, the patient had completely recovered and was discharged from the hospital.

CASE FOUR
SUMMERHEAT WARMTH WITH DAMPNESS (EPIDEMIC ENCEPHALITIS B)
暑温挟湿(流行性乙型脑炎)

The patient, a 6-year-old female, was an in-patient at the Héběi Provincial Hospital in the Department of Communicable Diseases. Her initial examination date was August 1st, 1971.

CHIEF COMPLAINT

High fever and somnolence for six days and, on the day of the initial examination, convulsions.

INQUIRY EXAMINATION

For six days the patient presented with an unabated high fever of 38–40°C, spirit-affect indifference, a frontal headache, somnolence, and scant yellow urine. The bowels were normal. The day before the initial examination, the child was treated at the hospital emergency room where a lumbar puncture and examination of the cerebrospinal fluid were performed. The conclusive diagnosis was encephalitis B, and she was admitted to the Department of Communicable Diseases. Upon admission, the child's body emitted heat, and her hands were very hot, but there was no evidence of sweating and she was unconscious. On the next morning, reverse-flow of the limbs occurred, the hands and feet were cold, her neck was rigid, and there were occasional convulsions, which stopped only after the patient received sedative drugs. At this point, the family requested diagnosis and treatment from a Chinese medical physician.

INSPECTION EXAMINATION

Her development was good, and her nutrition appeared normal. She was, however, unconscious and speechless, and her face was slightly red in color. Still, the tongue body was not red and the tongue fur was slightly white.

LISTENING AND SMELLING EXAMINATION

Her respiration was rough.

PALPATION EXAMINATION

Her limbs were cold as far up as the elbows and knees, her neck was inflexible, and the thoracic area was hot to the touch with no evidence of sweating. The pulse was stringlike and rapid.

PATTERN IDENTIFICATION

This disease happened at the time of the hot summer weather, and dampness and heat were steaming together. Summerheat warmth accompanied by damp evil injured the patient. Dampness is by nature clammy and viscous; it is persistent and difficult to cure. Thus, it caused a high fever that for many days did not abate, along with headache, absence of sweating, body heat, and very hot hands. Summerheat warmth clouds the heart orifice; thus, the patient was unconscious and speechless. Since extreme heat stirs wind, convulsions occurred, and the pulse had a stringlike manifestation. Since depressed and blocked summerheat warmth was not resolved, clear yáng could not penetrate to the four limbs, causing cold limbs due to reverse flow. After correlating the four examinations, I diagnosed summerheat warmth with dampness.

TREATMENT METHOD

Clear and resolve summerheat warmth, open the orifices and extinguish wind, assisted by transforming dampness.

PRESCRIPTION

shēng shí gāo (生石膏 raw gypsum, Gypsum Crudum) 15 g (pre-
decocted)

gé gēn (葛根 pueraria, Puerariae Radix) 6 g

cāng zhú (苍术 atractylodes, Atractylodis Rhizoma) 3 g

xiāng rú (香薷 mosla, Moslae Herba) 3 g

jīn yín huā (金银花 lonicera, Lonicerae Flos) 12 g

lián qiáo (连翘 forsythia, Forsythiae Fructus) 9 g

huáng lián (黄连 coptis, Coptidis Rhizoma) 3 g

shí chāng pú (石菖蒲 acorus, Acori Tatarinowii Rhizoma) 6 g

dà qīng yè (大青叶 isatis leaf, Isatidis Folium) 18 g

tiān zhú huáng (天竹黄 bamboo sugar, Bambusae Concretio Silicea)
4.5 g

quán xiē (全蝎 scorpion, Scorpio) 3 g

wú gōng (蜈蚣 centipede, Scolopendra) 1 piece

gōu téng (钩藤 uncaria, Uncariae Ramulus cum Uncis) 12 g

The patient received one packet of this prescription, and in addition to this, I prescribed two pills of *niú huáng zhèn jīng wán* (Bovine Bezoar Fright-Settling Pill), one pill twice a day, to be taken following the decoction.

FORMULA EXPLANATION

As chief medicinals, *shēng shí gāo* (raw gypsum) resolves the flesh and clears heat, and *dà qīng yè* (isatis leaf) resolves toxins and clears heat.

As support medicinals, *gé gēn* (pueraria) resolves the flesh and outthrusts heat; *xiāng rú* (mosla) resolves the exterior, dispels summerheat, and transforms dampness; *cāng zhú* (atractylodes) transforms and dispels dampness with aroma; and *jīn yín huā* (lonicera) and *lián qiáo* (forsythia) clear heat and resolve toxins.

As assistant medicinals, *huáng lián* (coptis) clears the heart and eliminates heat; *tiān zhú huáng* (bamboo sugar) clears the heart and transforms phlegm; *shí chāng pú* (acorus) clears the heart and opens the orifices; *quán xiē* (scorpion) dispels wind and stabilizes convulsions; and *wú gōng* (centipede) extinguishes wind and settles tetany.

The courier is *gōu téng* (uncaria); this medicinal frees and penetrates the four limbs, clears heart heat, extinguishes liver wind, and stops convulsions.

Furthermore, this formula was paired with *niú huáng zhèn jīng wán* (Bovine Bezoar Fright-Settling Pill) to clear the heart and open the orifices and to transform phlegm and extinguish wind. Thus, the two formulas together outthrust and clear summerheat and abate fever while opening the orifices and extinguishing wind.

FOLLOWUP TREATMENT

Second visit on August 2, 6:00 A.M.: The high fever reached 40°C yesterday at noon, so both prescriptions were started, the decoction and the pills. After finishing the daytime dose of the Chinese medicinals, the patient was relatively quiet. Then at the time of the nighttime dose, I added *ān gōng niú huáng wán* (Peaceful Palace Bovine Bezoar Pill), only one pill, and throughout this period of time, there was no recurrence of the convulsions and no need to administer Western sedative drugs. On the morning on August 2, the patient had already opened her eyes, and her spirit-affect was very good. The fever had abated to some extent, but still bordered on 38 °C. The pulse was still rapid. I stayed with the above-mentioned prescription, but I removed *cāng zhú* (atractylodes) and added 3 grams of *jīng jiè* (schizonepeta). I also changed the dosage of *shēng shí gāo* (raw gypsum) to 30 grams. I gave the patient one packet of this prescription along with one pill of *ān gōng niú huáng wán* (Peaceful Palace Bovine Bezoar Pill), to be divided in half and to be taken twice a day after the decoction.

Third visit on August 3: The patient had opened her eyes and the eyeballs themselves were active. Since the administration of the prescription yesterday, there had been no recurrence of convulsions. The fever had clearly abated and her body temperature was 37.3 °C. The four limbs were quite warm and without any sign of reverse-flow. The stools and urine were normal. The tongue body was no longer red, and the tongue fur was slightly white; the pulse was rapid. I modified the previous prescription as follows:

> *shēng shí gāo* (生石膏 raw gypsum, Gypsum Crudum) 24 g (pre-decocted)
>
> *dà qīng yè* (大青叶 isatis leaf, Isatidis Folium) 18 g
>
> *gé gēn* (葛根 pueraria, Puerariae Radix) 4.5 g
>
> *jīn yín huā* (金银花 lonicera, Lonicerae Flos) 12 g
>
> *lián qiáo* (连翘 forsythia, Forsythiae Fructus) 12 g
>
> *tiān zhú huáng* (天竹黄 bamboo sugar, Bambusae Concretio Silicea) 4.5 g
>
> *quán xiē* (全蝎 scorpion, Scorpio) 3 g
>
> *wú gōng* (蜈蚣 centipede, Scolopendra) 1 piece
>
> *tiān huā fěn* (天花粉 trichosanthes root, Trichosanthis Radix) 9 g
>
> *shí chāng pú* (石菖蒲 acorus, Acori Tatarinowii Rhizoma) 3 g
>
> *gōu téng* (钩藤 uncaria, Uncariae Ramulus cum Uncis) 12 g

I prepared one packet for the patient. Again, I prescribed *niú huáng zhèn jīng wán* (Bovine Bezoar Fright-Settling Pill), two pills, to be taken following the decoction, one pill each time.

Fourth visit on August 4: Her spirit-mind was wide awake. She was able to eat and drink, the generalized fever had abated, her body temperature was 37.1°C, and stools and urine were regular. The tongue body was normal and the fur white; the pulse was soggy and slippery. On the basis of this evidence, I had to clear the remaining evil and dispel summerheat dampness by using the center-regulating and heart-clearing method. This was the prescription:

> *shēng shí gāo* (生石膏 raw gypsum, Gypsum Crudum) 15 g (pre-decocted)
> *zhú yè* (竹叶 bamboo leaf, Lophatheri Folium) 3 g
> *jīn yín huā* (金银花 lonicera, Lonicerae Flos) 9 g
> *lián qiáo* (连翘 forsythia, Forsythiae Fructus) 9 g
> *tiān zhú huáng* (天竹黄 bamboo sugar, Bambusae Concretio Silicea) 3 g
> *huáng lián xū* (黄连 fibrous coptis, Coptidis Rhizoma Tenuis) 3 g
> *qīng hāo* (青蒿 sweet wormwood, Artemisiae Annuae Herba) 6 g
> *ròu dòu kòu yī* (肉豆蔻衣 nutmeg aril, Myristicae Arillus) 1.5 g
> *shí chāng pú* (石菖蒲 acorus, Acori Tatarinowii Rhizoma) 4.5 g
> *jiāo shén qū* (焦神曲 scorch-fried medicated leaven, Massa Medicata
>   Fermentata Usta) 6 g
> *gōu téng* (钩藤 uncaria, Uncariae Ramulus cum Uncis) 15 g

I prepared another packet for the patient together with *niú huáng zhèn jīng wán* (Bovine Bezoar Fright-Settling Pill), two pills, to be administered exactly as before. I coordinated the treatment with my Western medical colleagues for an intramuscular injection of 2 ml *bǎn lán gēn* (isatis root) liquid preparation.

Fifth examination on August 5: The patient had essentially regained her health. I found nothing abnormal concerning her cognition and also found no disease sequelae, so I continued prescribing the above-mentioned formula.

Sixth examination on August 6: Due to excessive eating and drinking, a slight low-grade fever had developed. I added the following medicinals to the above-mentioned prescription and gave the patient one packet:

> *jiāo shān zhā* (焦山楂 scorch-fried crataegus, Crataegi Fructus Ustus) 6 g
> *jiāo mài yá* (焦麦芽 scorch-fried barley sprout, Hordei Fructus
>   Germinatus Ustus) 6 g
> *jiāo bīng láng* (焦槟榔 scorch-fried areca, Arecae Semen Ustum) 6 g

Seventh examination on August 7: The body temperature stabilized at 36.2°C. Her essence-spirit had improved, her speech was clear and distinct, and her physical activities were normal. The child had completely recovered from her illness and was discharged from the hospital.

CASE FIVE
HEAD WIND (SHEEHAN'S SYNDROME)
头风(席汉氏综合征)

The patient was a 31-year-old female who had come from the provinces to Běijīng for treatment. Her initial examination date was April 12, 1968.

CHIEF COMPLAINT
A roaring, booming sound of insects inside the patient's head and generalized headache for more than a year.

INQUIRY EXAMINATION
Early last year, the patient went to a local medical school hospital and received a diagnosis of Sheehan's syndrome. She received treatment there at the hospital and at a Chinese medical hospital, and she also spent time in recovery at the adjacent sanitarium. She received both Chinese and Western medical treatments, but without any good results. Finally, she came to Běijīng for treatment.

This disease was due to her post-partum condition, and the symptoms were as follows: the sound of insects inside the head together with a booming, rumbling noise as if someone were starting an engine or running machinery, and aching pain and clouding oppression of the entire head. Every day the patient took painkillers to ease the pain, usually 6–7 pills, but sometimes even more. She suffered from generalized fatigue and could only get up from bed and walk around her room; she could not leave the house or go to the market. Whenever she had to leave the house, her entire body became powerless, she was without strength, and her legs ached so badly that she could not return home on foot. She was constantly tired and weak and wanted only to stay in bed and sleep. Her menses were very scant in amount.

INSPECTION EXAMINATION
Her development and nutrition appeared normal. Her complexion was slightly jaundiced and lacked luster and sheen. The tongue fur was thin and white.

LISTENING AND SMELLING EXAMINATION
No abnormalities noted.

PALPATION EXAMINATION
The pulse was slightly slippery and slightly fine. No other abnormalities were seen.

PATTERN IDENTIFICATION
Since the pulse demonstrated a fine manifestation, I knew that this was blood vacuity. Since post-partum blood vacuity had occurred, blood could not

ascend to provide luxuriance to the head; therefore, sounds occurred inside the head. Blood vacuity also engendered wind, and wind combined with phlegm turbidity to invade the upper body. Thus, there were symptoms such as headache, cloudy oppression, and roaring and rumbling sounds. Since blood vacuity could not give luxuriance and nourishment to the entire body, generalized bodily weakness occurred, and the menses appeared very scant in amount. After correlating the four examinations, I diagnosed head pain and head wind caused by post-partum blood vacuity.

TREATMENT METHOD

Nourish blood and dispel wind, assisted by eliminating phlegm.

PRESCRIPTION

I gave the patient six packets of the following prescription to be decocted in water:

> *dāng guī* (当归 Chinese angelica, Angelicae Sinensis Radix) 12 g
> *shú dì huáng* (熟地黄 cooked rehmannia, Rehmanniae Radix Praeparata) 12 g
> *chuān xiōng* (川芎 chuanxiong, Chuanxiong Rhizoma) 9 g
> *chì sháo yào* (赤芍药 red peony, Paeoniae Radix Rubra) 12 g
> *fáng fēng* (防风 saposhnikovia, Saposhnikoviae Radix) 12 g
> *bái jí lí* (白蒺藜 tribulus, Tribuli Fructus) 12 g
> *jú huā* (菊花 chrysanthemum, Chrysanthemi Flos) 9 g
> *jīng jiè* (荆芥 schizonepeta, Schizonepetae Herba) 9 g
> *hé shǒu wū* (何首乌 flowery knotweed, Polygoni Multiflori Radix) 12 g
> *qiāng huó* (羌活 notopterygium, Notopterygii Rhizoma et Radix) 9 g
> *chén pí* (陈皮 tangerine peel, Citri Reticulatae Pericarpium) 6 g
> *zhì fù piàn* (制附片 sliced processed aconite, Aconiti Radix Lateralis Praeparata Secta) 6 g

FORMULA EXPLANATION

As chief medicinals, *dāng guī* (Chinese angelica) warms yáng and supplements blood, and *shú dì huáng* (cooked rehmannia) enriches yīn and supplements blood. These two medicinals strengthen the blood-supplementing effect.

As support medicinals, *hé shǒu wū* (flowery knotweed) nourishes blood and boosts essence, thereby treating post-partum blood vacuity and causing essence-blood to ascend and provide luxuriance to the upper body. *Chì sháo yào* (red peony) quickens blood and moves stasis. *Chuān xiōng* (chuanxiong) moves blood and tracks down wind. *Fáng fēng* (saposhnikovia) and *qiāng huó* (notopterygium) dispel wind and overcome dampness.

As assistant medicinals, *bái jí lí* (tribulus) and *jú huā* (chrysanthemum) regulate the liver and dispel wind; *chén pí* (tangerine peel) rectifies qì and transforms phlegm; *fù piàn* (sliced aconite) reinforces yáng, dries dampness, and dispels head wind.

The courier medicinal is *jīng jiè* (schizonepeta); it enters the blood aspect. It is effective for treating headache and post-partum blood disease and wind disease, and it conducts the other medicinals up to the head.

FOLLOWUP TREATMENT

<u>Second visit on April 18</u>: The patient felt that the headache and head wind insect sounds had lessened, and every day she took 1–2 fewer pills of pain-killers; however, she was still fatigued and the other symptoms were the same as before. Because this was a case of chronic disease, I increased the dosage of blood-quickening medicinals; because of the intermittent occurrence of insect roaring in the head, I increased the dosage of phlegm-eliminating medicinals. Consequently, I gave her the following prescription:

dāng guī (当归 Chinese angelica, Angelicae Sinensis Radix) 12 g

shú dì huáng (熟地黄 cooked rehmannia, Rehmanniae Radix Praeparata) 12 g

chuān xiōng (川芎 chuanxiong, Chuanxiong Rhizoma) 9 g

hé shǒu wū (何首乌 flowery knotweed, Polygoni Multiflori Radix) 12 g

chì sháo yào (赤芍药 red peony, Paeoniae Radix Rubra) 9 g

guì zhī (桂枝 cinnamon twig, Cinnamomi Ramulus) 9 g

tiān nán xīng (天南星 arisaema, Arisaematis Rhizoma) 6 g

zhì fù piàn (制附片 sliced processed aconite, Aconiti Radix Lateralis Praeparata Secta) 7.5 g

xià kū cǎo (夏枯草 prunella, Prunellae Spica) 9 g

hóng huā (红花 carthamus, Carthami Flos) 9 g

bái jí lí (白蒺藜 tribulus, Tribuli Fructus) 12 g

fáng fēng (防风 saposhnikovia, Saposhnikoviae Radix) 9 g

jīng jiè (荆芥 schizonepeta, Schizonepetae Herba) 9 g

I gave the patient three packets to be decocted in water, and I advised her to take another three packets if the first three were effective.

<u>Third visit on May 6</u>: Altogether the patient had taken ten packets of the above-mentioned prescription. The headache was alleviated and the fatigue had improved. The patient felt that the insect sounds in the head had also improved, but the tongue and pulse signs were without any notable changes. I made some modifications and gave the patient three packets of the following, to be decocted in water:

dāng guī (当归 Chinese angelica, Angelicae Sinensis Radix) 9 g

shú dì huáng (熟地黄 cooked rehmannia, Rehmanniae Radix Praeparata) 15 g

hóng huā (红花 carthamus, Carthami Flos) 9 g

táo rén (桃仁 peach kernel, Persicae Semen) 9 g

chì sháo yào (赤芍药 red peony, Paeoniae Radix Rubra) 12 g

fáng fēng (防风 saposhnikovia, Saposhnikoviae Radix) 12 g

tiān nán xīng (天南星 arisaema, Arisaematis Rhizoma) 7.5 g

xì xīn (细辛 asarum, Asari Herba) 3 g

zhì fù piàn (制附片 sliced processed aconite, Aconiti Radix Lateralis Praeparata Secta) 9 g

bái zhǐ (白芷 Dahurian angelica, Angelicae Dahuricae Radix) 9 g

qiāng huó (羌活 notopterygium, Notopterygii Rhizoma et Radix) 6 g

jīng jiè (荆芥 schizonepeta, Schizonepetae Herba) 9 g

Fourth visit May 9: The patient had taken the medicinals, but the symptoms had not changed at all. I again carefully reexamined the signs and symptoms. I thought that the intermittent roaring sounds in the head belonged to a pattern of blood vacuity, and then on the other hand, I saw the pattern of head wind. In the previous prescriptions, I had used blood-nourishing, blood-quickening, wind-dispelling, and phlegm-transforming medicinals to treat these two patterns. Although these were effective to some extent, the disease was so profoundly enduring that clear yáng was unable to ascend; therefore, turbid yīn could not descend.

Consequently, I completely changed the prescription to *qīng zhèn tāng* (Clearing Invigoration Decoction) to ascend the clear yáng qì. I reevaluated the prescription and substituted *shēng má* (cimicifuga) for *jīng jiè* (schizonepeta) and *bái zhǐ* (Dahurian angelica), and substituted *cāng zhú* (atractylodes) for *tiān nán xīng* (arisaema) and *qiāng huó* (notopterygium), then I added *hé yè* (lotus leaf); this was the principle of *qīng zhèn tāng* (Clearing Invigoration Decoction). So, I added 9 grams of *hé yè* (lotus leaf) to the previous prescription and gave the patient three packets, to be decocted in water. If these packets proved to be effective, then the patient would receive more packets.

Fifth visit on May 23: The patient felt that the insect sounds with the head had greatly improved after taking this last prescription, and the headache had been greatly reduced. Now everyday she took only 1–2 pills of painkillers and continued taking ten packets of the original prescription. Her physical strength and essence-spirit clearly improved, and she was outdoors walking again. The tongue fur was thin and white, and the fine manifestation of the pulse had taken a turn for the better. Thus, I advised her to continue with six packets of this prescription.

<u>Sixth visit on May 27</u>: The patient felt that the insect sounds in the head and the headache had been even further alleviated. It was enough for her to take the painkillers only once in two or three days. At this time, her chief complaint was dizziness and some pain at the lateral end of both superciliary ridges on her forehead. She was physically strong without any feeling of fatigue; she was not sleeping at all during the daytime, but rather spending her time strolling about in the streets. She even went shopping and walked up and down the stairs at the department stores. She was in high spirits and her confidence had doubled. She had a somewhat dry throat, mouth, and eyes. Her menses arrived and the amount and color had improved compared to her previous periods. There were no changes in the tongue signs, and the pulse manifestation was slightly slippery. Because there was an appearance of some internal heat, I removed *zhì fù piàn* (sliced processed aconite) from the prescription and gave her three packets of the following:

> *dāng guī wěi* (当归尾 tangkuei tail, Angelicae Sinensis Radicis Extremitas) 9 g
>
> *shú dì huáng* (熟地黄 cooked rehmannia, Rehmanniae Radix Praeparata) 15 g
>
> *qiāng huó* (羌活 notopterygium, Notopterygii Rhizoma et Radix) 9 g
>
> *hé yè* (荷叶 lotus leaf, Nelumbinis Folium) 9 g
>
> *bái zhǐ* (白芷 Dahurian angelica, Angelicae Dahuricae Radix) 9 g
>
> *xì xīn* (细辛 asarum, Asari Herba) 4.5 g
>
> *tiān nán xīng* (天南星 arisaema, Arisaematis Rhizoma) 9 g
>
> *jú huā* (菊花 chrysanthemum, Chrysanthemi Flos) 9 g
>
> *bò hé* (薄荷 mint, Menthae Herba) 6 g (added after)
>
> *xīn yí* (辛夷 magnolia flower, Magnoliae Flos) 9 g
>
> *hóng huā* (红花 carthamus, Carthami Flos) 9 g
>
> *chì sháo yào* (赤芍药 red peony, Paeoniae Radix Rubra) 9 g
>
> *gǎo běn* (藁本 Chinese lovage, Ligustici Rhizoma) 3 g
>
> *jīng jiè* (荆芥 schizonepeta, Schizonepetae Herba) 9 g

<u>Seventh visit on May 30</u>: All the symptoms continued to improve even further; in general her physical strength increased and she was no longer taking painkillers. I modified the prescription even further and gave her 6–9 more packets of the following:

> *dāng guī wěi* (当归尾 tangkuei tail, Angelicae Sinensis Radicis Extremitas) 9 g
>
> *shú dì huáng* (熟地黄 cooked rehmannia, Rehmanniae Radix Praeparata) 15 g
>
> *hóng huā* (红花 carthamus, Carthami Flos) 9 g

chì sháo yào (赤芍药 red peony, Paeoniae Radix Rubra) 9 g

fáng fēng (防风 saposhnikovia, Saposhnikoviae Radix) 12 g

bái zhǐ (白芷 Dahurian angelica, Angelicae Dahuricae Radix) 9 g

huáng qín (黄芩 scutellaria, Scutellariae Radix) 12 g

rěn dōng téng (忍冬藤 lonicera stem, Lonicerae Caulis) 24 g

tiān nán xīng (天南星 arisaema, Arisaematis Rhizoma) 5 g

hé yè (荷叶 lotus leaf, Nelumbinis Folium) 9 g

jú huā (菊花 chrysanthemum, Chrysanthemi Flos) 9 g

xì xīn (细辛 asarum, Asari Herba) 3 g

dǎng shēn (党参 codonopsis, Codonopsis Radix) 12 g

jīng jiè (荆芥 schizonepeta, Schizonepetae Herba) 9 g

<u>Eighth visit on June 10</u>: The patient had taken nine packets of the above prescription and afterwards all of the subjective symptoms were eliminated. Every day she was out of the house to go shopping without becoming tired; her essence-spirit was good, she was not sleepy at all, and she had not taken painkillers for many days. She wanted to have the prescription in pill form to take with her, since she planned to return to her home province and go back to work. So I prepared the following prescription for her:

dāng guī (当归 Chinese angelica, Angelicae Sinensis Radix) 9 g

shú dì huáng (熟地黄 cooked rehmannia, Rehmanniae Radix Praeparata)
    15 g

hóng huā (红花 carthamus, Carthami Flos) 9 g

chì sháo yào (赤芍药 red peony, Paeoniae Radix Rubra) 9 g

fáng fēng (防风 saposhnikovia, Saposhnikoviae Radix) 12 g

bái zhǐ (白芷 Dahurian angelica, Angelicae Dahuricae Radix) 9 g

cāng zhú (苍术 atractylodes, Atractylodis Rhizoma) 6 g

chén pí (陈皮 tangerine peel, Citri Reticulatae Pericarpium) 6 g

xì xīn (细辛 asarum, Asari Herba) 3 g

tiān nán xīng (天南星 arisaema, Arisaematis Rhizoma) 4.5 g

hé yè (荷叶 lotus leaf, Nelumbinis Folium) 9 g

dǎng shēn (党参 codonopsis, Codonopsis Radix) 12 g

jú huā (菊花 chrysanthemum, Chrysanthemi Flos) 9 g

huáng qín (黄芩 scutellaria, Scutellariae Radix) 12 g

rěn dōng téng (忍冬藤 lonicera stem, Lonicerae Caulis) 24 g

jīng jiè (荆芥 schizonepeta, Schizonepetae Herba) 9 g

Because the climate in her home province was more humid than that of Běijīng, I added *cāng zhú* (atractylodes) to the prescription. I also added *chén pí* (tangerine peel) to transform phlegm and to prevent the supplementing medicinals from causing stagnation in the stomach. I advised her to decoct and take at least three packets of the above-mentioned prescription during the time in which the pill prescription was being compounded.

The ingredients for the pill prescription were ground into a fine powder and mixed with refined honey to form pills weighing 9 g each. During this time she took five packets of the prescription. The dosage was one pill 2–3 times a day, to be taken with boiled water. The patient happily took the pills with her and returned home.

EMPIRICAL KNOWLEDGE

Treatment based on a Western medical diagnosis of a traditional disease category produces unsatisfactory results.

Chinese medicine and Western medicine each have their own characteristics. Certainly, Chinese medicine recognizes symptoms and diseases and classifies them for diagnosis and treatment. Yet as defined by Chinese medicine, these diseases are not the same as in Western medicine; although their names may be identical, the implications and concepts are distinctly different. Some examples of this are malaria, dysentery, and the common cold. Consider the diseases malaria and dysentery. Western medicine diagnoses malaria by seeking to find and identify the various types of malarial parasites, and the Western medical model diagnoses bacterial dysentery by identifying the various types of cultured bacilli associated with it. Thus the most important concern for Western medical treatment is the elimination of the protozoa or bacteria.

In Chinese medicine, the diagnostic criteria for the diseases of malaria and dysentery are based upon the following conditions: whether the patient experiences heat effusion and aversion to cold at fixed times or regular intervals; whether heat effusion is greater than aversion to cold or vice-versa; whether heat effusion precedes aversion to cold or vice-versa; and whether there is heat effusion without aversion to cold or vice-versa. Concerning dysentery, Chinese medicine considers whether it is red or white, whether there is tenesmus or not, whether there is a liking for cold or hot foods and drink, whether red is more predominant than white or vice-versa, whether the stools resemble an azuki bean drink or fish brains. Furthermore, examination of the entire body is required, together with examination of the tongue and pulse. Inspection of the complexion is conducted, and listening and smelling must also be performed to obtain definitive diagnostic information.

On the basis of these criteria, diseases categories include: true malaria, pure-heat malaria, female malaria, and miasmic malaria; damp-heat dysentery, vacuity-cold dysentery, and epidemic toxic dysentery. The Chinese medical treatment method is not directed at the protozoa or the bacteria, even though these are recognized as factors in the cause of disease. Rather, the chief principle follows a pattern and selects a treatment method such as harmonizing and resolving the lesser yáng (*shào yáng*), harmonizing construction and defense, clearing and disinhibiting damp-heat, or regulating qì and harmonizing blood. Thus, as disease arises and develops along its pathological course, Chinese medicine assists the human body to overcome damage from disease and enhances the body's ability to resist disease and to compensate or balance itself. Chinese medicine regulates and adjusts the organism so that the dynamic equilibrium of yīn and yáng and of qì and blood is balanced, and it promotes the organism's recovery from illness. Consequently, whether medicinals are used in the treatment of malaria and dysentery, or whether acupuncture and moxibustion are used, either method will be effective.

If Chinese medicine were to treat Western medically diagnosed hepatitis, it would by no means specifically treat the liver. If it were to treat anemia, it would by no means treat just the blood. To treat pneumonia, it would by no means treat just the lung. To treat nephritis, it would by no means treat just the kidney.

Thus, we can clearly see that Chinese and Western medical models recognize and classify symptoms and disease by different means, and diagnosis and treatment methods vary between the two modalities. If Chinese medicine were only concerned with the Western medical diagnosis of disease, then no particular attention would be given to applying principles and treatment methods based on pattern identification or to analyzing and drawing conclusions from pattern identification. Furthermore, treatments would not be holistic, and that which is perceived as hepatitis would simply imply treatment of the liver; nephritis would simply imply treatment of the kidney; cholecystitis would simply imply treatment of the gallbladder. In the end, two medical modalities with different viewpoints on recognition and classification of diseases would be just mixed together.

In all my years of clinical experience, I have seen many cases that are frequently called effective, but are less than ideal. For example, in Case 1 of this chapter, at the time of the initial visit, I right away made the mistake of basing treatment on a Western medical diagnosis instead of a traditional disease category. I relied on an already known prescription that had been proven to be useful in the treatment of chorea, but I did not use the Chinese medical principles of pattern identification to determine treatment. As a result, the treatment was ineffective. Later, I applied Chinese medical principles by conducting pattern identification to determine treatment, and good results were obtained very quickly.

At the initial visit of the patient in Case 2, I took into account the fact that the patient had already received a Western medical diagnosis of acute myocarditis. Therefore, at the time of the initial examination, I prescribed blood-nourishing heart-quieting medicinals together with medicinals that reinforced yáng and opened impediment. But this was not enough, and the symptoms such as chest pain and oppression, flusteredness, shortness of breath, and fatigue did not improve. In all the subsequent visits, I increased the dosage of yáng-assisting impediment-opening medicinals and readjusted the prescription. Thus, I gradually obtained a satisfactory result when I paid more attention to treating holistically.

I learned from experience with this case that it is not at all appropriate to treat only from the viewpoint of "cardiac" or "inflammation" alone, but rather to apply the method of pattern identification to determine treatment. Consequently, I directed the treatment to reinforce yáng and open impediment, simultaneously taking into account the condition of the kidney, spleen and stomach, and thoroughfare (chōng) and controlling (rèn) vessels. I then administered a holistic treatment and obtained results. This not only eliminated the patient's symptoms of chest pain, flusteredness, and palpitations, but also successfully treated the aching weak lumbus, the excessive menses, the poor appetite, and the fatigue. All the symptoms were addressed and the patient was restored to health.

For the patient in Case 3 with the diagnosis of acute jaundice from infectious hepatitis, I treated from the beginning according to the principle of pattern identification to determine treatment. In this case, I selected the method of disinhibiting dampness and clearing heat, regulating and harmonizing the liver and stomach, and freeing the intestine. I did not by any means determine treatment based on the liver alone. In the final two cases, Case 4 and Case 5, I again applied the principle of pattern identification to determine treatment and obtained very good results for these patients as well.

Never conduct a Chinese medical treatment based solely on a Western medical disease name.

Because Chinese medicine and Western medicine each have their own characteristics, their theoretical systems are different also. Therefore, when Chinese medicine is used to treat a disease that has been diagnosed by Western medical methods, the treatment should not be based solely on the "disease name" provided by Western medical diagnosis. You cannot just focus on lowering blood pressure, for instance, for the patient with hypertension; or simply consider raising the platelet count for a case of thrombocytopenic purpura; or just dispel wind-damp for cases of rheumatic heart disease. Treatment directions such as these often bring unsatisfactory results.

A good example of this concept is Case 1. At the time of his first visit, the treatment began with just one disease name: pediatric chorea. Western medicine holds the view that the majority of pediatric chorea cases are caused by rheumatism. When I attempted to equate the Western medical idea of rheumatism or wind-damp with the Chinese medical idea of wind-damp, I noticed in the prescription the use of several wind-damp-dispelling medicinals such as *guì zhī* (cinnamon twig), *fáng fēng* (saposhnikovia), *qín jiāo* (large gentian), and *fáng jǐ* (fangji). I simply went along with the use of these medicinals. I did not use Chinese medical theory to conduct pattern identification or to analyze which viscus or bowel was involved with the disease, and I did not consider whether the symptoms were associated with vacuity or repletion, cold or heat, or question whether the wind was internal or external. So, as a consequence, the treatment had no therapeutic effect at all.

At the time of the second visit, I used Chinese medical theory to identify the hyperactive tongue symptom as belonging to the heart and liver channels. Moreover, I used the liver-settling, yáng-subduing, heart-clearing, and wind-extinguishing treatment method. The results, of course, were clearly different than the results of the first visit when the prescribed medicinals and assumed patterns were inconsistent with each other. Interestingly enough, the two prescriptions from the first and second visits both used medicinals to treat wind. The first prescription used many medicinals that treat exterior wind and dispel wind-damp; the second prescription included medicinals that treat interior wind. Even more importantly, the liver-settling, yáng-subduing, heart-clearing, and convulsion-settling treatment method was chosen. Thus, the patient received a holistic treatment.

As seen from this example, the use of the Chinese medical theory of pattern identification to determine treatment provides a more positive treatment outcome than reliance solely on the Western medical disease name and treatment methodology. From my own experience, I believe that when Chinese medical physicians diagnose and treat patients who have already received a Western medical diagnosis, those physicians are well advised to conduct a pattern identification to determine treatment and not establish their treatment method based solely on a Western medical disease name and protocol.

For this first case, there are still some remaining thoughts. My Western medical colleague and I copied the first prescription from a book, and if we had used the method of pattern identification to determine treatment for our analysis, then the method would have been consistent and the medicinals and patterns compatible, and the outcome would have been effective. Thus it is not the prescription itself that brings unsatisfactory results, but rather it is the mechanical copying and indiscriminate application of Western medical protocols when treating the patient.

Prior to his Chinese medicine consultation, the patient in Case 5 had already seen several Western medical physicians for his diagnosis of "Sheehan's syndrome." Nevertheless, I used the method of pattern identification to determine treatment. I did not simply emphasize a Western diagnosis of "endocrinopathy or endocrine imbalance"; instead, I treated him effectively with the method of nourishing blood and dispelling wind, assisted by the method of transforming phlegm. Later, after further analysis, I thought that his pattern was head wind disease, so I prescribed *qīng zhèn tāng* (Clearing Invigoration Decoction) to raise the clear yáng qì, which clearly improved his condition. This method very quickly obtained ideal results. This is another example that demonstrates how Chinese medicine should be used to treat patients who already have a Western medical diagnosis. Chinese medical physicians should still conduct pattern identification to determine treatment for each and every patient since that strengthens the ability to be effective. Chinese medical physicians should never stubbornly cling to the idea of treatment based upon Western medical disease name protocols, but instead should always determine treatment by pattern identification.

Biomedical application of Chinese medicinals often produces results that are not ideal.

In recent years both in China and the West, medical professionals have conducted pharmacological studies and scientific research on many Chinese medicinals with very positive results. We have discovered, for instance, the anti-bacterial action of many Chinese medicinals and the anti-viral properties of others; we now know that some medicinals can expand the coronary artery and increase the amount of coronary blood flow; some medicinals have anti-carcinogenic action, and still others possess "adaptogenic" properties, which means that the medicinal can enhance the organism's natural defense capability and can enable the organism to adjust to changes in its environment. All these investigations have produced very gratifying achievements and have helped to promote the modernization of Chinese medicine.

However, along with the assimilation and utilization of these scientific achievements came the emergence of a different set of methods. For example, some people think that in the process of Western medical diagnosis, if a disease is thought to be caused by the existence of bacteria, then it is fitting to use large dosages of anti-bacterial medicinals to treat the patient. If the disease is diagnosed due to the presence of a virus, then some people pile on the medicinals known to have anti-viral properties in their effort to treat the patient. In the same way, these people treat their patients diagnosed with cancer by using only those medicinals shown to have anti-carcinogenic effects. In the final analysis, they abandon the patterns of Chinese medicine, and they prescribe medicines based on the specific Western medically-defined disease. The individuals who follow this line of thinking do not integrate the method of pattern identification to determine treatment; they merely identify the Western medical disease cause, the pathology, and the Western disease name, and excessively prescribe the called-for medicinals. This method is called "the biomedical application of Chinese medicinals."

My own clinical experience during recent years has proven that the method of "biomedical application of Chinese medicinals" is inferior to the method of prescribing medicinals based on pattern identification. However, the latter method may, at the time of selecting medicinals for a prescription, take into account modern scientific research of a particular medicinal and evaluate it for inclusion in a prescription. This provides another way to organize the prescription for better treatment efficacy. A clear example of this concept can be seen in the treatment of infectious hepatitis. If the physician does not consider the specific patterns of this disease and instead only uses large quantities of heat-clearing toxin-resolving medicinals such as *pú gōng yīng* (dandelion), *bài jiàng cǎo* (patrinia), *bǎn lán gēn* (isatis root), and *dà qīng yè* (isatis leaf), which are known to have anti-viral properties, then frequently the symptoms of hepatitis do not improve and other symptoms, such as stomach discomfort, poor appetite, sloppy stools, and a thick white tongue fur, will also appear. Such symptoms appear because of stomach injury caused by the inappropriate use of large quantities of cold, bitter medicinals.

There was some interesting information that emerged several years ago regarding the use of medicinals for treating hepatitis. One of the medicinals, *wǔ wèi zǐ* (schisandra), had been used in research as a single powdered substance to lower the glutamic-pyruvate transaminase level, and at first it appeared to be quite effective. Later, when the medicinal powder was discontinued and 2–3 weeks had passed, the transaminase level gradually began to rise again. Another medicinal was *chuān xiōng* (chuanxiong), a blood-quickening stasis-transforming medicinal that proved effective for dilating blood vessels; however, its flavor is aromatic and its nature is mobile and penetrating; it is acrid and warm, and as a consequence, can dry blood. Therefore, if *chuān xiōng* is used as a single medicinal in large quantities, it frequently causes symptoms such as red tongue and dry mouth, vexation and thirst, constipation, and agitation. When *chuān xiōng* is used continuously to treat the patient with internal heat or blood vacuity and liver effulgence, the condition of the patient worsens and the disease becomes serious.

As another example, we can discuss the "adaptogenic" properties of *rén shēn* (ginseng). If a physician prescribes *rén shēn* to "enable the organism to adjust to changes in its environment," and by following the notion of "the more the better," prescribes large quantities of *rén shēn* over a long period of time, but does not use the principles and method of pattern identification to determine treatment, then the outcome will not be ideal. On the contrary, side-effects will occur, and the patient will suffer such symptoms as headache, toothache, thirst, dry stools, nosebleed, insomnia, and agitation. In other words, patterns of qì exuberance, fire, and heat will arise. I once treated a patient who had been ill for eighteen months after he had taken a soup made with a whole chicken and six *liǎng* of *rén shēn* (ginseng). This event was a consequence of not prescribing according to principles, method, formulas, and medicinals and was the result of the "the biomedical application of Chinese medicinals."

Another good example of this concept is Case 1 in this chapter. When the patient had his first examination, I simply prescribed medicinals without conducting thorough pattern identification. Actually, my diagnosis at that time followed the notion of biomedical application of Chinese medicinals, and the desired therapeutic effect was not achieved. In Case 3, I certainly did use medicinals such as *huáng bǎi* (phellodendron), *shān zhī zǐ* (gardenia), and *huáng qín* (scutellaria), which possess anti-bacterial and anti-viral properties, but nevertheless I also followed the principle of pattern identification to determine treatment and composed a prescription that was guided by the method of disinhibiting dampness, clearing heat, and regulating and harmonizing the liver and stomach. As a result, the therapeutic effect for this patient was ideal.

Although medicinals such as *jīn yín huā* (lonicera), *lián qiáo* (forsythia), and *dà qīng yè* (isatis leaf) were included in the prescription for the patient in Case 4, these medicinals were not at all the focus of the prescription; instead, the composition of the prescription was guided by the principle of pattern identification to determine treatment, and I used these medicinals together with other appropriate medicinals to clear heat and resolve summerheat and to open the orifices and extinguish wind while simultaneously transforming dampness. I obtained good results.

Thus, I have learned from experience that when a Chinese medical physician diagnoses and treats a patient who already has a Western medical diagnosis, they should not only apply the method of pattern identification to determine treatment, but they should also be careful to avoid the method of "biomedical application of Chinese medicinals" when composing prescriptions. The Chinese medical physician should hold fast to principles, methods, formulas, and medicinals. One should assimilate the achievements of modern scientific research when it is appropriate; and should analyze and choose new advancements when possible. Physicians should also be able to organically integrate all this material with the specific symptoms and circumstances of each individual patient, closely combine them with the condition of the patient, and then select medicinals according to the pattern. This procedure not only enhances treatment efficacy, but also lays a sound foundation for Western and Chinese medical integration and the modernization of Chinese medicine.

Concerning the identification of disease and the identification of patterns

Medical journals often put forward the view that Western medicine disease identification and Chinese medicine pattern identification must be integrated. This opinion is meant to convince us that these two medical modalities are indeed mutually linked, and that their integration is beneficial to understanding of the nature of disease and advantageous to enhanced diagnostic proficiency and treatment efficacy. Therefore, the integration of Chinese medicine and Western medicine is promoted. Such opinions are positive and worthwhile. However, there are other individuals who hold the opinion that Chinese medicine should focus exclusively on pattern identification and not pay attention to Western disease identification; they even suggest that Chinese medical physicians be allowed only to conduct pattern identification and not disease identification. This viewpoint is quite incorrect. Chinese medicine diagnosis and treatment of disease is accomplished by pattern identification and the recognition of symptoms of disease — namely, disease identification; the physician must have knowledge of disease fundamentals and must distinguish the reasons why certain disease manifestations emerge. When that is accomplished, the treatment method follows based on the pattern, then the selection and application of formula and medicinals is made, followed by the treatment itself.

For example, the *Jīn Guì Yào Lüè* ("Essential Prescriptions of the Golden Coffer") mentions, "chest impediment disease with panting, coughing and spitting, pain the chest and back, shortness of breath, and an inch opening pulse [that is] sunken and slow," and further, "When the yang2 [pulses] are slight, and the yin1 [pulses] are stringlike, this is chest impediment and chest pain." On the basis of these pulse signs alone, the diagnosis is chest impediment disease, and *guā lóu xiè bái bái jiǔ tāng* (Trichosanthes, Chinese Chive, and White Liquor Decoction) governs the treatment. If the condition is accompanied by "inability to lie down and heart pain stretching through to the back," then chest impediment disease is complicated by a pattern of phlegmdrool congestion within the chest. *Guā lóu xiè bái bàn xià tāng* (Trichosanthes, Chinese Chive, and Pinellia Decoction) governs this treatment by freeing yáng and dissipating binds while eliminating rheum and downbearing counterflow. If chest impediment disease is accompanied by "glomus qì in the heart, qì bind in the chest, chest fullness, and counterflow under the rib-side prodding the heart," then chest impediment is complicated by patterns of qì stagnation in the chest and liver-stomach counterflow qì; so the treatment method frees yáng, dissipates binds, and downbears counterflow to calm the surging. *Zhǐ shí xiè bái guì zhī tāng* (Unripe Bitter Orange, Chinese Chive, and Cinnamon Twig Decoction) governs the treatment in this case. If chest impediment disease is accompanied by "glomus in the heart, counterflow, and heart suspended pain," then chest impediment is complicated by a pattern of cold-rheum collecting internally. *Guì zhī shēng jiāng zhǐ shí tāng* (Cinnamon Twig, Fresh Ginger, and Unripe Bitter Orange) governs the treatment here by using a treatment method to free yáng and dissipate cold, warm and transform water-rheum, and open binds and downbear qì. These examples illustrate how to distinguish between the types of chest impediment disease, how to recognize the various differences between the patterns involved, and how each distinct pattern is associated with a treatment method and its formula.

There are still others who ask why Chinese medicine must conduct a disease identification process at all if, indeed, pattern identification can already distinguish all the elements (yīn, yáng, exterior, interior, vacuity, repletion, cold, heat, heart vacuity, liver yáng effulgence, exuberant stomach fire, etc.) necessary to arrive at the treatment method, to select formulas and apply medicinals, and finally to treat the patient. Because pattern identification can only realize the most current phase of the transformation of the patient's condition, it cannot possibly realize every different type of disease in every stage of etiology, development, transformation, and change — in other words, the course of pathology as a whole and the transformations thereof. For example, if the patient presents with symptoms such as headache and painful stiff nape of the neck, aversion to cold with heat effusion, no sweating, panting, and a floating, tight pulse, then pattern identification reveals that these symptoms belong to an exterior pattern, but these symptoms actually indicate an exterior pattern of cold damage disease. Since I know this is a cold damage disease, I can go a step further and be even more definitive with pattern identification and inquire whether this is a pattern of exterior vacuity, exterior repletion, or half-exterior half-interior, whether the evil has entered the interior and transformed into heat, or if these symptoms are the result of inappropriate treatment of chest bind or glomus. I can also determine a pattern of greater yáng (*tài yáng*) evil passing to the yáng brightness (*yáng míng*) channel, or greater yáng evil passing to the lesser yīn (*shào yīn*) channel, or yáng brightness evil passing to the greater yīn (*tài yīn*) channel, or greater yáng evil passing to the lesser yáng (*shào yáng*) channel. I can also investigate further into combination disease and drag-over disease in which an evil remains in one channel, but passes to another channel as well. I can also explore the particular characteristics of how cold evil may easily damage yáng.

Now if the patient presents with symptoms such as headache, slight aversion to wind and cold, or no aversion to wind and cold, heat effusion and thirst, and a floating, rapid pulse, the pattern is an exterior one, but very specifically an exterior pattern of warm disease. There are several patterns associated with the treatment of warm disease, such as defense-aspect patterns; qì-aspect patterns; construction-aspect patterns; and blood-aspect patterns. Each of these patterns is different from the other. Furthermore, there are significant passages and shifts between the aspects of warm disease. For example, disease in the qì-aspect may enter the construction-aspect, and disease in the defense-aspect may enter the qì-aspect. Disease in the construction-aspect may shift to the qì-aspect or both qì and construction may be ablaze. There may also be abnormal passage to the pericardium. However, the characteristic trait of warm disease is the pattern of heat evil damaging yīn. Therefore, on one hand there is pattern identification and on the other is disease identification; consider integrating them by comparing and contrasting them in a comprehensive manner to better understand disease and its symptoms.

Consider Case 2 in this chapter. At the time of the initial visit, the patient suffered from chest impediment disease with patterns of insufficient heart-blood and devitalization of chest yáng, but I did not thoroughly investigate one characteristic of chest impediment disease: "slight yáng [pulse], stringlike yīn [pulse]," in other words, yáng vacuity with yīn exuberance. It was not enough to simply prescribe yáng-assisting medicinals, and as a consequence, the patient's symptoms of chest oppression, flusteredness, and chest and back pain did not improve. Then at the second visit, I increased the dosage of *guì zhī* (cinnamon twig) and *bàn xià* (pinellia), and, taking the principles of *zhǐ shí xiè bái guì zhī tāng* (Unripe Bitter Orange, Chinese Chive, and Cinnamon Twig Decoction) and *guā lóu xiè bái bàn xià tāng* (Trichosanthes, Chinese Chive, and Pinellia Decoction), I modified the formula according to the pattern. Only then were the symptoms of chest oppression, flusteredness, and chest and back pain alleviated and gradually eliminated.

In contrast to Case 2 was the jaundiced patient in Case 3 (Chinese medicine does identify jaundice as a disease). From the very beginning, I paid particular attention to the characteristics of this yáng jaundice pattern due to damp-heat brewing in the center burner and its influence on the liver and stomach. When organizing the prescription, I was determined to unite these theories, and consequently, I obtained satisfactory results. In Case 4, in compliance with the transformation theories of summerheat warmth and in consideration of the characteristic traits of summerheat, heat, and dampness, I prescribed and modified a formula according to the pattern to disperse summerheat, transform dampness, open the orifices, and extinguish wind. The patient recovered. I prescribed *qīng zhèn tāng* (Clearing Invigoration Decoction) for the patient in Case 5 according to Chinese medical theory, and good results were clearly accomplished. As for the young patient in Case 1, I did not consider that wind alone was the pattern to treat; I specifically recognized that hyperactive tongue wind disease was present and that this involved such patterns as exuberant heart heat and the stirring of liver wind. At the time of treatment, I used a liver-settling, yáng-subduing, heart-clearing, and wind-extinguishing method, and only this approach obtained good results.

These examples clearly illustrate that in the diagnosis and treatment of disease, Chinese medicine closely integrates the characteristic traits of each type of disease and selects formulas and medicinals for treatment based on the pattern. It is important to have a comprehensive treatment viewpoint and never disregard any symptom at the time of diagnosis. In famous medical books such as the *Shāng Hán Lùn* ("On Cold Damage") and *Jīn Guì Yào Lüè* ("Essential Prescriptions of the Golden Coffer") written during the Hàn dynasty, there are references that "identify a certain disease with its associated pulse, patterns, and treatment."

From these references, it can be seen how since ancient times Chinese medicine has paid attention to the integration of pattern identification with disease identification. I believe that even now in the modern world the diagnosis and treatment methods of past physicians still demonstrate the integration of these concepts of pattern identification and disease identification. It remains to us to understand in depth and to study intensively the content of these valuable ancient texts. Of course, Chinese medicine has many disease patterns that remain at the level of pattern identification and do not reach the level of combined disease and pattern identification. These should be subject to further observation and analysis so that the level of our understanding can be raised.

There is a great difference between Chinese medicine disease identification and Western medicine disease identification. If a Chinese physician cannot identify nameable diseases, then this individual can only conduct a treatment by pattern identification. Thus, an integration of Chinese medicine pattern identification and Western medicine disease identification is formulated with the intent to improve both modalities. However, you cannot simply equate Western medical diseases and Chinese medical diseases with each other. If these two modalities could simply be equated with each other, then you would arrive at the concept of "one disease, one method." There would be no need to modify according to the pattern, and you could simply disregard the characteristics of the Chinese medical system of pattern identification to determine treatment. It is important to understand that this approach cannot obtain very good therapeutic results.

Thus, from the achievements of Chinese medicine, we must first learn to emulate the Chinese medical concept of pattern identification to determine treatment — in other words, Chinese medical diagnosis and treatment methods based on the integration of Chinese medical pattern and disease identification. With this as a foundation, the occasion may arise to study the disease identification of Western medicine, to integrate the content of this together with pattern identification, to investigate more thoroughly according to the very essence of pattern identification to determine treatment, and to explore new methods of identification and treatment. Such activity would improve diagnostic proficiency and medical efficacy, promote the integration of Chinese and Western modalities, and accelerate a beneficial modernization of Chinese medicine. However, it is crucial at all times to practice the Chinese medicine characteristic of treatment based on pattern identification because, even with the current proficiency level of medical science, Western medicine identifies certain diseases quite distinctly but is sometimes without an effective treatment method. Some examples are: neurosis, hysteria, autonomic nerve function disorder, rheumatoid arthritis, and aplastic anemia. When Chinese medicine treats diseases such as these using the method of pattern identification to determine treatment, even though all cases obtain treatment efficacy, some results are comparatively ideal. For this reason, I propose that the concepts of Western medicine disease identification and Chinese medicine pattern identification be integrated, for this is actually how we practice.

Furthermore, it is worth pondering deeply the valuable experience and theories that past physicians have accumulated concerning the issues of integrated pattern and disease identification and their medical system of pattern identification to determine treatment. In some cases, ancient insights are similar to the modern understanding of pathophysiological changes and their management. A good example is the modern understanding and management of the biomedical disease called "DIC" or disseminated intravascular coagulation. Based on pattern identification to determine treatment, some physicians have successfully employed the method of quickening blood and dispelling stasis while clearing heat and resolving toxin, and the therapeutic results have been very good. In recent years, there was a Western medical researcher who discovered that when treating hypertension, strong regulation to lower blood pressure would sometimes produce the opposite effect, so he proposed that the treatment positively reinforce the organism's homeostatic ability. This idea is compatible with the Chinese medical principles:

> "Excess causes harm, preventing its development brings order, and order engenders transformation."

> "To treat disease, first seek the root."

> "Keep to the pathomechanisms, for each has its own category, then course, regulate, and harmonize qì and blood."

This method of thinking is extremely similar to the example above. Therefore, since it is already necessary to identify the disease based on the requirements and integration of Western medicine, we can supplement Chinese medicine in the treatment of certain diseases where we recognize insufficiencies, but we should never lose sight of the characteristics of pattern identification to determine treatment.

It is also essential to realize the differences between Chinese medical disease and pattern identification and Western medical disease and pattern identification. The latter also holds the idea of pattern identification, but in comparison to Chinese medicine the idea is very limited. Both modalities have methods to recognize and treat disease. Western medical diagnosis and treatment of disease has merit and should be actively studied and assimilated, and we should use it to supplement the shortcomings of Chinese medicine and to lay a foundation for Chinese-Western medical integration.

Case 2 illustrates this idea. Before and after treatment, the patient on many occasions had undergone an electrocardiogram examination, which proved to be of great assistance in revealing the change in the patient's condition and in confirming the treatment effect. Furthermore, Chinese medical treatment based on pattern identification cannot forever remain at the original level of proficiency, but should progress along with modern science and continually develop in a forward direction.

CHAPTER SIX

A brief discussion on the Chinese medical statement, "Treating different diseases with the same method and treating same diseases with different methods."

The statement, "treating different diseases with the same method, and treating same diseases with different methods" is an important component of Chinese medical theory and is also an important rule when determining treatment based on pattern identification. It is important to apply this concept at all times when diagnosing and treating in clinic to enhance treatment efficacy. I submit here five clinical cases, together with a discussion on several points based on my experience with this concept.

CASE STUDIES

CASE ONE
ABDOMINAL PAIN (ACUTE GASTRITIS)
腹痛(急性胃炎)

The patient was a 38-year-old male worker in Běijīng, whose initial examination date was December 14, 1961.

CHIEF COMPLAINT
Abdominal pain for the last two days.

INQUIRY EXAMINATION

On the evening of December 12, the patient made a return trip to Běijīng and, since he was very hungry, he ate half a pan of steamed rice-flour cakes. After eating, he wanted to sleep without a cover and during the night took a chill. The next morning he had pain in his upper abdomen and in the area to the left of his umbilicus. There was glomus, distention, and fullness in the stomach duct, and the patient had no appetite, short voidings of reddish colored urine, and no bowel movements for three days. When he came in for treatment on December 14, the pain was severe.

INSPECTION EXAMINATION

His development was normal, but his nutrition was insufficient. He presented with acute pain and suffering, and he stooped, holding his abdomen with his hands. His tongue fur was white.

LISTENING AND SMELLING EXAMINATION

His speech was clear and distinct and his breathing and voice were normal.

PALPATION EXAMINATION

The upper abdomen and the area to the left of the umbilicus were painful when pressed. The abdominal wall was soft and the painful sites refused pressure. The pulse was stringlike and slippery. The WBC was $11,700/ml^3$ and neutrophils were 86%.

PATTERN IDENTIFICATION:

The *Huáng Dì Nèi Jīng* ("The Yellow Emperor's Inner Canon") says, "Great amounts of food and drink damage the stomach and intestines." Excessive fullness after eating damages the stomach, so the center burner cannot transport food and drink; water and grains are then blocked, and qì and blood become obstructed. Thus, the patient suffered pressure-resisting pain in the stomach duct and to the left of the umbilicus. Upbearing and downbearing were abnormal, so there was no desire for food and drink and the bowels did not move. This patient had white tongue fur, which was the chief indicator of center burner stagnation. The stringlike pulse is the chief indicator of pain, and the slippery pulse is the chief indicator of food stagnation. After correlating the four examinations, I diagnosed food stagnation abdominal pain.

TREATMENT METHOD

Disperse food and abduct stagnation.

PRESCRIPTION

I prescribed one packet of *dà chéng qì tāng* (Major Qì-Infusing Decoction) with modifications according to the pattern:

jiǔ dà huáng (酒大黄 wine-processed rhubarb, Rhei Radix et Rhizoma cum Vino Preparati) 12 g *zhǐ shí* (枳实 unripe bitter orange, Aurantii Fructus Immaturus) 12 g

hòu pò (厚朴 officinal magnolia bark, Magnoliae Officinalis Cortex) 9 g

máng xiāo (芒硝 mirabilite, Natrii Sulfas) 6 g

jiāo bīng láng (焦槟榔 scorch-fried areca, Arecae Semen Ustum) 9 g

jiāo sān xiān (焦三仙 scorch-fried three immortals, Tres Immortales Usti) 9 g

FORMULA EXPLANATION

As the chief medicinal, *jiǔ dà huáng* (wine-processed rhubarb) shifts accumulation and stagnation.

As support medicinals, *zhǐ shí* (unripe bitter orange) descends qì and eliminates glomus, and *hòu pò* (officinal magnolia bark) moves qì and disperses distention. These are further assisted by *jiāo bīng láng* (scorch-fried areca) and *jiāo sān xiān* (scorch-fried three immortals), which disperse food and abduct stagnation.

Máng xiāo (mirabilite) is the courier medicinal. It has a bitter nature and salty flavor and has an upwelling and draining action; thus, it reinforces the dispersing, abducting, and shifting action of other medicinals.

This was a food-dispersing, stagnation-abducting prescription to expel food and remove stagnation.

I also immediately treated him with acupuncture needles to eliminate the abdominal pain as quickly as possible. I used the following acupuncture points bilaterally: LI-4 (*hé gǔ*), LI-1 (*shāng yáng*), PC-6 (*nèi guān*), and ST-25 (*tiān shū*). I used a strong stimulation method, but did not retain the needles. After the acupuncture treatment, the pain in the stomach duct and umbilical area was alleviated to some extent.

FOLLOWUP TREATMENT

On a follow-up visit on May 17, 1962, the patient said he had passed malodorous stools after taking the prescription. The pain in the stomach duct and abdomen had completely disappeared; he made a full recovery and there had been no relapse since his initial examination.

CASE TWO
STOMACH DUCT PAIN (ACUTE GASTRITIS)
胃脘痛(急性胃炎)

The patient was a 33-year-old male from a small village in a county of Gānsù province. His initial examination date was December 2, 1967.

CHIEF COMPLAINT

Severe upper abdominal pain for more than two days.

INQUIRY EXAMINATION

Two days ago, after eating an excessive amount of boiled sugar beets, the patient had taken a chill and afterwards had severe abdominal pain. He had already visited his local provincial physician, who gave him atropine tablets among other medications. Moreover, he had twice received intravenous injections of atropine, but neither of these methods was effective for alleviating the pain. On the evening of the day before his initial visit, the patient requested diagnosis and treatment from the medical staff physician and immediately received 100 mg of atropine, which finally relieved the pain. However, the pain recurred on the morning of the initial examination day, and there was again glomus, oppression, distention, and fullness in the upper abdomen. The patient had no desire for food and drink, and the pain was severe; he tossed and turned and his bowels had not moved for three days. Due to these difficulties, he requested treatment from a Chinese medical physician.

INSPECTION EXAMINATION

His development was normal. He presented with acute pain and suffering. He was lying on his side, wrapped in a blanket, and holding a heated brick to his abdomen with both hands to keep it warm. The tongue fur was white and full and was slightly yellow in color behind the center area.

LISTENING AND SMELLING EXAMINATION

His speech was low and he groaned occasionally.

PALPATION EXAMINATION

There was glomus and fullness in the stomach duct and abdomen, and the pain resisted pressure and preferred warmth. He presented no other abnormal signs and symptoms. The pulse was stringlike and slippery [and forceful].

PATTERN IDENTIFICATION

The patient lived in a cold region of China and at a high altitude, and his illness occurred during a severe winter; he had overeaten and afterwards took a chill. Consequently, food had stagnated in the center burner, cold and food had aggravated each other, and downbearing of stomach qì and blood was obstructed; thus, there was stomach duct pain. I knew this was a pattern of cold evil because the stomach area desired warmth; since the pain refused pressure, I knew this was also a repletion pattern. The stringlike pulse was the chief indicator of pain, and the slippery forceful pulse indicated food stagnation. The tongue fur was white and thick overall, which also indicated stagnation in the center burner. After correlating the four examinations, I diagnosed stomach duct pain caused by stomach cold with food stagnation.

TREATMENT METHOD

Warm the center and abduct stagnation.

PRESCRIPTION

I gave the patient the following prescription with instructions to decoct immediately and take in two doses:

> *gāo liáng jiāng* (高良姜 lesser galangal, Alpiniae Officinarum Rhizoma) 9 g
>
> *gān jiāng* (干姜 dried ginger, Zingiberis Rhizoma) 6 g
>
> *wú zhū yú* (吴茱萸 evodia, Evodiae Fructus) 9 g
>
> *mù xiāng* (木香 costusroot, Aucklandiae Radix) 5 g
>
> *zhǐ shí* (枳实 unripe bitter orange, Aurantii Fructus Immaturus) 9 g
>
> *hòu pò* (厚朴 official magnolia bark, Magnoliae Officinalis Cortex) 9 g
>
> *jiǔ dà huáng* (酒大黄 wine-processed rhubarb, Rhei Radix et Rhizoma cum Vino Preparati) 9 g
>
> *jiāo bīng láng* (焦槟榔 scorch-fried areca, Arecae Semen Ustum) 12 g
>
> *jiāo shén qū* (焦神曲 scorch-fried medicated leaven, Massa Medicata Fermentata Usta) 12 g
>
> *sān léng* (三棱 sparganium, Sparganii Rhizoma) 9 g
>
> *yán hú suǒ* (延胡索 corydalis, Corydalis Rhizoma) 12 g

FORMULA EXPLANATION

As chief medicinals, *gāo liáng jiāng* (lesser galangal) and *wú zhū yú* (evodia) warm the stomach and dispel cold.

As support medicinals, *gān jiāng* (dried ginger) warms the center and dispels cold. *Zhǐ shí* (unripe bitter orange) disperses glomus and descends qì. *Hòu pò* (official magnolia bark) moves qì and eliminates fullness. *Jiǔ dà huáng* (wine-processed rhubarb) expels accumulation and stagnation. These medicinals powerfully warm the center and abduct stagnation.

As assistant medicinals, *yán hú suǒ* (corydalis) quickens blood, moves qì, and dispels pain, while *shén qū* (medicated leaven) and *sān léng* (sparganium) transform food, disperse accumulation, and abduct stagnation.

The couriers are *mù xiāng* (costusroot) and *bīng láng* (areca); these medicinals respectively move stagnated qì in the intestines and stomach and disperse food and abduct qì downward.

By using these medicinals together, the prescription warms the center and dispels cold, disperses food and abducts stagnation, and frees qì and blood to relieve pain.

FOLLOWUP TREATMENT

<u>Second visit on December 3</u>: The stomach duct pain was alleviated, the glomus and fullness in the duct was eliminated, and no pressure pain was evident. The patient was able to eat some thin porridge, and he desired warm

food and drink. There was still a slight feeling of pain when heavy pressure was applied on the area to the left of the umbilicus, and the stool had not yet moved. The tongue fur had already transformed and had become thin and white, and the pulse was slippery and forceful when heavily pressed. Through analysis of the pulse signs, I knew center cold had already been dispelled, and stagnated food had moved downward. Therefore, I used the warm precipitation method to flush evil out of the body. I used the above-mentioned prescription with a few modifications, combining in principle *dà huáng fù zǐ tāng* (Rhubarb and Aconite Decoction) and *dāng guī tōng yōu tāng* (Chinese Angelica Dark-Gate–Freeing Decoction) with modifications according to the pattern. Thus, I gave the patient one packet of the following prescription:

wú zhū yú (吴茱萸 evodia, Evodiae Fructus) 6 g

gān jiāng (干姜 dried ginger, Zingiberis Rhizoma) 6 g

jiǔ dà huáng (酒大黄 wine-processed rhubarb, Rhei Radix et Rhizoma cum Vino Preparati) 6 g

fù piàn (附片 sliced aconite, Aconiti Radix Lateralis Praeparata Secta) 6 g

zhǐ shí (枳实 unripe bitter orange, Aurantii Fructus Immaturus) 9 g

dāng guī (当归 Chinese angelica, Angelicae Sinensis Radix) 9 g

táo rén ní (桃仁泥 crushed peach kernel, Persicae Semen Tusum) 9 g

jiāo bīng láng (焦槟榔 scorch-fried areca, Arecae Semen Ustum) 12 g

jiāo shén qū (焦神曲 scorch-fried medicated leaven, Massa Medicata Fermentata Usta) 10 g

jī nèi jīn (鸡内金 gizzard lining, Galli Gigeriae Endothelium Corneum) 9 g

yán hú suǒ (延胡索 corydalis, Corydalis Rhizoma) 9 g

<u>Third visit on December 4</u>: The bowels had finally moved, the stomach duct pain had not returned, and the abdominal area was without discomfort. The tongue fur was now normal, and the pulse was harmonious and moderate. I advised him to discontinue the medicinals and to take better care of his dietary needs. The patient had follow-up visits on December 6th and 8th, but he had already recovered.

CASE THREE

GREATER YÁNG AND YÁNG BRIGHTNESS COMBINATION DISEASE (SALMONELLA INFECTION)

太阳、阳明合病(沙门氏菌属感染)

The patient was a 38-year-old male whose initial examination date was April 21, 1961.

CHIEF COMPLAINT

An unabated high fever for the last three to four days.

INQUIRY EXAMINATION

The patient ate some steamed wild vegetables on the afternoon of April 16th, and later felt discomfort in the upper abdomen. By midnight he had distention, fullness, and pain in the upper abdomen, and three times he passed watery diarrhea that contained undigested food. There was neither pus nor blood in the stool, but after defecation, he had a sagging sensation in the abdomen. The patient was nauseous and wanted to vomit, but could not. At 5 AM the following morning, he was rushed to the hospital emergency room where blood tests were taken and a bowel examination was done. The diagnosis was acute enteritis, and he was admitted to the hospital.

The Western drug treatment and intravenous injections that he received in the hospital quickly relieved his abdominal pain and diarrhea. However, his body temperature, which had been between 37.5–37.8 °C (99.5–100.0 °F), rose sharply to 39.5 °C (103.1 °F) after the morning of April 18, and the high fever would not abate. He used antibiotics, alcohol rub baths, ice packs, bowel purges, injections of quinine, oral doses of an analgesic drug, aspirin, and many other treatments, but still the fever did not abate. Then on the night of April 20th, the patient experienced clouded spirit and delirium; he picked at his bedclothes and was not able to sleep peacefully. His WBC was 9000/ml^3, neutrophils were 85%, erythrocyte sedimentation rate was 26 mm/hour, Widal's agglutination test and Weil-Felix test were (-). The diagnosis was (1) salmonella infection and (2) high fever of undetermined cause. On the afternoon of April 21st, the patient requested a Chinese medical diagnosis.

At the time of the initial examination, the patient had a headache, head distention, vexation and agitation, high fever with thirst, desire for cold drinks, glomus and fullness in the chest and stomach duct, desire to vomit yet inability to do so, and inability to eat. He had constipation for four days and reddish-yellow urine. He developed an unclear spirit after 4:00 PM with delirious speech at night, and he did not recognize anyone. Sometimes he even picked at his bedclothes, and he had not slept for two nights.

INSPECTION EXAMINATION

His development was normal, but his complexion and eyes were red. He had a high fever and a sickly appearance and his spirit-mind was slightly unclear. The tongue fur was thick and yellow with scant moisture, and the center of the tongue was brownish-yellow and slightly black. He desired cooling and was unwilling to cover himself with blankets. His head was sweating.

LISTENING AND SMELLING EXAMINATION

His breathing was rough with a high pitch and his breath was hot and foul-smelling.

PALPATION EXAMINATION

There was glomus, fullness, and aversion to pressure in the stomach duct and abdomen, the abdomen was distended, and the liver and spleen could not be touched. His limbs were normal. The pulse was surging, slippery, and rapid.

The *Huáng Dì Nèi Jīng* ("The Yellow Emperor's Inner Canon") says, "In yáng brightness disease, yáng is exuberant and causes a person to talk wildly, curse, and avoid other people. This person will have no desire to eat, and instead will wander and act rashly."

The *Shāng Hán Lùn* ("On Cold Damage") states, "In yáng brightness disease, the stomach domain (stomach and intestines) is replete."

The *Wēn Bìng Tiáo Biàn* ("Systematized Identification of Warm Diseases") explains further:

> In yáng brightness warm disease, the complexion and eyes are red, speech sounds are low and deep, respiration is rough, and there is constipation and difficult urination. The tongue fur appears old and yellow; if severe, [the tongue is] black and has prickles. However, there is aversion to heat, not to cold. When the disease becomes worse in the late afternoon, it will pass to the center burner."

This patient had a red complexion and vigorous heat, aversion to heat not to cold, bowels that had not moved for several days, thirst and desire for cool drinks, and stomach fullness with no desire for food. The patient had an unclear or clouded spirit by the afternoon and delirium at night while picking at his bedclothes. His tongue fur was thick and yellow and the pulse was surging and rapid. I knew from these signs that the pattern was yáng brightness repletion heat. Furthermore, there were other symptoms such as nausea with a desire to vomit, headache, head distention, glomus oppression in the chest and stomach duct, head sweating, and a surging pulse. On the basis of these symptoms, I knew that the exterior evil and the yáng brightness channel heat evil were both not completely cleared and resolved, and the repletion evil that had transformed into heat was still not completely bound in the center burner yáng brightness bowel. By correlating the four examinations, I diagnosed yáng brightness heat repletion due to incompletely resolved exterior evil.

TREATMENT METHOD

Clear heat and resolve the exterior with cool-acridity, followed with emergency precipitation to preserve yīn.

PRESCRIPTION

I gave the patient one packet of the following:

jīn yín huā (金银花 lonicera, Lonicerae Flos) 12 g
lián qiáo (连翘 forsythia, Forsythiae Fructus) 12 g
sāng yè (桑叶 mulberry leaf, Mori Folium) 9 g
jú huā (菊花 chrysanthemum, Chrysanthemi Flos) 6 g
jīng jiè (荆芥 schizonepeta, Schizonepetae Herba) 6 g
bò hé (薄荷 mint, Menthae Herba) 3 g (add at end)
shēng shí gāo (生石膏 raw gypsum, Gypsum Crudum) 30 g (pre-decoct)
zhī mǔ (知母 anemarrhena, Anemarrhenae Rhizoma) 6 g
huáng qín (黄芩 scutellaria, Scutellariae Radix) 9 g
shān zhī zǐ (山栀子 gardenia, Gardeniae Fructus) 9 g
jiāo sān xiān (焦三仙 scorch-fried three immortals, Tres Immortales
    Usti) 9 g each
jiāo bīng láng (焦槟榔 scorch-fried areca, Arecae Semen Ustum) 6 g

FORMULA EXPLANATION

As chief medicinals, *jīn yín huā* (lonicera), *lián qiáo* (forsythia), *sāng yè* (mulberry leaf), and *jú huā* (chrysanthemum), together with *jīng jiè* (schizonepeta) and *bò hé* (mint), are acrid, cool, gentle and balanced. They scatter the remaining unresolved evil in the exterior with their coolness and acridity.

I prescribed a heavy dosage of *shēng shí gāo* (raw gypsum) and *zhī mǔ* (anemarrhena) to clear heat in the yáng brightness channel; these support medicinals are acrid and cooling.

As assistant medicinals, *huáng qín* (scutellaria) and *shān zhī zǐ* (gardenia) clear heat.

Jiāo sān xiān (scorch-fried three immortals) and *jiāo bīng láng* (scorch-fried areca) are the couriers; they reinforce the dispersing and transforming medicinals and stimulate the stomach qì.

FOLLOWUP TREATMENT

Second visit on April 22: After taking the acrid-cooling medicinals to clear heat and resolve evil, the patient said that his entire body had perspired and his headache disappeared. At one point, his body temperature had lowered to 37 °C, but rose again to 37.8 °C. He was still thirsty with a desire for fluids, and the glomus and fullness in the abdomen still resisted pressure. Spontaneous sweating occurred on his hands and feet, and the bowels had not yet moved. On the morning of the examination he managed to eat a small bowl of thin rice gruel. The tongue fur was yellow, thick, and slimy, and the pulse was slippery, slightly rapid, and forceful when heavily pressed. On the basis of the pulse and symptoms, I used the method of emergency precipitation to preserve yīn, and I treated him with *dà chéng qì tāng* (Major Qì-Infusing Decoction) with added medicinals.

PRESCRIPTION

I gave him one packet of the following:

shēng dà huáng (生大黄 raw rhubarb, Rhei Radix et Rhizoma Crudi) 24 g
hòu pò (厚朴 officinal magnolia bark, Magnoliae Officinalis Cortex) 15 g
zhǐ shí (枳实 unripe bitter orange, Aurantii Fructus Immaturus) 21 g
máng xiāo (芒硝 mirabilite, Natrii Sulfas) 21 g (add at end)
jiāo sān xiān (焦三仙 scorch-fried three immortals, Tres Immortales
    Usti) 12 g each
chuān lián (川连 Sichuan coptis, Coptidis Rhizoma Sichuanense) 9 g
bīng láng (槟榔 areca, Arecae Semen) 12 g
qīng bàn xià (清半夏 purified pinellia, Pinelliae Tuber Depuratum) 15 g
chén pí (陈皮 tangerine peel, Citri Reticulatae Pericarpium) 12 g

The patient decocted one packet in 400 ml of water and divided it into two doses. I advised his family that if there was precipitation of watery stools within four hours of the first dose, then the patient should not take the second dose. But if he passed no stool, then he should take the second dose immediately.

Third visit on April 23: After taking the first dose, the patient had a bowel movement, but it was very small in amount. The family telephoned me, and I advised them to give him the second half of the prescription. The bowels moved three times after taking the second dose. His body temperature dropped to normal, he could sleep at night, he had a meal, and he regained a normal taste in his mouth. Sometimes he still belched, and his urine was dark yellow in color. The tongue fur had gradually transformed. The right pulse was slippery, but no longer rapid, and slightly larger than the left pulse, which was almost normal. I again focused on regulating and harmonizing the center burner. The patient received two packets of the following:

shēng dài zhě shí (生代赭石 crude hematite, Haematitum Crudum) 18 g
    (pre-decocted)

xuán fù huā (旋覆花 inula flower, Inulae Flos) 9 g (wrapped in cloth)

qīng bàn xià (清半夏 purified pinellia, Pinelliae Tuber Depuratum) 9 g

jiāo sān xiān (焦三仙 scorch-fried three immortals, Tres Immortales
    Usti) 9 g each

chǎo zhǐ shí (炒枳实 stir-fried unripe bitter orange, Aurantii Fructus
    Immaturus Frictus) 9 g

chén pí (陈皮 tangerine peel, Citri Reticulatae Pericarpium) 6 g

zhú rú (竹茹 bamboo shavings, Bumbusae Caulis in Taenia) 9 g

hòu pò (厚朴 officinal magnolia bark, Magnoliae Officinalis Cortex) 6 g

zhī mǔ (知母 anemarrhena, Anemarrhenae Rhizoma) 6 g

chǎo huáng qín (炒黄芩 stir-fried scutellaria, Scutellariae Radix Fricta) 9 g

shēng gān cǎo (生甘草 raw licorice, Glycyrrhizae Radix Cruda) 3 g

<u>Fourth visit on April 27</u>: The patient said his body temperature was completely normal, but there was still some oppression in the stomach duct when heavy pressure was applied. Occasionally he had a cloudy headed-sensation on the right side. His bowels moved twice a day now; they were still yellow in color, but the stool was formed. His appetite was returning to normal, yet the urine remained dark yellow. The tongue fur on the right half of the tongue was white and thick and the pulse was slightly slippery.

Again, I prescribed medicinals to regulate and rectify the center burner and to enhance the recovery rate. The patient received two packets of the following prescription:

hòu pò (厚朴 officinal magnolia bark, Magnoliae Officinalis Cortex) 6 g

zhǐ shí (枳实 unripe bitter orange, Aurantii Fructus Immaturus) 9 g

zhǐ qiào (*ké*) (枳壳 bitter orange, Aurantii Fructus) 9 g

chén pí (陈皮 tangerine peel, Citri Reticulatae Pericarpium) 6 g

zhú rú (竹茹 bamboo shavings, Bumbusae Caulis in Taenia) 9 g

qīng bàn xià (清半夏 purified pinellia, Pinelliae Tuber Depuratum) 6 g

shí hú (石斛 dendrobium, Dendrobii Herba) 9 g

gé gēn (葛根 pueraria, Puerariae Radix) 9 g

chǎo huáng lián (炒黄连 stir-fried coptis, Coptidis Rhizoma Frictum) 3 g

xiāng fù (香附 cyperus, Cyperi Rhizoma) 6 g

jú huā (菊花 chrysanthemum, Chrysanthemi Flos) 6 g

dà fù pí (大腹皮 areca husk, Arecae Pericarpium) 9 g

By April 29, the patient had completely recovered and was discharged from the hospital. I saw the patient twice on follow-up visits in the middle of

May and at the end of June that year. The patient remained in good health after leaving the hospital and had already returned to work.

CASE FOUR
WHEEZING AND PANTING (ASTHMA)
哮喘

The patient was a 17-year-old female student whose initial examination date was August 14, 1958.

CHIEF COMPLAINT

Panting disease for the last ten years; at the time of the initial examination, the patient was at an acute stage of the disease.

INQUIRY EXAMINATION

When she was seven years of age, the patient experienced a critical episode of asthma, and since that time, every year during autumn, winter, and early spring, or whenever the weather changed, the illness would recur. During the last several months, this cycle occurred more frequently. On the morning of the examination, she had a feeling of oppression in the chest and throat, and she was panting. She was aware that a relapse was imminent, so she immediately came to the clinic for diagnosis. Whenever she took a walk, she felt flustered and had palpitations, and she complained about fatigue. The patient was unable to sleep since the panting was more severe at night; she was thirsty and had a desire for cool drinks, and she was fearful of heat. Inhalation was more difficult for her than exhalation. Her appetite was still good, and urine and stool were normal. Because of the wheezing and panting, she had given up her studies and suspended school for the last ten months.

INSPECTION EXAMINATION

Her development and nutrition were normal, but her complexion was dark and somber. She appeared worried, confused, and fearful. Her tongue fur was thin and white but the root of the tongue had thick and slimy fur.

LISTENING AND SMELLING EXAMINATION

She was mildly panting and slightly short of breath, but her speech was normal. Heart auscultation was normal; lung auscultation revealed rough breathing bilaterally together with panting rale.

PALPATION EXAMINATION

The pulses were overall slippery and slightly rapid; the cubit pulse was weak. The abdomen was soft and supple, without any pressure pain. The liver and spleen did not appear enlarged, and the four limbs looked normal. Her body temperature was 36.6°C, the pulse was 80 beats per minute, and the blood pressure was 95/50 mm/Hg.

PATTERN IDENTIFICATION

I knew this was a pattern of lung heat, since whenever the patient had a panting attack, she also had symptoms of aversion to heat and thirst with desire for cool drinks. Inhalation that was more difficult than exhalation and a weak cubit pulse indicated kidney vacuity with qì absorption failure. After correlating the four examinations, I diagnosed panting disease due to lung heat and kidney vacuity.

TREATMENT METHOD

Clear the lung and eliminate phlegm, simultaneously assisted by boosting the kidney.

PRESCRIPTION

I gave the patient two packets of the following prescription:

má huáng (麻黄 ephedra, Ephedrae Herba) 3 g

xìng rén (杏仁 apricot kernel, Armeniacae Semen) 6 g

shēng shí gāo (生石膏 raw gypsum, Gypsum Crudum) 15 g (pre-decocted)

gān cǎo (甘草 licorice, Glycyrrhizae Radix) 4.5 g

zhī mǔ (知母 anemarrhena, Anemarrhenae Rhizoma) 9 g

huáng qín (黄芩 scutellaria, Scutellariae Radix) 9 g

bái qián (白前 willowleaf swallowwort, Cynanchi Stauntonii Rhizoma) 4.5 g

zhè bèi mǔ (浙贝母 Zhejiang fritillaria, Fritillariae Thunbergii Bulbus) 9 g

shēng mǔ lì (生牡蛎 raw oyster shell, Ostreae Concha Cruda) 9 g (pre-decocted)

nǚ zhēn zǐ (女贞子 ligustrum, Ligustri Lucidi Fructus) 9 g

líng cí shí (灵磁石 magnetic loadstone, Magnetitum Magneticum) 12 g (pre-decocted)

jié gěng (桔梗 platycodon, Platycodonis Radix) 4.5 g

FORMULA EXPLANATION

As chief medicinals, *má huáng* (ephedra) diffuses lung qì and calms panting, and *xìng rén* (apricot kernel) depurates and downbears lung qì, and thereby calms panting.

As support medicinals, *shēng shí gāo* (raw gypsum), *zhī mǔ* (anemarrhena), and *huáng qín* (scutellaria) clear lung heat and check vexing thirst; *zhè bèi mǔ* (Zhejiang fritillaria) and *bái qián* (willowleaf swallowwort) downbear counterflow qì and transform phlegm-heat.

As assistant medicinals, *nǔ zhēn zǐ* (ligustrum) supplements the kidney and eliminates phlegm; *líng cí shí* (magnetic loadstone) supplements the kidney to absorb qì; and *shēng mǔ lì* (raw oyster shell) boosts the kidney and transforms phlegm.

As courier medicinals, *jié gěng* (platycodon) guides the other medicinals to the lung, and *gān cǎo* (licorice) regulates and harmonizes all the medicinals in the formula.

As a whole, this formula clears the lung and eliminates heat, boosts the kidney and transforms phlegm, and calms panting.

FOLLOWUP TREATMENT

Second visit on August 16: The patient said that no symptoms remained at all after taking the prescription. There was no panting and no oppressive feeling in the chest, and she felt normal. However, the patient had contracted wind damage common cold on the day before; she presented with symptoms of nasal congestion and runny nose, thirst with a desire for fluids, a moist tongue without fur, and a slippery, rapid, and slightly floating pulse. This time, I used the exterior-resolving method with acrid-cooling medicinals and gave the patient two packets of the following:

> *jīn yín huā* (金银花 lonicera, Lonicerae Flos) 9 g
>
> *lián qiáo* (连翘 forsythia, Forsythiae Fructus) 9 g
>
> *bò hé* (薄荷 mint, Menthae Herba) 3 g (add at end)
>
> *jié gěng* (桔梗 platycodon, Platycodonis Radix) 4.5 g
>
> *tiān huā fěn* (天花粉 trichosanthes root, Trichosanthis Radix) 9 g
>
> *dàn zhú yè* (淡竹叶 lophatherum, Lophatheri Herba) 6 g
>
> *zhè bèi mǔ* (浙贝母 Zhejiang fritillaria, Fritillariae Thunbergii Bulbus)
> 9 g
>
> *xiān lú gēn* (鲜芦根 fresh phragmites, Phragmititis Rhizoma Recens) 24 g
>
> *shēng gān cǎo* (生甘草 raw licorice, Glycyrrhizae Radix Cruda) 3 g

Third visit on August 18: The patient had recovered from the wind damage common cold. There had been no relapse of the panting, and she was without any significant symptoms. The patient wanted to prevent a relapse of the wheezing and panting so she requested a daily pill prescription to eliminate the disease root. The tongue was moist without fur and the pulse slightly slippery and rapid. On the basis of this evidence, I prescribed the following in pill form:

> *zhì má huáng* (炙麻黄 mix-fried ephedra, Ephedrae Herba cum Liquido
> Fricta) 24 g
>
> *nán xìng rén* (南杏仁 southern apricot kernel, Armeniacae Semen
> Australis) 45 g

shēng shí gāo (生石膏 raw gypsum, Gypsum Crudum) 120 g

zhī mǔ (知母 anemarrhena, Anemarrhenae Rhizoma) 60 g

bái qián (白前 willowleaf swallowwort, Cynanchi Stauntonii Rhizoma) 36 g

huáng qín (黄芩 scutellaria, Scutellariae Radix) 60 g

zhè bèi mǔ (浙贝母 Zhejiang fritillaria, Fritillariae Thunbergii Bulbus)
    75 g

jié gěng (桔梗 platycodon, Platycodonis Radix) 36 g

huà jú hóng (化橘红 Huazhou pomelo rind, Citri Grandis Exocarpium
    Rubrum) 30 g

shēng dì huáng (生地黄 dried rehmannia, Rehmanniae Radix Exsiccata)
    90 g

shēng mǔ lì (生牡蛎 raw oyster shell, Ostreae Concha Cruda) 75 g

nǔ zhēn zǐ (女贞子 ligustrum, Ligustri Lucidi Fructus) 75 g

líng cí shí (灵磁石 magnetic loadstone, Magnetitum Magneticum) 90 g

chǎo zhī zǐ (炒栀子 stir-fried gardenia, Gardeniae Fructus Frictus) 30 g

shēng gān cǎo (生甘草 raw licorice, Glycyrrhizae Radix Cruda) 75 g

These medicinals were ground together into a fine powder and then mixed with refined honey to form pills that weighed 9 grams each. The dosage was one pill twice a day. I advised her to increase the dosage if necessary to 2 pills 2–3 times a day, and to take the pills with boiled water.

<u>Fourth visit on August 29</u>: There had been no relapse of panting after taking the pill prescription. The patient felt that this prescription had been successful in preventing a wheezing-panting relapse. Her essence-spirit had greatly improved, her breathing was stronger, her appetite increased, and her complexion was lustrous. She was ready to resume her interrupted studies and pursue her certificate. I examined her tongue and pulse, auscultated her heart and lungs, and found no abnormalities. I agreed that she should resume her studies and she joyfully went back to school.

On New Year's Day 1959, I saw her at her family home for a follow-up visit. The patient was engaged in her studies and the panting had not recurred.

CASE FIVE
WHEEZING AND PANTING (ASTHMA)
哮喘

The patient was a 61-year-old male whose initial examination date was June 3, 1972. He was an outpatient from the Héběi provincial hospital.

CHIEF COMPLAINT

Asthma for four to five years; recently the symptoms had become more serious.

INQUIRY EXAMINATION

His asthma had flared up during the spring and winter seasons every year for the last four years. The wheezing and panting had become worse in the last few days, and he presented with symptoms of cough with expectoration of white phlegm, throat rale, and panting. When he encountered cold, the symptoms worsened, so he was referred from the Tángshǎn hospital in Héběi to my hospital for diagnosis.

INSPECTION EXAMINATION

His development was normal, but he was short of breath and panting. His tongue fur was white and slimy.

LISTENING AND SMELLING EXAMINATION

Speech was clear and distinct, but in his throat was a wheezing and ringing sound. Auscultation of the lung area revealed rough respiration in both lungs and wheezing, but without a damp rale sound.

PALPATION EXAMINATION

The pulse was slippery and rapid, but there were no other abnormalities noted.

PATTERN IDENTIFICATION

Based on the symptoms of white, thick, and slimy tongue fur, the slippery pulse, and expectoration of white phlegm, I knew this was exuberant phlegm obstructing the lung. Since the symptoms worsened whenever the patient encountered cold, I knew this was a case of cold panting. After correlating the pulse and the symptoms, I diagnosed repletion panting due to cold phlegm obstructing the lung.

TREATMENT METHOD

Warm and transform phlegm-turbidity, and diffuse and downbear lung qì.

PRESCRIPTION

The patient received two packets of the following prescription:

má huáng (麻黄 ephedra, Ephedrae Herba) 5 g

xìng rén (杏仁 apricot kernel, Armeniacae Semen) 9 g

chén pí (陈皮 tangerine peel, Citri Reticulatae Pericarpium) 9 g

bàn xià (半夏 pinellia, Pinelliae Rhizoma) 9 g

fú líng (茯苓 poria, Poria) 9 g

zǐ sū zǐ (紫苏子 perilla fruit, Perillae Fructus) 9 g

hòu pò (厚朴 officinal magnolia bark, Magnoliae Officinalis Cortex) 9 g

zǐ wǎn (紫菀 aster, Asteris Radix) 9 g

sāng bái pí (桑白皮 mulberry root bark, Mori Cortex) 9 g

FORMULA EXPLANATION

This prescription was my empirical formula, *má xìng èr sān tāng* (Ephedra and Apricot Kernel Two-Three Decoction) with modifications. As chief medicinals, *má huáng* (ephedra) warms and diffuses lung qì and calms panting, and *xìng rén* (apricot kernel) downbears lung qì to calm panting.

As support medicinals, *bàn xià* (pinellia), *chén pí* (tangerine peel), and *fú líng* (poria) warm and transform phlegm and dampness, and downbear qì and harmonize the center. These medicinals are essential components of the formula *èr chén tāng* (Two Matured Ingredients Decoction).

As assistant medicinals, *zǐ sū zǐ* (perilla fruit) and *hòu pò* (officinal magnolia bark) downbear qì and loosen the chest; they also disperse distention and calm panting.

As the courier medicinal, *sāng bái pí* (mulberry root bark) drains phlegm-damp in the lung.

FOLLOWUP TREATMENT

Second visit on June 5: The patient said that his wheezing and panting had greatly improved after taking the medicinals, but his mouth had become dry. His tongue fur was white and his pulse was stringlike. Auscultation still revealed dry rale in both lungs. I again chose the original formula and considered the reasons for the mouth dryness. Then, I added 9 grams of *huáng qín* (scutellaria) to the prescription and gave the patient two packets.

Third visit on June 7: After taking the previous prescription from June 5, the patient experienced some discomfort at night, the wheezing and panting became worse, and he did not sleep peacefully. The tongue fur was still white and the pulse was stringlike. Auscultation again revealed dry rale in both lungs. Consequently, I removed *huáng qín* (scutellaria) from the prescription and gave him two more packets. I asked him to bring back the one remaining packet so that *huáng qín* (scutellaria) could be removed and the dosage given as before.

Fourth visit on June 9: After taking the prescription without *huáng qín* (scutellaria), the patient recovered from the wheezing and panting, and he slept well through the entire night. The tongue fur was white and the pulse was still stringlike. This time auscultation revealed no panting rale, and his respiration sounded only slightly rough. The patient believed he had already recovered, and he returned to Tángshān carrying several packets of the decoction prescription with him.

EMPIRICAL KNOWLEDGE

Regarding the expression, "Treating different diseases with the same method and treating same diseases with different methods"

The expression, "Treating different diseases with the same method, and treating same diseases with different methods," is a Chinese medical treatment principle, and the earliest reference to it is cited in the *Huáng Dì Nèi Jīng* ("The Yellow Emperor's Inner Canon"). It says:

> "When the physician treats disease, he uses different treatments for one disease, yet every patient recovers; why is this so?"

> Qí Bó replied, "The geographic terrain is the reason for this. The sage-like physician mixes and combines different treatments, for each treatment has its own appropriate role to play; thus, the treatment uses different methods, yet the patient always recovers from illness. If the physician understands the circumstances and condition of the patient, then he grasps the main principle of the treatment."

The *Nèi Jīng* ("Inner Canon") further explains:

> "To treat patients in the western and northern climate regions, use the dissipating and cooling method. To treat patients in the southern and eastern climate regions, use the contracting and warming method. This is the meaning of "treating different diseases with the same method, and treating same diseases with different methods."

For several thousand years, this single treatment principle has been an important component of the Chinese medical system of determining treatment based on pattern identification. Once you have considered the interior-exterior factors of disease and have identified the pattern, then you should pay attention to the diversity of the treatment methods, for identical diseases may transform under a different set of conditions; thus, each disease is atypical. At the time of identifying patterns to determine treatment, you should not only distinguish the circumstances surrounding the five viscera and six bowels and the conditions of vacuity and repletion and heat and cold; you must also take into consideration the situation of the patient with regard to the climate and region of the country where he lives, the seasons, life-style and personal habits, diet, and physical constitution. These factors should be carefully considered even though the diseases of patients may be the same. Since "each method has an appropriate role to play," you should devise treatments methods that are different from one another. By doing so, you can easily effect recovery from illness and enhance treatment efficacy.

A good example of this principle is demonstrated by Case 1 and Case 2. Both patients were middle-aged men almost equal in their physical constitutions. They both fell ill during the month of December, and in both cases the cause of the illness was food damage. Their chief symptoms were similar: abdominal pain, white tongue fur, and a stringlike and slippery pulse. On the basis of these symptoms, I saw that they suffered from the same disease. However, the patient in Case 1 was a resident of Běijīng, and although the onset of his illness occurred during the winter, the weather was moderate and warm when compared to Gānsù province; furthermore, he was able to stay warm indoors quite easily. Thus, although he had overeaten and had caught cold, the cold symptoms had not yet presented. For that reason, besides treating him with acupuncture needles to stop pain, I also chose *dà chéng qì tāng* (Major Qì-Infusing Decoction) to offensively precipitate with bitter and salty medicinals, and to shift the food accumulation. He recovered. In Case 2, the patient was a resident of Gānsù province in the western rural region of the country, and the onset of his illness occurred during the dead of winter when the weather was bitterly cold. Although he had an indoor stove, he nevertheless suffered cold, and because cold evil made a sneak attack on him, a cold pattern presented with symptoms of abdominal pain that preferred warmth and a desire for hot food and drink. Therefore, I chose acrid, warming medicinals to precipitate and to warm the stomach and disperse food, and he recovered as well. The treatment method and medicinals were different in both cases, but the results were the same.

Another example concerns the patients from Case 4 and Case 5. Both of these patients suffered from asthma. The disease of the patient in Case 4 was due to lung heat with symptoms at the onset such as thirst, a desire for cold drinks, and fear of heat. Whenever the patient in Case 5 encountered cold, his symptoms worsened, and the diagnosis was a lung cold pattern. Although these two cases had the same disease, the presentation of the illness was different in each patient. Consequently, I treated them differently; one I treated with the clearing method, and the other with the warming method, and both methods obtained very good results.

From these examples, we can readily see the great flexibility of Chinese medicine treatment methods and the extraordinary clarity of its principles. For instance, the prescriptions in Case 1 and Case 2 were different; one prescription used the offensively precipitating method with bitter and cold medicinals, and the other used a precipitating method with acrid and warm medicinals. Yet, in their treatment principle, both prescriptions represent the precipitating and abductive-dispersion methods, which are among the eight methods of treatment. You must write prescriptions that correspond to a specific method; you cannot recklessly act outside the principles.

The legacy of time has allowed Chinese physicians to accumulate extensive clinical experience that gives ample verification to the principle of "treating different diseases with the same method," as well as the principle of "treating same diseases with different methods." Diseases may differ, yet if they possess the same pathological process and are accompanied by the same patterns, you may apply the principle of "treating different diseases with the same method" and select identical treatment methods for different diseases.

A good example of this principle is the comparison of the two patients in Case 3 and Case 1. The former patient had a heat pattern with symptoms of high fever that would not abate, thirst with a desire for cold drinks, clouded spirit in the evening and at night, delirious speech, and picking at bedclothes. The latter had an interior pattern with abdominal pain and no desire for food and drink. One patient suffered from cold damage and the other from a miscellaneous disease, so it could be said that both patients suffered from different diseases. Yet, in the process of disease development, both patients had yáng brightness (stomach and intestine) disease that was identical in its pathology. Even though one patient had a pattern of yáng brightness heat accumulation and the other had yáng brightness food stagnation, the clinical presentation for both was a pattern of yáng brightness interior repletion. They did have the following symptoms in common: abdominal glomus and stagnation that refused pressure, bowels that had not moved for several days, thick tongue fur, and a slippery and forceful pulse. On the basis of this evidence, I chose for both patients a precipitation method using acrid, salty, bitter, down-bearing medicinals, and prescribed *dà chéng qì tāng* (Major Qì-Infusing Decoction) with modifications according to their individual pattern. This method obtained very good results for both patients.

In the *Shāng Hán Lùn* ("On Cold Damage"), yáng brightness bowel pattern is associated with yáng brightness disease, and in the *Wēn Bìng Tiáo Biàn* ("Systematized Identification of Warm Diseases"), yáng brightness heat accumulation is associated with center burner warm disease; the former is caused by cold damage, and the latter is a warm disease. Yet, in the process of disease development and transformation, the pathological process and the symptom presentation appear to be the same. For this reason, I chose the precipitation method and used *dà chéng qì tāng* (Major Qì-Infusing Decoction) as the guiding treatment. This is the principle of "treating different diseases with the same method."

While we have paid attention to the sense of principle and precision of the treatment method, we should also give equal time to its flexibility and variability. For instance, both the yáng brightness bowel repletion pattern associated with cold damage disease and the yáng brightness heat accumulation pattern associated with center burner warm disease use the offensive-precipitation method of *dà chéng qì tāng* (Major Qì-Infusing Decoction). But in the former pattern, cold evil has already transformed into heat, and since enduring heat can damage yīn, *dà chéng qì tāng* uses emergency precipitation to preserve yīn through the use of acrid, bitter, salty, and cold medicinals. However, in center burner warm disease, the characteristic trait is that warm evil has already begun to damage yīn. Therefore, by the time evil enters the qì aspect and a yáng brightness heat accumulation pattern emerges, the yīn of the patient has already been damaged; thus, when using the precipitation method in these cases, I frequently add sweet, cold, moistening, and nourishing medicinals to the prescription, such as *shēng dì huáng* (dried rehmannia), *xuán shēn* (scrophularia), and *mài mén dōng* (ophiopogon). When these are combined with *máng xiāo* (mirabilite) and *dà huáng* (rhubarb), the formula becomes a sweet, cold, moistening precipitation formula. This is how *zēng yè chéng qì tāng* (Humor-Increasing Qì-Infusing Decoction) was originally developed for exactly this kind of use as a precipitation formula in the treatment of warm and hot diseases.

As you can see from my experience in the above-mentioned examples, when identifying patterns to determine treatment in clinic, you should not only adhere at all times to the principle of "treating different diseases with the same method, and treating same diseases with different methods," you should also comply with the rules for writing prescriptions. You should always observe that things that appear to be identical may be different, and that things that appear different may indeed be identical. You should stick with a flexible method of prescribing medicinals.

The statement, "treating different diseases with the same method, and treating same diseases with different methods" is an important component of Chinese medical theory and is also an important treatment rule within the system of identifying patterns to determine treatment. Constantly strive to integrate the application of these concepts in the clinic to enhance treatment efficacy.

Further applications of the principle of "Treating different diseases with the same method and treating same diseases with different methods"

In current clinical practice, we often see patients who have been previously diagnosed and treated by our biomedical colleagues. Regardless of the outcome of any such diagnosis and treatment, we must nevertheless focus on integrating the principle of "treating different diseases with the same method, and treating same diseases with different methods." Since we study the diagnosis and treatment methods of Western medicine, we should combine Western and Chinese medical modalities because there is great advantage in doing so. For instance, if we consider all cases of peptic ulcers, we must distinguish that some have a liver-stomach disharmony pattern, some have a center burner vacuity cold pattern, and still other cases have a pattern of liver overwhelming spleen vacuity. This same principle applies to other diseases such as dysentery, for example, because some cases of dysentery have a damp-heat pattern, some have a vacuity cold pattern, and still others have a cold-heat complex pattern. These examples demonstrate that the same disease can have different patterns, and this fact indicates that a different treatment method is appropriate.

However, if we consider this argument conversely, then it is immaterial which biomedically diagnosed disease we discuss, whether it is cerebral arterial thrombosis, angio-neurotic headache, angina pectoris, or myocardial infarction; provided that the clinical presentation is static blood obstruction, we know immediately that the blood-quickening stasis-transforming method is appropriate. If the clinical presentation is qì stagnation with blood stasis, then use the qì-moving blood-quickening method. For a qì vacuity blood stasis pattern, use the qì-boosting blood-quickening method; for a phlegm turbidity congestion pattern, use the phlegm turbidity downbearing and transforming method. When the condition presents as a pattern of impeded chest yáng, then the yáng-assisting impediment-opening method is appropriate; when the condition presents as wind-phlegm obstruction, then use the method of dispelling wind and transforming stasis while quickening the blood and freeing the network vessels. When we consider these different diseases, but distinguish the same pattern among them, then we know that using the same treatment method is appropriate.

Consider Case 1 and 2 in this chapter. The patients were both diagnosed with acute gastritis. Because the patient in Case 2 very clearly had a cold pattern, I used the stomach-warming center-harmonizing precipitation method. Since the patient in Case 1 did not present with a cold pattern, but instead had a food stagnation pattern, I used the food-dispersing stagnation-abducting precipitation method. The patients in Cases 4 and 5 were diagnosed with bronchial wheezing and panting. I used a method of clearing the lung and eliminating phlegm while simultaneously boosting the kidney to treat Case 4, because the pattern was lung heat and kidney vacuity. However, I used the method to warm and transform phlegm-turbidity and to diffuse and downbear the lung qì to treat Case 5 because that pattern was cold phlegm obstruction. The treatment method in all these cases obtained ideal results, and the patients recovered.

The Chinese medical treatment principle of "treating different diseases with the same method, and treating same diseases with different methods" is exactly what is needed to treat each individual patient, given their differences in place, time, and constitution. We should simultaneously apply this principle and combine this approach with the characteristics of biomedical diagnosis and treatment, as well as the fruits of modern scientific research. In this way, medical professionals in combined Chinese and biomedical fields would benefit greatly.

CHAPTER SEVEN

Important issues when applying pattern identification to determine treatment

Presented below are several case studies with discussions that illustrate some important points concerning the application of "pattern identification to determine treatment."

CASE STUDIES

CASE ONE

JOINT-DEFORMITY IMPEDIMENT (RHEUMATOID ARTHRITIS)
痹证(尪痹)(类风湿性关节炎)

The patient was a 14-year-old female student from a commune in Liáoníng province. Her initial examination date was October 18, 1976.

CHIEF COMPLAINT
Joint pain and deformity, with an inability to walk for the last three years.

INQUIRY EXAMINATION
The illness had first occurred three years ago with symptoms of foot pain and swelling, and then gradually the right wrist joint had also become swollen and painful, but there had been no change in skin color. She had gone to the local provincial hospital, where the diagnosis was rheumatoid arthritis. How-

ever, the treatment she received there produced no positive results. She had also gone to the People's Liberation Hospital 204 (PLA 204) for an x-ray examination and blood tests, including an ESR (erythrocyte sedimentation rate) test. The result of the ESR was 108 mm/hour. She again received a diagnosis of rheumatoid arthritis at this hospital, and by this time she was unable to walk at all. In 1975, she came to the orthopedic surgical department of a hospital in Běijīng, where the diagnosis was still rheumatoid arthritis, but the physicians advised her to seek the help of a Chinese medical physician for diagnosis and treatment.

At her initial examination, she was unable to walk, and both ankles were swollen and painful. There was no change in skin color. Both wrists were also swollen and painful, and she could not even hold a bowl level with both hands or hold chopsticks, which made eating very difficult. Because both knees were swollen and severely deformed, she could not walk, and had to be carried wherever she needed to go. Urine was profuse, her bowels were normal, and she had not as yet experienced her menarche.

INSPECTION EXAMINATION

Her development was inadequate, but nutrition seemed normal. Her spirit-mind was clear, but she presented with acute pain and suffering. Both wrist joints were very swollen, and were so painful that the patient did not even want them touched for examination. Both knee joints were very swollen and deformed, and the left knee was in worse condition than the right. The ankle joints were extremely swollen, but the skin color unchanged. She could not walk on her own and was carried to the examination on her father's back. Her tongue fur was thin and white.

LISTENING AND SMELLING EXAMINATION

Her speech was clear, but her voice was slightly low.

PALPATION EXAMINATION

All the above-mentioned joints were extremely swollen and inflexible and could not tolerate touch or pressure; however, they showed no sign of heat and were not red in color. The pulse was stringlike and slippery; the cubit pulse was sunken.

PATTERN IDENTIFICATION

"When the three qì of wind, cold, and dampness arrive in combination, they unite to form impediment." The *Huáng Dì Nèi Jīng* ("The Yellow Emperor's Inner Canon") discusses qì and blood impediment and network vessel obstruction, both of which deprive the joints of luxuriance. With further contraction of wind, cold, and damp evils, cold evil enters the bones, and over time shrinks the sinews and impedes the bones. The patient suffers gradual worsening of lameness and emaciation.

The kidney governs bone, and it governs the feet and knees. Because the condition of the patient was relatively severe in the lower limbs, the cubit pulse was sunken, and the menarche had not arrived, I knew that cold evil had entered the bones and had caused bone impediment and sinew hypertonicity, deformed joints, and blocked menses. After correlating the four examinations, I diagnosed joint-deformity pattern. I developed this pattern name, which refers to impediment pattern with osseous tissue joint deformity. [Editor's note: Dr. Jiao appears to be the first doctor to introduce this pattern name, which has now become commonly used in Chinese medical theory.]

TREATMENT METHOD

Supplement the kidney and dispel cold, quicken blood and free the network vessels, strengthen sinew and bone, and disinhibit the joints.

PRESCRIPTION

bǔ gǔ zhī (补骨脂 psoralea, Psoraleae Fructus) 9 g

gǔ suì bǔ (骨碎补 drynaria, Drynariae Rhizoma) 10 g

shú dì huáng (熟地黄 cooked rehmannia, Rehmanniae Radix Praeparata) 12 g

zhì fù piàn (制附片 sliced processed aconite, Aconiti Radix Lateralis Praeparata Secta) 6.5 g

guì zhī (桂枝 cinnamon twig, Cinnamomi Ramulus) 12 g

chì sháo yào (赤芍药 red peony, Paeoniae Radix Rubra) 9 g

bái sháo yào (白芍药 white peony, Paeoniae Radix Alba) 9 g

zhī mǔ (知母 anemarrhena, Anemarrhenae Rhizoma) 10 g

fáng fēng (防风 saposhnikovia, Saposhnikoviae Radix) 6 g

niú xī (牛膝 achyranthes, Achyranthis Bidentatae Radix) 10 g

cāng zhú (苍术 atractylodes, Atractylodis Rhizoma) 6 g

wēi líng xiān (威灵仙 clematis, Clematidis Radix) 12 g

má huáng (麻黄 ephedra, Ephedrae Herba) 3 g

hóng huā (红花 carthamus, Carthami Flos) 6 g

zhì shān jiǎ (炙山甲 mix-fried pangolin scales, Manis Squama cum Liquido Fricta) 6 g

sōng jié (松节 knotty pine wood, Pini Nodi Lignum) 15 g

qiāng huó (羌活 notopterygium, Notopterygii Rhizoma et Radix) 9 g

dú huó (独活 pubescent angelica, Angelicae Pubescentis Radix) 9 g

tòu gǔ cǎo (透骨草 speranskia/balsam, Speranskiae seu Impatientis Herba) 25 g

yì yǐ rén (薏苡仁 coix, Coicis Semen) 30 g

zhì hǔ gǔ (炙虎骨 mix-fried tiger bone, Tigris Os cum Liquido Frictum) 10 g (decoct separately and then add)

The patient received 10–15 packets of this prescription, to be decocted in water. When these proved effective, I advised her to take more.

FORMULA EXPLANATION

I formulated this prescription from two classic formulas: *hŭ gŭ săn* (Tiger Bone Powder) by Zhāng Jǐng-Yuè and *guì zhī sháo yào zhī mŭ tāng* (Cinnamon Twig, Peony, and Anemarrhena Decoction) from the *Jīn Guì Yào Lüè* ("Essential Prescriptions of the Golden Coffer").

As chief medicinals, *bŭ gŭ zhī* (psoralea), *gŭ suì bŭ* (drynaria), *guì zhī* (cinnamon twig), and *fù piàn* (sliced aconite) supplement the kidney and dissipate cold while dispelling bone wind.

As support medicinals, *shú dì huáng* (cooked rehmannia), *chì sháo yào* (red peony), *bái sháo yào* (white peony), *fáng fēng* (saposhnikovia), *wēi líng xiān* (clematis), *qiāng huó* (notopterygium), and *dú huó* (pubescent angelica) supplement the kidney and nourish blood while quickening stasis and dispelling wind.

As assistant medicinals, *má huáng* (ephedra), *cāng zhú* (atractylodes), *yì yǐ rén* (coix), *sōng jié* (knotty pine wood), and *tòu gŭ căo* (speranskia/balsam) dissipate cold and dispel dampness, and relax the sinews and disinhibit the joints. *Hóng huā* (carthamus) and *chuān shān jiǎ* (pangolin scales) quicken blood and free the network vessels. *Zhī mŭ* (anemarrhena) nourishes yīn and clears heat and prevents *guì zhī* (cinnamon twig) and *fù piàn* (sliced aconite) from engendering heat and damaging yīn liquid.

As courier medicinals, *niú xī* (achyranthes) guides the other medicinals downward to enter the kidney and the knees and feet; *hŭ gŭ* (tiger bone) dispels wind, strengthens the sinews and bone, and guides the medicinals to the kidney. [Editor's note: This case history describes the consistent administration of tiger bone, totaling over 2.5 kilograms over the course of treatment. Beyond the ethical issues involved with the use of tiger bone, its expense alone makes one question whether the medicinal used in this case was actually true tiger bone versus a substitute product.]

The prescription as a whole supplements the kidney and dissipates cold, dispels wind and disinhibits dampness, frees the channels and quickens the network vessels, and strengthens sinews and invigorates bone.

FOLLOWUP TREATMENT

<u>Second visit on August 28, 1977</u>: After taking the initial 10–15 packets of the above-mentioned prescription and having good results, the patient continued with approximately 100 packets in succession. The symptoms were alleviated; there was no swelling or pain in either wrist joint, although the fingers were still crooked and slanted laterally. The left ankle joint had recovered

its normal condition with no swelling or pain. The right ankle joint was still slightly swollen; the right knee joint still appeared very swollen, but was not painful. The patient was now able to walk around on her own accord, and she was able to walk as far as one mile on a level surface and to climb three flights of stairs. Urine and stools were normal, her tongue fur was thin and white, and her pulse was stringlike and slippery with the right side being slightly larger. I added the following medicinals to the above-mentioned prescription:

> *fáng jǐ* (防己 fangji, Stephaniae Tetrandrae Radix) 9 g
>
> *huáng bǎi* (黄柏 phellodendron, Phellodendri Cortex) 6 g
>
> *zé xiè* (泽泻 alisma, Alismatis Rhizoma) 9 g
>
> *xún gǔ fēng* (寻骨风 mollissima, Aristolochiae Mollissimae Herba) 12 g
>
> *quán xiē* (全蝎 scorpion, Scorpio) 6 g
>
> *xì xīn* (细辛 asarum, Asari Herba) 3 g

I then changed the dosage amount of the following medicinals in the first prescription:

> *fáng fēng* (防风 saposhnikovia, Saposhnikoviae Radix) 9 g
>
> *fù piàn* (附片 sliced aconite, Aconiti Radix Lateralis Praeparata Secta) 7.5 g
>
> *niú xī* (牛膝 achyranthes, Achyranthis Bidentatae Radix) 12 g
>
> *cāng zhú* (苍术 atractylodes, Atractylodis Rhizoma) 9 g
>
> *hóng huā* (红花 carthamus, Carthami Flos) 7.5 g
>
> *zhì shān jiǎ* (炙山甲 mix-fried pangolin scales, Manis Squama cum Liquido Fricta) 9 g

The dosage of the remaining medicinals was unchanged. I gave the patient 30 packets of this prescription and again told her to continue with the prescription as long as there was a good effect.

Third visit on November 21, 1978: After more than 100 packets, all the signs and symptoms were alleviated to some extent. She could write again, and she attended school once more. Although both hands were still bent slightly outward, they were mobile and flexible. She was completely without pain and could do her laundry and attend to her daily chores. Her legs were as strong as before her illness, and she could walk the two kilometers to her school. The right ankle joint was no longer swollen, but she still felt pain if she walked for a long time. Her right knee joint was still relatively swollen, and pain recurred when walking on it too much. Her health was restored as before, and her complexion was relatively bright and lustrous. Her essence-spirit had also taken a turn for the better, but the menses still had not arrived. Her tongue fur was normal and her pulse was slightly slippery. Since the above-mentioned prescription had produced the desired effect, I made just a few modifications as follows:

> *guì zhī* (桂枝 cinnamon twig, Cinnamomi Ramulus) 15 g
>
> *gǔ suì bǔ* (骨碎补 drynaria, Drynariae Rhizoma) 10 g
>
> *bǔ gǔ zhī* (补骨脂 psoralea, Psoraleae Fructus) 10 g
>
> *xù duàn* (续断 dipsacus, Dipsaci Radix) 15 g
>
> *sāng jì shēng* (桑寄生 mistletoe, Loranthi seu Visci Ramus) 25 g
>
> *zhì fù piàn* (制附片 sliced processed aconite, Aconiti Radix Lateralis
>   Praeparata Secta) 9 g
>
> *chì sháo yào* (赤芍药 red peony, Paeoniae Radix Rubra) 9 g
>
> *bái sháo yào* (白芍药 white peony, Paeoniae Radix Alba) 9 g
>
> *wēi líng xiān* (威灵仙 clematis, Clematidis Radix) 14 g
>
> *má huáng* (麻黄 ephedra, Ephedrae Herba) 4 g
>
> *fáng fēng* (防风 saposhnikovia, Saposhnikoviae Radix) 8 g
>
> *hóng huā* (红花 carthamus, Carthami Flos) 7 g
>
> *zhì shān jiǎ* (炙山甲 mix-fried pangolin scales, Manis Squama cum
>   Liquido Fricta) 10 g
>
> *sōng jié* (松节 knotty pine wood, Pini Nodi Lignum) 15 g
>
> *qiāng huó* (羌活 notopterygium, Notopterygii Rhizoma et Radix) 10 g
>
> *dú huó* (独活 pubescent angelica, Angelicae Pubescentis Radix) 10 g
>
> *shēng yǐ mǐ* (生苡米 raw coix seed, Coicis Semen Crudum) 30 g
>
> *bái jiè zǐ* (白芥子 white mustard, Sinapis Albae Semen) 5 g
>
> *tòu gǔ cǎo* (透骨草 speranskia/balsam, Speranskiae seu Impatientis
>   Herba) 25 g
>
> *shú dì huáng* (熟地黄 cooked rehmannia, Rehmanniae Radix Praeparata)
>   12 g
>
> *zhī mǔ* (知母 anemarrhena, Anemarrhenae Rhizoma) 10 g
>
> *zé lán* (泽兰 lycopus, Lycopi Herba) 10 g
>
> *niú xī* (牛膝 achyranthes, Achyranthis Bidentatae Radix) 12 g
>
> *cāng zhú* (苍术 atractylodes, Atractylodis Rhizoma) 8 g
>
> *zhì hǔ gǔ* (炙虎骨 mix-fried tiger bone, Tigris Os cum Liquido Frictum)
>   10 g (decoct separately and add later)

I gave the patient 30–50 packets of this prescription to be decocted in water. Afterwards, she was advised to continue with four more packets, in which the ingredients were ground into a fine powder. The dosage was 3 g twice a day with boiled water. This relatively long-term treatment was the optimal approach to consolidate the therapeutic effect and hopefully to eliminate the disease root.

In the winter of 1979 on a follow-up visit with her family in Běijīng, I received a letter from her stating that her condition was very good, and she did not feel any need to visit the city again for diagnosis and treatment.

CASE TWO
HEMILATERAL HEADACHE (ANGIO-NEUROTIC HEADACHE)
偏头痛(血管神经性头痛)

The patient was a 65-year-old female, an employee at the Běijīng bus company. Her initial examination date was August 10, 1980.

CHIEF COMPLAINT

Hemilateral (right-sided) headache for more than a year.

INQUIRY EXAMINATION

Sometimes the headache was mild and sometimes severe. During the last three to four months, her headache had become more severe, with an intermittent onset every day, and the right side of her face and jaw was excruciatingly painful. Several episodes of severe pain occurred daily, so each day she took 8–10 pills of painkillers for the discomfort. In the past, she had visited the local Běijīng hospital, where an x-ray examination had been done by the neurological department, but the results were negative and the x-rays revealed nothing. The diagnosis was angio-neurotic headache, and treatments such as injections, block therapy, and drug medications produced no positive results. Therefore, she requested a diagnosis from a Chinese medical physician.

At the initial examination, in addition to the hemilateral headache, she was also agitated and irascible. Her appetite, urine, and stools were normal. At times she also experienced pain in both temples of the head.

INSPECTION EXAMINATION

Her development was normal, and her nutrition was good. She was slightly overweight, and she presented with acute pain and suffering. Her tongue fur was thin and white.

LISTENING AND SMELLING EXAMINATION

There were no abnormalities in her speech and respiration.

PALPATION EXAMINATION

Examination of the head revealed nothing unusual; the abdomen was soft and flat. Examination also showed that the spleen and liver were normal in size. The pulse was stringlike.

PATTERN IDENTIFICATION

The pulse of the liver channel ascends to both sides of the head. Because the headache was right-sided, the pulse was stringlike, and the patient was agitated, I knew that this was exuberant liver yáng and liver wind harassing the upper body. Wind is a yáng evil; when it endures and is not resolved, it damages yīn liquids. If liver yīn is vacuous, liver yáng becomes effulgent. Thus, yīn and yáng had influenced each other and caused continual hemilateral headache that did not improve. After correlating the pulse with the symptoms, my diagnosis was hemilateral headache caused by yīn vacuity and liver effulgence.

TREATMENT METHOD

Nourish yīn and emolliate the liver while quickening blood and extinguishing wind.

PRESCRIPTION

The patient received 6–10 packets of the following prescription, to be decocted in water:

> *shēng dì huáng* (生地黄 dried rehmannia, Rehmanniae Radix Exsiccata) 12 g
>
> *bái sháo yào* (白芍药 white peony, Paeoniae Radix Alba) 12 g
>
> *shēng shí jué míng* (生石决明 raw abalone shell, Haliotidis Concha Cruda) 30 g (pre-decocted)
>
> *shēng dài zhě shí* (生代赭石 crude hematite, Haematitum Crudum) 30 g (pre-decocted)
>
> *chuān xiōng* (川芎 chuanxiong, Chuanxiong Rhizoma) 9 g
>
> *sū mù* (苏木 sappan, Sappan Lignum) 20 g
>
> *jīng jiè* (荆芥 schizonepeta, Schizonepetae Herba) 9 g
>
> *bái jiāng cán* (白僵蚕 silkworm, Bombyx Batryticatus) 9 g
>
> *wú gōng* (蜈蚣 centipede, Scolopendra) 3 pieces
>
> *bái fù zǐ* (白附子 typhonium, Typhonii Rhizoma) 6 g
>
> *xiāng fù* (香附 cyperus, Cyperi Rhizoma) 10 g
>
> *huáng qín* (黄芩 scutellaria, Scutellariae Radix) 10 g

FORMULA EXPLANATION

As chief medicinals, *shēng dì huáng* (dried rehmannia) and *shēng shí jué míng* (raw abalone shell) simultaneously nourish liver yīn and subdue liver yáng.

As support medicinals, *shēng dài zhě shí* (crude hematite) settles the liver and downbears counterflow; *bái sháo yào* (white peony) nourishes blood and emolliates the liver; *chuān xiōng* (chuanxiong) and *sū mù* (sappan) resolve depression, quicken blood, and free the network vessels; and *bái jiāng cán* (silkworm) and *wú gōng* (centipede) dispel wind and dissipate binds.

As assistant medicinals, *xiāng fù* (cyperus) and *huáng qín* (scutellaria) course the liver and clear heat.

As courier medicinals, *jīng jiè* (schizonepeta), a wind medicinal, guides the other medicinals by its ascending and outthrusting action to the head; and *bái fù zǐ* (typhonium) is effective for dispelling wind from the face and head.

FOLLOWUP TREATMENT

<u>Second visit on August 24</u>: After taking the above-mentioned prescription, the hemilateral headache was clearly alleviated. Basically, she no longer needed to take the painkillers, and only on certain days did she take 1–2 pills, which seemed to be enough. The tongue and pulse signs were the same as before, so I made a few modifications to the prescription and gave her the following:

shēng dì huáng (生地黄 dried rehmannia, Rehmanniae Radix Exsiccata) 15 g

shēng shí jué míng (生石决明 raw abalone shell, Haliotidis Concha Cruda) 30 g (pre-decocted)

bái sháo yào (白芍药 white peony, Paeoniae Radix Alba) 12 g

shēng dài zhě shí (生代赭石 crude hematite, Haematitum Crudum) 30 g (pre-decocted)

chuān xiōng (川芎 chuanxiong, Chuanxiong Rhizoma) 9 g

sū mù (苏木 sappan, Sappan Lignum) 20 g

wú gōng (蜈蚣 centipede, Scolopendra) 3 pieces

bái jiāng cán (白僵蚕 silkworm, Bombyx Batryticatus) 9 g

bái fù zǐ (白附子 typhonium, Typhonii Rhizoma) 6 g

màn jīng zǐ (蔓荆子 vitex, Viticis Fructus) 10 g

xiāng fù (香附 cyperus, Cyperi Rhizoma) 10 g

huáng qín (黄芩 scutellaria, Scutellariae Radix) 10 g

bái zhǐ (白芷 Dahurian angelica, Angelicae Dahuricae Radix) 9 g

fáng fēng (防风 saposhnikovia, Saposhnikoviae Radix) 9 g

The patient received ten packets of this prescription with instructions to take ten more if the first ten proved to be effective.

<u>Third visit on September 14</u>: In the end, the patient took altogether twenty packets of this prescription, and afterwards said that her head was no longer painful. Her teeth also felt light and relaxed without discomfort. (I mention the teeth in passing since they were not particularly painful; the headache had been more severe, so the issue of the teeth was not present in our initial discussion.) She had discontinued the painkillers twenty days ago. Whenever she was greatly fatigued or she walked too far in the mountains, she sometimes

felt a slight discomfort in the temples or on the top of the head, but after rest-ing for awhile, this feeling disappeared. Her tongue fur was normal and her pulse was slightly slippery. She no longer appeared agitated. Therefore, I again modified the prescription and advised her to continue with several more packets, one packet every other day. I gave her 6–20 packets of the following prescription, to be decocted in water:

> *shēng dì huáng* (生地黄 dried rehmannia, Rehmanniae Radix Exsiccata) 15 g
>
> *bái sháo yào* (白芍药 white peony, Paeoniae Radix Alba) 12 g
>
> *shēng shí jué míng* (生石决明 raw abalone shell, Haliotidis Concha Cruda) 30 g (pre-decocted)
>
> *shēng dài zhě shí* (生代赭石 crude hematite, Haematitum Crudum) 30 g (pre-decocted)
>
> *xiāng fù* (香附 cyperus, Cyperi Rhizoma) 10 g
>
> *chǎo huáng qín* (炒黄芩 stir-fried scutellaria, Scutellariae Radix Fricta) 10 g
>
> *jīng jiè* (荆芥 schizonepeta, Schizonepetae Herba) 9 g
>
> *sū mù* (苏木 sappan, Sappan Lignum) 20 g
>
> *quán xiē* (全蝎 scorpion, Scorpio) 8 g
>
> *bái fù zǐ* (白附子 typhonium, Typhonii Rhizoma) 8 g
>
> *màn jīng zǐ* (蔓荆子 vitex, Viticis Fructus) 10 g
>
> *chuān xiōng* (川芎 chuanxiong, Chuanxiong Rhizoma) 10 g
>
> *bái zhǐ* (白芷 Dahurian angelica, Angelicae Dahuricae Radix) 9 g
>
> *bái jiāng cán* (白僵蚕 silkworm, Bombyx Batryticatus) 9 g
>
> *fáng fēng* (防风 saposhnikovia, Saposhnikoviae Radix) 9 g
>
> *gǎo běn* (藁本 Chinese lovage, Ligustici Rhizoma) 5 g

In November 1980 on a follow-up visit, I learned from her son that, after taking the medicinals, the patient never again had any recurrence of a head-ache. Her teeth had also improved, and she was eating once again with pleas-ure. After the third visit, she took one packet of the prescription every other day and never suffered a relapse. After the national holiday, she happily re-turned to her home.

CASE THREE
INTESTINAL WELLING-ABSCESS (ACUTE APPENDICITIS)
肠痈(急性阑尾炎)

The patient, an 18-year-old male student; was initially examined Decem-ber 22, 1969 in the surgical department of a Hénán provincial hospital.

CHIEF COMPLAINT

Abdominal pain for the last two days, gradually becoming more severe.

INQUIRY EXAMINATION

In the morning two days previous, the patient had experienced sudden abdominal pain that started in the area surrounding the umbilicus. The pain had gradually moved to the lower right abdomen and had been accompanied by vomiting. There had been no bowel movement for two days. He was immediately rushed to the emergency room for diagnosis, which was acute appendicitis, and he was admitted to the surgical department hospital ward. He wanted to take Chinese medicinals for his illness, so he had requested a consultation with a Chinese medical physician.

INSPECTION EXAMINATION

His development was normal, his spirit-mind was clear, but he presented with acute abdominal pain. His tongue fur was white.

LISTENING AND SMELLING EXAMINATION

Speech, voice, and respiration were all normal.

PALPATION EXAMINATION

All six pulses were slippery and rapid. The lower abdomen on the right side refused pressure, and while lying on his back, he held his leg flexed and could only slightly extend it.

Western medical examination revealed that the heart and lungs were normal. There was obvious pain at McBurney's point in the lower right abdomen. Rebound pain was (++), psoas muscle reflex was (+), and muscle hypertonicity was (+++). Blood tests: leukocyte count was 13,000/mm^3; differentials were: neutrophil granulocytes 95% and lymphocytes 5%.

PATTERN IDENTIFICATION

The following symptoms were present: the lower right quadrant of the abdomen was painful, the patient flexed his leg while lying down, the tongue fur was white, the pulse was slippery and rapid, and the bowels had not moved for two days. These symptoms indicated accumulation in the intestines and qì-blood congestion and stasis all brewing internally and transforming into heat; this was a pattern of intestinal welling-abscess.

TREATMENT METHOD

Free the intestines and abduct stagnation while quickening the blood and dissipating stasis.

PRESCRIPTION

I gave the patient the following prescription, to urgently decoct and take:

shēng dà huáng (生大黄 raw rhubarb, Rhei Radix et Rhizoma Crudi) 12 g

mǔ dān pí (牡丹皮 moutan, Moutan Cortex) 12 g

dōng guā zǐ (冬瓜子 wax gourd seed, Benincasae Semen) 24 g

lián qiáo (连翘 forsythia, Forsythiae Fructus) 12 g

dāng guī wěi (当归尾 tangkuei tail, Angelicae Sinensis Radicis Extremitas) 12 g

chì sháo yào (赤芍药 red peony, Paeoniae Radix Rubra) 15 g

jīn yín huā (金银花 lonicera, Lonicerae Flos) 12 g

shēng yǐ mǐ (生苡米 raw coix seed, Coicis Semen Crudum) 21 g

huáng qín (黄芩 scutellaria, Scutellariae Radix) 12 g

huáng bǎi (黄柏 phellodendron, Phellodendri Cortex) 12 g

yuán míng fěn (元明粉 refined mirabilite, Natrii Sulfus Exsiccatus) 18 g (divided in half and taken drenched)

This prescription is a modification of *dà huáng mǔ dān pí tāng* (Rhubarb and Moutan Decoction), which is cited in the *Jīn Guì Yào Lüè* ("Essential Prescriptions of the Golden Coffer").

As chief medicinals, *dà huáng* (rhubarb) and *yuán míng fěn* (refined mirabilite) shift intestinal accumulation and stagnation and eliminate congestion.

As support medicinals, *mǔ dān pí* (moutan) and *chì sháo yào* (red peony) quicken stasis and clear heat. *Dōng guā zǐ* (wax gourd seed) disinhibits the intestines and eliminates congestion; it is an important medicinal in the treatment of intestinal welling-abscess. *Dāng guī wěi* (tangkuei tail) frees the channels and quickens blood.

As assistant medicinals, *jīn yín huā* (lonicera) and *lián qiáo* (forsythia) clear heat and resolve toxins. *Huáng qín* (scutellaria) clears heat and cools blood, and *yì yǐ rén* (coix) disinhibits dampness and expels pus.

As the courier, *huáng bǎi* (phellodendron) clears lower burner damp-heat.

FOLLOWUP TREATMENT

Second visit on December 23: The patient took the prescription, and afterwards he had diarrhea seven or eight times. The lower right quadrant abdominal pain was alleviated, and he could get up from bed and walk around. When hand pressure was applied to the lower right quadrant, there was some tenderness, but rebound pain was not present. The tongue fur was white and the pulse stringlike and rapid. Using the above-mentioned prescription, I removed *yuán míng fěn* (refined mirabilite) and changed the dosage of *shēng dà huáng* (raw rhubarb) to 9 grams. I added 30 grams of *bài jiàng cǎo* (patrinia) and gave the patient another packet.

Third visit on December 24: The patient was not aware of any lower right quadrant abdominal pain, the pressure pain and tenderness had improved even further, and rebound pain tested at (+). His blood tests taken the day before revealed the following results: leukocytes 6,800/mm^3, and differentials of 80% for neutrophil granulocytes and 20% for lymphocytes. The tongue and pulse signs were the same as before; therefore, I again modified the previous prescription. I gave the patient two packets of the following, to be decocted in water:

shēng dà huáng (生大黄 raw rhubarb, Rhei Radix et Rhizoma Crudi) 12 g

mǔ dān pí (牡丹皮 moutan, Moutan Cortex) 12 g

lián qiáo (连翘 forsythia, Forsythiae Fructus) 12 g

dōng guā zǐ (冬瓜子 wax gourd seed, Benincasae Semen) 30 g (crushed)

huáng qín (黄芩 scutellaria, Scutellariae Radix) 12 g

chì sháo yào (赤芍药 red peony, Paeoniae Radix Rubra) 21 g

dāng guī wěi (当归尾 tangkuei tail, Angelicae Sinensis Radicis Extremitas) 12 g

táo rén (桃仁 peach kernel, Persicae Semen) 9 g

shēng yǐ mǐ (生苡米 raw coix seed, Coicis Semen Crudum) 30 g

huáng bǎi (黄柏 phellodendron, Phellodendri Cortex) 12 g

yuán míng fěn (元明粉 refined mirabilite, Natrii Sulfus Exsiccatus) 9 g
    (divided in half and taken drenched)

Fourth visit on December 25: The patient took three doses of the medicinals that he received yesterday and half a packet still remained. He experienced no pain in the lower right quadrant. He frequently got out of bed to walk around in his room, and he was completely without any sign of pain. His bowels moved once a day. The lower right quadrant abdominal wall was soft and without any sign of tenderness. The patient felt mild pain only when the heaviest pressure was applied. The tongue fur was thin and white and the pulse was slightly sunken and slippery. Again, I modified the prescription and put together two packets of the following:

shēng dà huáng (生大黄 raw rhubarb, Rhei Radix et Rhizoma Crudi) 9 g

mǔ dān pí (牡丹皮 moutan, Moutan Cortex) 9 g

jīn yín huā (金银花 lonicera, Lonicerae Flos) 12 g

lián qiáo (连翘 forsythia, Forsythiae Fructus) 12 g

dōng guā zǐ (冬瓜子 wax gourd seed, Benincasae Semen) 24 g (crushed)

huáng qín (黄芩 scutellaria, Scutellariae Radix) 12 g

dāng guī (当归 Chinese angelica, Angelicae Sinensis Radix) 9 g

chì sháo yào (赤芍药 red peony, Paeoniae Radix Rubra) 15 g

bái sháo yào (白芍药 white peony, Paeoniae Radix Alba) 15 g

shēng yǐ mǐ (生苡米 raw coix seed, Coicis Semen Crudum) 30 g

yán hú suǒ (延胡索 corydalis, Corydalis Rhizoma) 9 g

chǎo chuān liàn zǐ (炒川楝子 stir-fried toosendan, Toosendan Fructus
   Frictus) 9 g

jiāo bīng láng (焦槟榔 scorch-fried areca, Arecae Semen Ustum) 9 g

At the end of December, I went to the surgical department hospital ward for a follow-up examination with him, but the nurse told me that the patient had fully recovered and had been already discharged two or three days ago.

CASE FOUR

LATENT DAMP-HEAT IN THE LESSER YÁNG (*SHÀO YÁNG*) (FEVER, ETIOLOGY UNKNOWN)

湿热伏于少阳 （发热待查）

The patient, a 48-year-old female, was a worker in a textile factory in the town of Dānchéng in Hénán Province. Her initial examination date was May 31, 1980.

CHIEF COMPLAINT

A fever that had continued for 50 days.

INQUIRY EXAMINATION

In the beginning of April 1980, the patient had suddenly experienced the onset of a high fever; her body temperature had reached as high as 39°C and she had a sore throat. During the day, her body temperature dropped and then in the evening it would rise again. She had gone for a diagnosis to a small clinic affiliated with the factory. There she had had diagnostic tests performed that revealed the following: erythrocyte sedimentation rate (ESR) 80mm/hour and normal leukocyte count (WBC). The lymph nodes were enlarged on the left side of her neck, and the doctors had suspected tuberculosis of the lymph nodes. She was treated with aspirin and streptomycin, and the fever dropped to 37.8–38.5°C, but still would not abate. Then, in the beginning of May, she had been admitted to the hospital for diagnosis and treatment. At that time, she had received intramuscular penicillin and streptomycin along with orally administered erythromycin, aspirin, and hydrocortisone. Yet her body temperature still was not under control, and the ESR had risen to 102 mm/hour.

The blood tests also revealed hemoglobin 9.3 gm and leukocytes 11,400/mm^3. The differentials were neutrophil granulocytes 64%, lymphocytes 36%, and anti-streptolysin O test was 1:625. There was no evidence of lupus erythematosus. A routine urinalysis had shown 7–8 red blood cells and

5–7 white blood cells. The diagnostic tests for liver function were normal, as were the cardio-pulmonary tests. Etiology of the disease could not be definitely diagnosed, and at the end of May 1980, she was discharged from the hospital with a diagnosis of "fever, etiology unknown." On May 31, 1980, she arrived at my clinic and requested a diagnosis.

At this time, she had a daily fever; her body temperature dropped to 37.8–38.5°C during the day and then would rise in the evening to 38.5–39°C. Just before the onset of the fever, she first experienced fear of cold, and then the fever followed very quickly. She also had symptoms of a bitter taste in the mouth, nausea with a desire to vomit, sweating with an aversion to wind, chest oppression, loss of appetite, and dry stool.

INSPECTION EXAMINATION

Her development and nutrition were normal, but she presented with a high fever. Her mind was clear and she appeared physically fit. Her tongue fur was thick, slimy, and yellow.

LISTENING AND SMELLING EXAMINATION

Her speech and voice were slightly low, but respiration was normal. Auscultation of both lungs was negative.

PALPATION EXAMINATION

Lymph nodes were enlarged on the left side of the neck, and there was pressure pain. The liver and spleen were normal in size, but her body temperature was 38.5°C. The right pulse was slippery, and the left was sunken, slippery, and fine.

PATTERN IDENTIFICATION

Latent evil in the lesser yáng (shào yáng) and latent dampness in the membrane source was indicated by cold and heat occurring at set periods of time that was still unresolved after a month, thick and slimy tongue fur, a slippery pulse, poor appetite, chest oppression, and nausea with a desire to vomit. The swollen, painful nodulations on the left side of the laryngeal prominence (Adam's apple) indicated damp-heat brewing internally and engendering toxin that gathered and did not dissipate. By comprehensively correlating the pulse and the symptoms, I diagnosed latent damp-heat in the lesser yáng.

TREATMENT METHOD

Harmonize and resolve the lesser yáng while transforming dampness and clearing heat.

PRESCRIPTION

I modified two formulas according to the pattern: *chái hú guì zhī tāng* (Bupleurum and Cinnamon Twig Decoction) and *bái hǔ tāng* (White Tiger Decoction). I gave the patient three packets to decoct in water:

> *chái hú* (柴胡 bupleurum, Bupleuri Radix) 15 g
>
> *huáng qín* (黄芩 scutellaria, Scutellariae Radix) 10 g
>
> *bàn xià* (半夏 pinellia, Pinelliae Rhizoma) 10 g
>
> *dǎng shēn* (党参 codonopsis, Codonopsis Radix) 10 g
>
> *guì zhī* (桂枝 cinnamon twig, Cinnamomi Ramulus) 10 g
>
> *bái sháo yào* (白芍药 white peony, Paeoniae Radix Alba) 10 g
>
> *jiāo bīng láng* (焦槟榔 scorch-fried areca, Arecae Semen Ustum) 10 g
>
> *cǎo guǒ* (草果 tsaoko, Tsaoko Fructus) 10 g
>
> *shēng shí gāo* (生石膏 raw gypsum, Gypsum Crudum) 40 g (pre-decocted)
>
> *zhī mǔ* (知母 anemarrhena, Anemarrhenae Rhizoma) 10 g
>
> *shēng gān cǎo* (生甘草 raw licorice, Glycyrrhizae Radix Cruda) 3 g
>
> *gēng mǐ* (粳米 non-glutinous rice, Oryzae Semen) 12 g

FORMULA EXPLANATION

The chief formula is *chái hú guì zhī tāng* (Bupleurum and Cinnamon Twig Decoction) because it harmonizes and resolves latent evil in half exterior half interior conditions.

The assistant formula is *bái hǔ tāng* (White Tiger Decoction), which clears heat evil that has spread through the entire body.

As courier medicinals, *bīng láng* (areca) and *cǎo guǒ* (tsaoko) transform latent damp turbidity in the membrane source.

FOLLOWUP TREATMENT

Second visit on June 3: The fever had been alleviated. The patient felt that her body temperature was reduced in the afternoon and in the evening. The spontaneous sweating had stopped and alternating cold and heat had abated. The tongue fur was yellow and the center of the tongue was thick and slimy; the right pulse was slightly slippery and the left was sunken and slippery. The pulse was larger on the right side. The medicinals proved appropriate, and I made only a few modifications to the prescription. I gave the patient four packets of the following, to be decocted in water:

> *chái hú* (柴胡 bupleurum, Bupleuri Radix) 18 g
>
> *huáng qín* (黄芩 scutellaria, Scutellariae Radix) 10 g
>
> *bàn xià* (半夏 pinellia, Pinelliae Rhizoma) 10 g

dǎng shēn (党参 codonopsis, Codonopsis Radix) 6 g

cǎo guǒ (草果 tsaoko, Tsaoko Fructus) 12 g

xuán shēn (玄参 scrophularia, Scrophulariae Radix) 15 g

zǎo xiū (蚤休 paris, Paridis Rhizoma) 12 g

shēng shí gāo (生石膏 raw gypsum, Gypsum Crudum) 30 g (pre-
decocted)

pèi lán (佩兰 eupatorium, Eupatorii Herba) 10 g

qīng hāo (青蒿 sweet wormwood, Artemisiae Annuae Herba) 15 g

zhī mǔ (知母 anemarrhena, Anemarrhenae Rhizoma) 10 g

shēng gān cǎo (生甘草 raw licorice, Glycyrrhizae Radix Cruda) 3 g

gēng mǐ (粳米 non-glutinous rice, Oryzae Semen) 10 g

Third visit on June 6: In the last three days, the patient did not experience
a fever at all during the day, but she still had a low-grade fever (37.1–37.4°C)
in the evening after meals. Her sleeping had improved, the nausea was eliminated, and her appetite was good. The tongue fur was yellow, and the thick,
slimy fur on the center of the tongue had gradually receded. The pulse was
sunken and slippery, but had become more tranquil and slow. Again, I modified the prescription and gave her five packets of the following:

chái hú (柴胡 bupleurum, Bupleuri Radix) 15 g

huáng qín (黄芩 scutellaria, Scutellariae Radix) 10 g

jiāo bīng láng (焦槟榔 scorch-fried areca, Arecae Semen Ustum) 10 g

bàn xià (半夏 pinellia, Pinelliae Rhizoma) 10 g

dǎng shēn (党参 codonopsis, Codonopsis Radix) 6 g

cǎo dòu kòu (草豆蔻 Katsumada's galangal seed, Alpiniae Katsumadai
Semen) 6 g

cǎo guǒ (草果 tsaoko, Tsaoko Fructus) 10 g

xuán shēn (玄参 scrophularia, Scrophulariae Radix) 15 g

zǎo xiū (蚤休 paris, Paridis Rhizoma) 12 g

qīng hāo (青蒿 sweet wormwood, Artemisiae Annuae Herba) 15 g

pèi lán (佩兰 eupatorium, Eupatorii Herba) 10 g

dì gǔ pí (地骨皮 lycium root bark, Lycii Cortex) 9 g

shēng gān cǎo (生甘草 raw licorice, Glycyrrhizae Radix Cruda) 3 g

Fourth visit on June 10: The patient had no fever at all, her body temperature was normal, her complexion was lustrous, and her essence-spirit had improved. She was eating and drinking normally; however, she still had some fatigue. The tongue was slightly dark and the center root area was slightly yellow and thick, so I once again modified the prescription for her as follows and
gave her four packets, to be decocted in water:

chái hú (柴胡 bupleurum, Bupleuri Radix) 15 g

huáng qín (黄芩 scutellaria, Scutellariae Radix) 10 g

bàn xià (半夏 pinellia, Pinelliae Rhizoma) 10 g

dǎng shēn (党参 codonopsis, Codonopsis Radix) 9 g

cǎo guǒ (草果 tsaoko, Tsaoko Fructus) 10 g

cǎo dòu kòu (草豆蔻 Katsumada's galangal seed, Alpiniae Katsumadai
    Semen) 8 g

bīng láng (槟榔 areca, Arecae Semen) 10 g

qīng hāo (青蒿 sweet wormwood, Artemisiae Annuae Herba) 15 g

huò xiāng (藿香 patchouli, Pogostemonis Herba) 10 g

xuán shēn (玄参 scrophularia, Scrophulariae Radix) 20 g

zǎo xiū (蚤休 paris, Paridis Rhizoma) 12 g

dì gǔ pí (地骨皮 lycium root bark, Lycii Cortex) 10 g

Fifth visit on June 17: The patient's condition had stabilized and her body temperature remained normal. Her neck was no longer painful, and the swollen lymph node on the left side had disappeared; there was no swelling and no pain. Whenever she was active, she still felt tired and physically weak. The tongue was slightly dark and the sides were mildly spotted with stasis macules, but the tongue fur had become thin and white. The pulse was harmonious, moderate, and slightly sunken; both pulses were essentially identical. So, I added 10 grams of *hóng huā* (carthamus) to the prescription and formulated twelve more packets for her.

Sixth visit on July 4: Her complexion was lustrous and her essence-spirit was good. She felt that her physical strength was gradually improving. Her tongue and pulse had not changed remarkably, and I formulated seven more packets of the prescription for her.

Seventh visit on July 15: The fever had not returned. Her complexion was lustrous and her essence-spirit was good. She had no subjective symptoms at all, and her tongue fur was thin and white with only a slight yellow color in the center. The pulse was sunken and slightly stringlike. The exterior and interior were harmonized and resolved, and consequently, she had fully recovered from the fever. Moreover, she was preparing in a few days to return to her home in Dānchéng.

CASE FIVE
HEMILATERAL HEADACHE (CERVICAL SPONDYLOSIS)
偏头痛(颈椎病)

The patient was a 66-year-old retired man who lived on the third floor of a residential unit in Běijīng. His initial examination date was April 15, 1980.

CHIEF COMPLAINT

Hemilateral headache on the left side for the last seven to eight days.

INQUIRY EXAMINATION

During the week prior to the initial examination, the patient felt that his neck had become stiff. He had experienced a throbbing left-sided hemilateral headache. The pain was quite severe, and he could not sleep at night because of it. He was also dizzy. He had visited a local hospital for a head x-ray examination, had received a diagnosis of "cervical spondylosis and hyperosteogeny," and had received intramuscular injections of vitamins B₁ and B₁₂, but the treatment was ineffective. In the last two days, the pain had become more severe. especially at night, so the patient had returned to the hospital emergency room for consultation. He again had received medications and injections to relieve pain, but without success. Consequently, he arrived at my clinic and requested a consultation and diagnosis. In addition to the symptoms already mentioned, he also was constipated; his bowels had not moved for two days.

INSPECTION EXAMINATION

His development and nutrition were normal. He presented with acute pain and suffering, his tongue fur was yellow, and there were stasis macules present on the tongue body.

LISTENING AND SMELLING EXAMINATION

His speech and respiration were normal.

PALPATION EXAMINATION

The head and neck showed no abnormalities, and the pulse was stringlike.

PATTERN IDENTIFICATION

The foot lesser yáng gallbladder channel travels bilaterally to the head, and the liver and gallbladder stand in interior-exterior relationship. Because the onset of the left-sided headache was very rapid, the pain was throbbing, and the pulse was stringlike, I knew that the illness was caused by liver depression engendering wind and liver wind harassing the upper body. The liver governs wind. Liver wind harassed the upper body, depressing qì and blood and obstructing the network vessels; thus, headache and dizziness occurred. Since there were stasis macules on the tongue body, I knew that depression had also affected the blood aspect. The neck was stiff and had lost its flexibility, and all six pulses were stringlike; thus, exterior wind had simultaneously assailed the greater yáng (*tài yáng*) and lesser yáng (*shào yáng*) channels, and interior-exterior combined evil was present. A stringlike pulse is the chief indicator of wind, of pain, and of liver and gallbladder channel diseases. After correlating the pulse with the symptoms, I diagnosed hemilateral headache caused by liver wind harassing the upper body, exterior wind assailing the network vessels, and blood stasis in the channels and network vessels.

TREATMENT METHOD

Dispel wind and soothe the liver while quickening stasis and freeing the network vessels, assisted by moistening the intestines.

PRESCRIPTION

jīng jiè (荆芥 schizonepeta, Schizonepetae Herba) 10 g

fáng fēng (防风 saposhnikovia, Saposhnikoviae Radix) 10 g

màn jīng zǐ (蔓荆子 vitex, Viticis Fructus) 10 g

chuān xiōng (川芎 chuanxiong, Chuanxiong Rhizoma) 12 g

dāng guī (当归 Chinese angelica, Angelicae Sinensis Radix) 10 g

hóng huā (红花 carthamus, Carthami Flos) 10 g

xià kū cǎo (夏枯草 prunella, Prunellae Spica) 12 g

dān shēn (丹参 salvia, Salviae Miltiorrhizae Radix) 12 g

jú huā (菊花 chrysanthemum, Chrysanthemi Flos) 10 g

bái jí lí (白蒺藜 tribulus, Tribuli Fructus) 10 g

jiǔ dà huáng (酒大黄 wine-processed rhubarb, Rhei Radix et Rhizoma cum Vino Preparati) 4 g

guā lóu (栝楼 trichosanthes, Trichosanthis Fructus) 30 g

qiāng huó (羌活 notopterygium, Notopterygii Rhizoma et Radix) 10 g

I prescribed five packets for the patient and advised him to take the medicinals three times a day, half a packet each time, so that he would take three packets in two days.

FORMULA EXPLANATION

This prescription is a modification of the formula *chuān xiōng chá tiáo sǎn* (Tea-Blended Chuanxiong Powder). As chief medicinals, *chuān xiōng* (chuanxiong) dissipates depression and quickens blood, and soothes the liver and dispels wind. *Jīng jiè* (schizonepeta) and *fáng fēng* (saposhnikovia) course wind and dissipate evil, while simultaneously guiding medicinals upward to the head.

As support medicinals, *màn jīng zǐ* (vitex) dispels liver and gallbladder wind and wind evil in the lesser yáng; *jú huā* (chrysanthemum) and *bái jí lí* (tribulus) dispel liver wind; and *dāng guī* (Chinese angelica), *hóng huā* (carthamus), and *dān shēn* (salvia) nourish and quicken blood.

As assistant medicinals, *qiāng huó* (notopterygium) dispels wind in the greater yáng channels; *guā lóu* (trichosanthes) loosens the chest and moistens the intestines; and *jiǔ dà huáng* (wine-processed rhubarb) removes the old and institutes the new.

As the courier medicinal, *xià kū cǎo* (prunella) enters the liver channel, calms the liver, and dissipates depression, thereby relieving pain.

FOLLOWUP TREATMENT

<u>Second visit on April 18</u>: The headache and dizziness were alleviated, the bowels were free and regular, and his neck was as flexible as before the illness. For the last two weeks, his lower limbs had been weak and without strength. The tongue body was slightly dark and still had stasis macules, and the pulse was sunken and stringlike. The medicinals had already taken effect, and I again gave him six packets with the following modifications:

I removed *jiǔ dà huáng* (wine-processed rhubarb), *jú huā* (chrysanthemum), and *dāng guī* (Chinese angelica) from the prescription and added:

> *dǎn xīng* (胆星 bile arisaema, Arisaema cum Bile) 10 g
>
> *sāng jì shēng* (桑寄生 mistletoe, Loranthi seu Visci Ramus) 30 g
>
> *xù duàn* (续断 dipsacus, Dipsaci Radix) 15 g
>
> *gé gēn* (葛根 pueraria, Puerariae Radix) 12 g

<u>Third visit on April 25</u>: The hemilateral headache had been eliminated. One night when he slept for more than four hours, he noticed upon awakening that his neck was again slightly stiff. The tongue body was dark and stasis macules were still present. The pulse was slightly stringlike and the inch pulse was slightly slippery. The bowels were now normal. I modified the prescription and gave him seven packets of the following:

> *jīng jiè suì* (荆芥穗 schizonepeta spike, Schizonepetae Flos) 10 g
>
> *chuān xiōng* (川芎 chuanxiong, Chuanxiong Rhizoma) 12 g
>
> *fáng fēng* (防风 saposhnikovia, Saposhnikoviae Radix) 10 g
>
> *màn jīng zǐ* (蔓荆子 vitex, Viticis Fructus) 10 g
>
> *gé gēn* (葛根 pueraria, Puerariae Radix) 15 g
>
> *guì zhī* (桂枝 cinnamon twig, Cinnamomi Ramulus) 9 g
>
> *xù duàn* (续断 dipsacus, Dipsaci Radix) 15 g
>
> *sāng jì shēng* (桑寄生 mistletoe, Loranthi seu Visci Ramus) 20 g
>
> *xià kū cǎo* (夏枯草 prunella, Prunellae Spica) 12 g
>
> *dǎn xīng* (胆星 bile arisaema, Arisaema cum Bile) 10 g
>
> *qiāng huó* (羌活 notopterygium, Notopterygii Rhizoma et Radix) 10 g
>
> *dāng guī* (当归 Chinese angelica, Angelicae Sinensis Radix) 10 g
>
> *hóng huā* (红花 carthamus, Carthami Flos) 10 g

<u>Fourth visit on May 4</u>: He had not had a headache throughout this entire time of treatment. Two days before this visit, the patient had received a haircut. After washing his hair in cold water, he noticed a slight feeling of discomfort on the left side of his head, but no headache occurred. His neck was

mobile and flexible, urine and stools were normal, and he was sleeping well. The tongue body was less dark and the stasis macules appeared only on the left side. The pulse was stringlike and slippery, and the left was larger than the right. However, he still felt that he had weakness in both legs, and in passing he informed me of his scrotal dampness and told me that he wished this condition treated as well. He requested that I take this symptom into account when making up the prescription, so I included the principle of *sān miào wán* (Mysterious Three Pill) with modifications and gave him six packets of the following:

> *jīng jiè suì* (荆芥穗 schizonepeta spike, Schizonepetae Flos) 10 g
> *chuān xiōng* (川芎 chuanxiong, Chuanxiong Rhizoma) 6 g
> *màn jīng zǐ* (蔓荆子 vitex, Viticis Fructus) 10 g
> *fáng fēng* (防风 saposhnikovia, Saposhnikoviae Radix) 10 g
> *sāng jì shēng* (桑寄生 mistletoe, Loranthi seu Visci Ramus) 30 g
> *xù duàn* (续断 dipsacus, Dipsaci Radix) 15 g
> *chǎo huáng bǎi* (炒黄柏 stir-fried phellodendron, Phellodendri Cortex Frictus) 9 g
> *cāng zhú* (苍朮 atractylodes, Atractylodis Rhizoma) 9 g
> *niú xī* (牛膝 achyranthes, Achyranthis Bidentatae Radix) 12 g
> *gé gēn* (葛根 pueraria, Puerariae Radix) 15 g
> *guì zhī* (桂枝 cinnamon twig, Cinnamomi Ramulus) 9 g
> *qiāng huó* (羌活 notopterygium, Notopterygii Rhizoma et Radix) 10 g
> *xià kū cǎo* (夏枯草 prunella, Prunellae Spica) 10 g
> *hóng huā* (红花 carthamus, Carthami Flos) 10 g

Fifth visit on May 13: The patient had just been to the hospital for x-rays on his neck, and the results revealed that hyperosteogeny was evident in C4 to C7. Yet, it appeared that the headache had not recurred at all, and his neck remained mobile and flexible without any abnormal sensations. His essence-spirit was good; his complexion was lustrous. Therefore, I prepared six more packets for him to consolidate the therapeutic effect.

Follow-up visit on March 5, 1981: I learned that the patient's headache had never recurred, and his condition was very good indeed.

EMPIRICAL KNOWLEDGE

Discussion of several important academic perspectives

In learning how to apply pattern identification to determine treatment, you should first learn good examples of Chinese medical theories. Moreover, within Chinese medical theories are several important academic perspectives, and knowledge of these perspectives is required to deeply understand and grasp the principle of pattern identification to determine treatment. Here I present several perspectives based on my experience.

The organic concept of the human body

The most comprehensive characteristic of Chinese medical theory is the organic concept of the human body. This concept permeates the entire doctrine of yīn and yáng, qì and blood, viscera and bowels, and channels and network vessels. It unites into one integral whole the separate aspects of physiology and pathology, interior-exterior and upper-lower, structure and function, essence-spirit and substance, and organism and environment. For instance, in the interior, the "heart" resides in the chest, moves the construction qì, and governs blood. On the exterior, its bloom is in the face, and the hair on the head is the surplus of blood. In the upper body, the sprout or orifice of the heart is the tongue, and the heart governs the spirit-light and has a connection to the brain. In the lower body, the heart and small intestines stand in interior-exterior relationship, and the heart channel descends to net the small intestine. As for the essence-spirit, the heart stores the spirit, and joy damages the heart. As for substance, Míng dynasty physician Lǐ Chān said, "The shape of the heart is like an unopened lotus blossom." Its color is red and it governs blood vessels. Concerning the physiology of the heart, it moves blood and stores the spirit. All painful and itching sores are pathologies that belong to the heart.

Lastly, concerning the relationship between the organism and the climate, the pulse is stringlike in spring, surging in summer, downy in autumn, and stone-like in winter. All five of the viscera engage in analogies of their own, but I will not list them here. Moreover, you must be able to integrate the organism and its environment. For example, you should know how to identify when cold damages the kidney, dampness damages the spleen, heat damages the heart, or dryness damages the lung. You should understand why through-flux diarrhea improves in late summer and why wind malaria improves in autumn. Such a perspective reflects a simple organic concept of the human body; thus, it effectively guides the prevention and treatment of disease and directly addresses the improvement of health and the prevention of aging.

In clinic, when we encounter certain physical symptoms, essence-spirit symptoms, or visceral and bowel symptoms, we must take into consideration all aspects of physiology and pathology on the basis of an organic conception of the human body, and then conduct a detailed pattern identification. We should always understand the physical or local symptoms as a part of the greater whole. Just as the *Huáng Dì Nèi Jīng* ("The Yellow Emperor's Inner Canon") states:

> "Palpate the movement of the pulse and perceive its bright essence, observe the five colors, contemplate the five viscera for surplus or insufficiency and the six bowels for strength or weakness, consider exuberance and debilitation, and henceforth, by threes and fives [the pulse], distinguish life and death."

First, consider Case 1 in this chapter. The patient suffered joint deformity and inability to walk, but when I considered her case holistically, I thought that she suffered cold damage to the kidneys. Since the kidney governs bone and the lower burner, when yīn cold evil invaded the kidney, it led to sinew hypertonicity, bone impediment, and joint deformation. Therefore, I did not directly treat the joints alone, but instead I took a holistic approach and used the treatment method to supplement kidney and dissipate cold and to nourish blood and dispel wind. This approach treated the root. To treat the tip, I used the method of disinhibiting dampness and quickening blood to free and disinhibit the joints. Consequently, both root and tip of the disease were treated effectively.

In Case 3, I was not especially focused on the appendicitis itself, but rather on the Chinese medical theory. I thought that the intestines should be free and smooth. The large and small intestines belong to the six bowels, and the six bowels fulfill their purposes when there is free flow. Yet in this case, the six bowels were obstructed, and the intestinal pathway was congested and depressed with brewing and binding evil transforming into heat. Thus, conveyance through the intestines was inhibited, and binding congestion formed the abscess. To unblock the congestion, I chose a blood-cooling toxin-resolving precipitation method to dissipate the abscess. The disease was located in one particular area of the body, but my treatment addressed the body holistically; thus, the patient recovered very quickly.

For Case 2, the patient with the hemilateral headache, I did not just treat the headache symptoms, but rather I used the method of treating the liver by nourishing blood and emolliating the liver, settling and subduing liver yáng, and quickening blood and extinguishing wind. This achieved a successful recovery.

Although Case 5 was also a patient suffering from hemilateral headache, the treatment method was different from the one used in Case 2. For Case 5, I used the method of dispelling wind and regulating the liver while freeing the bowel and moistening the intestines, and the results were very good. This is the principle of treating upper body disease through the lower body. Fundamentally, both cases were approached with holistic considerations, so even though both patients suffered from hemilateral headaches, I used different methods of treatment, and both patients experienced very good results.

The patient in Case 4 suffered from a long-term fever that would not abate. A special characteristic of this case was the inability of any method to reduce the fever by itself. But after holistic consideration, I diagnosed evil lodged in the lesser yáng channel and subsequently used a treatment method to harmonize and resolve the lesser yáng and to transform dampness and clear heat. This method improved the patient's condition.

In summary of this section, everyone should understand the organic concept of the human body, for this is a very important concept in Chinese medical theory for learning and utilizing the principles of pattern identification to determine treatment. Constant attention to this point will ensure a higher level of proficiency in pattern identification to determine treatment.

The concept of restraining and engendering transformation

Chinese medical science applies the doctrine of yīn-yáng and five phases, and of five movements and six qì; this doctrine holds the viewpoint that in the world all matter is unceasingly in the process of movement and change. The biological phenomena of the human body is considered no differently and is, as all matter, also unceasingly in the process of movement and change. The human body and its environment influence each other in this process, and physiology and pathology are constantly struggling with each other in the process of change. This concept is explained in the *Huáng Dì Nèi Jīng* ("The Yellow Emperor's Inner Canon"):

> "The life of things comes about by transformation; the end of things comes from transmutation. Transmutation and transformation weaken each other and are the cause of success or failure."

> "The human conditions of life and death are engendered by movement, and since movement is endless, change occurs."

> Where there is no inward and outward movement, there is no birth, growth, prime, aging, and death; where there is no upward movement or downward movement, there is no growth, transformation, withdrawal, and storage. Therefore, without inward and outward movements, and ascending and descending movements, there is nothing. Transformations are great and small; durations of time may be near or far, but these are the four movements. They are valuable and should be constantly safeguarded, for where there is perversity, disaster follows!"

In the *Huáng Dì Nèi Jīng* ("The Yellow Emperor's Inner Canon"), there is also this passage from the chapter entitled *Tiān Yuán Jì Dà Lùn* ("Great Treatise on the Origins and Principles of Heaven"):

> "When movement and tranquility summon each other, when ascension and descension check each other, when yīn and yang balance each other, then transmutation is engendered."

Within the human body, these factors automatically engender and resolve all contradictory physical movements. Chinese medical theory holds the view that these physical movements are alone responsible for the mechanism of mutual counterbalance and mutual cooperation and regulation. These movements are also responsible for the preservation of normal transmutation and transformation and for the maintenance of developmental balance. This idea is expressed in the *Huáng Dì Nèi Jīng* ("The Yellow Emperor's Inner Canon") as "when excess causes harm, then preventing its development brings order," and "when yīn is calm and yáng is sound, then the essence-spirit is balanced." I agree with the concept of continuous physical movement of transmutation and transformation and call this concept "restraining and engendering transformation."

On the basis of restraining and engendering transformation, when conducting pattern identification, emphasis is placed particularly on the transformational shifts of the disease pattern. Cold damage greater yáng disease, for instance, may enter the lesser yáng or yáng brightness, or it may pass to the lesser yīn or greater yīn. A defense aspect pattern of warm disease may transform into a qì aspect pattern; a construction aspect pattern may transform from a qì aspect pattern and may sometimes quickly take an abnormal passage to the pericardium. The determination of treatment proceeds also from these ideas and holds the view that "when treating liver disease, you should know that the liver may pass its disease to the spleen, so the treatment should first replenish the spleen." Thus:

> "On the first day of cold damage, greater yáng contracts [the disease]. If the pulse is tranquil, this means no passage, but if there is agitation and vexation, a strong desire to vomit, and a rapid, urgent pulse, then passage has occurred."

> "If there is thirst after taking *xiǎo chái hú tāng* (Minor Bupleurum Decoction), then the disease belongs to the yáng brightness; use [the appropriate] method to treat it."

I believe that disease patterns are continuously moving and changing. Therefore, I maintain the following principles:

"Yáng disease is treated through yīn; yīn disease is treated through yáng."

"Vacuity is treated by supplementing the mother; repletion is treated by draining the child."

"All diseases of heat are treated with cold; apply treatment through yīn. All diseases of cold are treated with heat; apply treatment through yáng."

"Invigorate the governor of water to restrain the brilliance of yáng; boost the source of fire to disperse the shroud of yīn."

"Keep to the pathomechanisms; each belongs to a category. If something exists, seek why; if something does not exist, question it. Seek these and use the appropriate treatment for exuberance or vacuity. First determine the five overcomings; then course, regulate, and harmonize qì and blood."

In this chapter, at the time of the initial examination in Case 3, evil and right qì were in a fierce struggle. The patient suffered from abdominal pain, constipation, and vomiting, so it was important to use a prescription to urgently precipitate and to disperse and eliminate congestion. By the time of the second examination, the symptoms had clearly improved, the bowels were smooth, and abdominal pain was alleviated. Therefore, I reduced the dosage for *dà huáng* (rhubarb) and *yuán míng fěn* (refined mirabilite). The abdomen was no longer painful by the final visit, and all the symptoms had improved; therefore, I completely eliminated *yuán míng fěn* from the prescription because it is a salty, cold medicinal that induces draining precipitation.

The patient in Case 1, however, suffered a chronic illness of relatively long duration, and his pattern had transformed slowly over time. Therefore, I treated him also according to the particular characteristics of his illness, by giving him a prescription appropriately designed to address the transformed patterns. The results were good.

In summary, when studying and applying the principle of pattern identification to determine treatment, it is important at all times to focus on the idea of "restraining and engendering transformation," which is inherent in the theory of Chinese medicine.

Transformation is influenced by pre-existing states.

Chinese medicine focuses in detail not only on the development of disease transformation, but also on its quality or nature. From long observation of changes in the nature of disease, Chinese medicine has learned that different disease evils can give rise to different diseases, and in some cases, even the same evils can give rise to different diseases. Through long practical experience, the following basic laws of transformation have crystallized: Even when the evil is the same, there are different transformations resulting from the influence of pre-existing states. Heat forms under the influence of yáng, and cold forms under the influence of yīn.

Consider, for example, three individuals whose condition is one of good health, and who, under the same circumstances, contract cold evil and become ill. The first person manifests symptoms of a headache and painful stiff nape, aversion to cold and heat effusion, bodily pain without sweating, oppressed breathing and slight panting, and a floating, tight pulse. These symptoms belong to the greater yáng exterior repletion pattern of cold damage disease. The next person, however, manifests symptoms such as fear of cold and no heat effusion, abdominal fullness and vomiting, inability to get food down, intermittent pain in the abdomen, watery stool, no thirst, and a sunken pulse. These symptoms belong to the greater yīn interior cold pattern of cold damage disease. Finally, the onset of the disease in the third person manifests with symptoms of slight aversion to wind and cold accompanied very quickly by heat effusion and thirst, headache, no sweating, slight coughing, and a floating, rapid pulse. These symptoms, however, belong to the wind-warmth defense aspect pattern of warm disease. All three of these persons have contracted a "cold" evil, so why is it that each of them manifests different symptoms? Chinese medicine believes this is because after the cold invades, the existence of yīn-yáng vacuity or repletion in the different individuals will give rise to "different transformations."

There is a general rule that "heat is formed under the influence of yáng and cold is formed under the influence of yīn." For example, consider the third of the three individuals mentioned above. If he has a yáng nature or constitution, or if, at the time of disease contraction, he already has an internal condition of accumulated heat, then "heat is formed under the influence of yáng," and the illness becomes warm disease. The second person may have a yīn constitution or, at the time of contraction, may already have an internally hidden cold evil; "cold is formed under the influence of yīn," and the illness is due to an interior cold pattern of cold damage disease. The first person mentioned above has a robust constitution, so when cold evil suddenly invades the exterior, defensive qì at the exterior of the body immediately responds at the skin to resist cold evil. Thus, the illness is due to the greater yáng exterior repletion pattern of cold damage disease. I have chosen only the example of cold evil in this discussion, but there are many other kinds of disease evils which also possess the capability of "different transformations." There is, however, no reason to be repetitive here.

Disease evils do not only transform differently at the onset of disease, as we discussed in the examples above, they also change during the development and course of disease. An example is the lesser yīn pattern of cold damage disease. Within this pattern are two different transformations: the cold transformation pattern or *fù zǐ tāng* (Aconite Decoction) and *sì nì tāng* (Counterflow Cold Decoction) patterns, as well as the heat transformation pattern or *zhū líng tāng* (Polyporus Decoction) and *huáng lián ē jiāo jī zǐ huáng tāng* (Coptis, Ass Hide Glue, and Egg Yolk Decoction) patterns.

Another example is the reverting yīn pattern, which demonstrates changes between heat reversal entering and abating and yīn-yáng retaliation. This phenomenon of transformation is also present in warm disease and in miscellaneous disease. Depending on the internal and external differences in every organism, warm disease evil will also transform in different ways. This idea is succinctly stated in the *Yī Zōng Jīn Jiàn* ("The Golden Mirror of Medicine"):

> "Illness in the six channels is usually due to cold damage, and even though [the evil] qì is the same, the disease itself differs. How can this be? Qì affects the physical viscera not just in one way, but in many ways, because of the process of transformation. You must understand what it means to say that water and fire are mutually overcoming, and what difficulties lie in the principles of cold transformation and heat transformation. You may casually speak about the transmutation and transformation of a thousand conditions, but these are never removed from the realm of yīn-yáng and exterior-interior."

I have explained from the examples above how seriously Chinese medicine considers the constitution of the individual and the nature of its response to the environment. It also seriously considers how the process of disease can engender different circumstances in a thousand different ways. When identifying patterns to determine treatment, you should focus on the relationship between the disease evil, its damage to the human body, and the struggle of the body to resist damage, for these elements substantially differ. You should also pay attention to how the human body can, under certain circumstances, turn the symptoms of disease around and anticipate the tendencies of disease development, thus assisting and regulating the interior of the body to resist damage from disease and to defeat illness.

Earlier in this chapter, in my discussion of Case 4, I knew that the pattern was dampness formed with heat since the patient had symptoms of thick, slimy, yellow tongue fur, a slippery pulse, and more heat signs than cold. Dampness by nature is sticky and slimy, and it is not easy for the patient to recover from damp patterns. At the time of treatment, I integrated the damp-transforming method when formulating the prescription by including medicinals such as *cǎo guǒ* (tsaoko), *pèi lán* (eupatorium), *qīng hāo* (sweet wormwood), *cǎo dòu kòu* (Katsumada's galangal seed), and *huò xiāng* (patchouli), which transform dampness by means of their aromatic properties. This method is quite a different approach than simply resolving the lesser yáng, but by doing so, results were quickly obtained and were extremely satisfactory.

Case 2 concerned a patient with a pattern of yīn vacuity with liver effulgence. When yīn vacuity is coupled with liver effulgence, the relationship is one of mutual influence, and together they form a vicious cycle. If the link between them was not resolved quickly, the headache would have been difficult to heal. For this reason, I primarily selected the yīn-nourishing liver-emolliating treatment method; the headache was relieved and the patient easily recovered.

In summary, Chinese medicine attaches great importance to the diversity of transformations within the human body; furthermore, it probes deeply into the development and transformation of the patient's condition. Therefore, when learning and applying the principle of pattern identification to determine treatment, you should at all times analyze and take into account the theory of transformation. In so doing, you raise the standard of determining treatment by pattern identification, and this is always beneficial.

Seek the cause when identifying patterns; seek the root when treating disease.

For several thousand years, Chinese medicine has treated countless patients under the guidance of holistic concepts. It brought together each separate element of patient care and devised a method of using the patient's symptoms to further investigate the transformations of the body as a whole. Later generations of physicians called this process "seeking the cause when identifying patterns," and they associated pattern and cause as an integrated concept.

For example, the symptom of "wind" is swift and changeable; it is associated with itching, convulsions, shaking and dizzy vision; it is wandering by nature and is usually associated with the liver and with the stringlike pulse. The symptom of "dampness" is associated with heaviness in the body; it is enduring and difficult to treat; its symptoms are water swelling, chest oppression and torpid intake, generalized fever that does not easily abate, thick, slimy tongue fur, and a slippery pulse; it is usually associated with the spleen. From examples such as these, the physician correlates the pathocondition to its associated cause or "seeks the cause by following the pathocondition." By analyzing this interrelationship and the particular characteristics of symptoms, you can utilize a holistic viewpoint to recognize the true nature of disease.

Case 4 in this chapter illustrates this point. This patient manifested cold and heat at set periods of time, so I knew the pattern was evil in the lesser yáng. She also had symptoms such as thick, slimy tongue fur, a slippery pulse, and a generalized fever that was enduring and difficult to treat, so I knew from these symptoms that damp-heat evil was also present. Consequently, I selected the method of harmonizing and resolving the lesser yáng while transforming dampness and clearing heat, and obtained very good results.

Case 1 was also diagnosed in the same manner. On the basis of severe pain and swelling of the ankle and knee joints and deformity of the osseous tissue, I knew the disease was in the kidney channel. Cold by nature is congealing and inhibiting and is a chief cause of pain. The *Huáng Dì Nèi Jīng* ("The Yellow Emperor's Inner Canon") states, "When cold qì is exuberant, the patient suffers painful impediment." According to these characteristics, I knew the pattern was cold evil entering the bones, channels, and network vessels. This caused impediment and obstruction, which gradually developed into hypertonicity of the sinews and bone impediment with joint deformity. The kidney governs bone, so the treatment method supplemented the kidney and dispelled cold, and a very satisfactory result was obtained.

In summary, to apply pattern identification to determine treatment, you should focus on "seeking the cause by following the pathocondition." Do not just "treat the head when there is headache" or "treat the toe when there is pain in the toe;" in other words, do not just treat the symptoms. You should, instead, "treat in accordance with the pattern."

While "seeking the cause by following the pathocondition," you should also focus on "seeking the root to treat disease." The Míng dynasty physician, Lǐ Niàn-É, explains this topic:

> "Although the diseases of humans are varied, they only belong to vacuity or repletion, to heat or cold, to qì or blood, or to the viscera or bowels; all are subject to the principle of yīn and yáng. Therefore, you should know that the transformation of disease is infinite, and the principle of yīn and yáng is its root. ... When you clearly understand the principle of yīn and yáng, you directly perceive the root of disease and perhaps can influence destiny."

Clearly, Chinese medicine holds the view that the human body has many defined categories of structure and function. These categories are summarized as mutually controlling and mutually stimulating and belong to the two aspects that are unified yet opposite, namely, yīn and yáng. I believe that yīn and yáng maintain their dynamic equilibrium within the waxing and waning of physical movement, and within this process, the organism carries out its normal life activities. Disease occurs when yīn and yáng are unregulated and imbalanced. The goal of Chinese medicine is to treat the root of disease. Its concern is the regulation of yīn-yáng imbalances in the human body; that is, whether these imbalances are from exuberance or debility. In effect, this means the achievement of "calm yīn and sound yáng," or the recovery and preservation of the yīn-yáng relationship. Therefore, as a general principle in the treatment of disease, physicians in the past highly emphasized the essential importance of regulating yīn and yáng. This concept is explained in the *Huáng Dì Nèi Jīng* ("The Yellow Emperor's Inner Canon"):

> "Ascertain the yīn and yáng [within disease] to distinguish the yielding from the firm. For yáng disease, treat yīn; for yīn disease, treat yáng. Stabilize qì and blood, for each preserves its own domain."

The Táng dynasty physician Wáng Bīng said:

> "Boost the source of fire to disperse the shroud of yīn, and invigorate the governor of water to restrain the brilliance of yáng."

As the Míng dynasty physician Zhāng Jǐng-Yuè further explains:

> "Yīn is rooted in yáng and yáng is rooted in yīn. Not every disease can be treated effectively by straight treatment (using cold to treat heat, for instance). You should, instead, conduct yīn through yáng and conduct yáng through yīn; for each of these, seek its associations and weaken it."

In this chapter, for the patient in Case 2, the treatment method primarily supplemented liver yīn and subdued liver yáng, while simultaneously quickening blood and extinguishing wind, and the method brought good results. The treatment method in Case 4 was mainly aimed at harmonizing and resolving the lesser yáng, while simultaneously clearing and transforming damp-heat; this approach also achieved satisfactory results. The pattern in Case 3 was yáng exuberance transforming into heat; therefore, the prescription was formulated to drain heat and eliminate congestion. Case 1, on the other hand, concerned the patterns of kidney yáng vacuity and yīn cold exuberance; thus, the treatment method centered on supplementing kidney yáng while dispelling cold and quickening the network vessels; this treatment was also successful.

In summary, when applying the principle of pattern identification to determine treatment, you should always focus on the idea of this most essential principle: "To treat disease, you must seek its root."

The integration of treatment and nutrition

In the treatment of disease, Chinese medicine not only actively conducts a holistic treatment of disease, but also attends to the physical needs of recovery from illness. This idea is found in the *Huáng Dì Nèi Jīng* ("The Yellow Emperor's Inner Canon"):

> "When treating disease with medicinals, remove highly toxic medicinals when the patient has recovered six parts of ten; remove normally toxic medicinals when the patient has recovered seven parts of ten; remove mildly toxic medicinals when the patient has recovered eight parts of ten; and remove non-toxic medicinals when the patient has recovered nine parts of ten. [Advise the patient to] eat and freely nourish himself with grains, meat, fruit, and vegetables, without causing excess or damage to the right [qì]."

> "You should first comply with the weather characteristics of the year in question, and do not go against the harmony of heaven. … Strive to remove medicinals, but follow the principle of food therapy for recovery."

In the chapter "Methods of Treating Visceral Qì in Accordance with the Seasons," this concept is explained further:

> "Attack evils with toxic medicinals, but nourish with the five grains, assist with the five fruits, boost with the five animal meats, replenish with the five vegetables; combine qì (natures) and flavors and administer them to supplement essence and boost qì."

It is my opinion that the appropriate coordination of diet and medication is effective for supplementing essence and boosting qì and for strengthening the physique and preventing disease. I would also point out that when the patient is at the initial stages of recovery and a remnant of evil qì is still present, food and drink may be administered to nourish right qì; this action will in turn eliminate the remaining evil. If medicinal administration is excessive, then I fear that damage to right qì may occur. On the basis of these ideas, Chinese medicine maintains the view that certain foods and drinks are either appropriate for use or should be avoided. Patients and their families should always be encouraged to combine treatment with nutrition, for this will accelerate the recovery time. Physicians of the past accumulated an abundance of valuable experience on this topic and published many books that discuss the subject of nutrition. Some of those titles are: *Shí Liáo Běn Cǎo* ("Herbal Foundation of

Diet Therapy"), *Yĭn Shàn Zhèng Yào* ("Principles of Correct Diet"), *Suí Xī Jū Yĭn Shí Pŭ* ("Guide to Food and Drink by the Master of Living in Retirement"), and *Shí Jiàn Bĕn Cǎo* ("The Mirror of Dietary Materia Medica"). I offer these titles for clinical reference since this subject is important in Chinese medicine.

The patient in Case 4, for instance, was advised not to eat sticky, greasy types of food that assist the production of dampness; such foods are New Year's cakes, glutinous rice dumplings and other things made with glutinous rice flour, soft-shelled turtle, duck, fatty meats, butter, and fat. It was appropriate for her to eat a clear, bland diet. The Case 3 patient was unable to eat hot, spicy, acrid foods that assisted fire, such as hot peppers, noodles with black pepper, raw garlic, raw scallions, beef, and lamb. It was not appropriate for the patient in Case 2 to consume foods that assisted liver fire or assisted yáng and stirred wind. I advised this patient to avoid chicken, chicken soup, lamb, beef, hot peppers, raw garlic, and raw Chinese chives. I advised the patient in Case 1 to eat foods that would supplement the kidney, assist kidney yáng, and assist heat to dispel cold. These were: *shān yào* (dioscorea), dried ginger, brown sugar, dog meat, lamb, beef, cinnamon, fennel, *gŏu qĭ zĭ* (lycium), walnuts, venison, and the flower-stalk of Chinese chives. These foods kept the lower limbs and joints warm. In addition, the patient engaged in moderate physical activity and exercise.

There is an old Chinese proverb that says, "Three parts medicinals; seven parts nutrition"; this expression reflects the spirit of the integration of treatment and nutrition. In summary, when applying the principle of pattern identification to determine treatment, it is important to consider the integration of treatment and nutrition since nutrition is another special characteristic of Chinese medicine.

Several problems concerning pattern identification

To treat illness correctly, Chinese medicine maintains that you must first master "pattern identification" to distinguish why the disease has manifested certain "patterns" at that moment in time. Then, based on that "pattern" distinction, determine a corresponding treatment method. When this is accomplished, the physician may select the formulas, medicinals, and other treatment strategies according to the requirements of the treatment method at that time. One should vary the treatment according to the pattern presented.

These ideas have emerged from a holistic conception of the human body, and they rest on the notion of a very close relationship between "pattern" and "treatment." This relationship is the basis of the entire methodology and is known as treatment based on pattern identification. It is the single greatest characteristic of Chinese medicine, for it constitutes a unique and distinctive medical treatment system. "Pattern identification" and "treatment determination" are two closely related concepts that can never be completely separated from each other. In this chapter, however, for the sake of convenience, I will relate some problems and issues concerning pattern identification and treatment determination, and I will discuss these concepts separately.

WHAT IS A "PATTERN"?

A "pattern" emerges from an organic conception of the human body and is based on the information derived from the inquiry, inspection, listening and smelling, and palpation examination methods. These examinations are conducted, the material is collected and analyzed, and then one of the following pattern identification theories is applied: eight-principle, six-channel, bowel and viscera, channel and network, disease cause, or four-aspect. The theory is then combined with factors such as the specific circumstances of the patient, the objective conditions, and other relevant information. At this point, by analysis, induction, inference, and discrimination, the disease symptoms are processed by "separating the grain from the chaff, by distinguishing the true from the false, by proceeding step-by-step, and from exterior to interior." After that, what emerges in any specified stage of disease observable at that moment is the synthesized result that we recognize as the pattern.

It can be said that a "pattern" is a defined process of disease recognition that progresses from perception to rational understanding. Therefore, a "pattern" is not just a pile of enumerated phenomena, but rather it is a method to gain knowledge of the various kinds of internal conditions in the human body relevant to disease management. The pattern is the process of analysis to understand the struggle between evil and right at any given time in the course of disease, and to obtain a predicated outcome; thus, the various categories of "pattern" concepts are formulated.

Therefore, we say that a "pattern" is the prerequisite to "treatment determination," since treatment determination is based on the pattern. Through our knowledge of patterns and observation of their rules of transformation, we can further gain an overall understanding of "diseases" in terms of numerous laws of pattern transformation and their special characteristics.

The patient in Case 1 of this chapter suffered bone impediment with sinew hypertonicity, known as joint-deformity impediment, which was caused by cold evil deeply invading the kidney channel. The patient in Case 2 had a pattern of yīn vacuity with liver effulgence and liver wind harassing the upper body. Case 3 was a patient who suffered intestinal welling-abscess disease that manifested, at its onset, as a pattern of qì-blood congestion and stasis brewing in the intestine and transforming into heat. Case 4 involved a damp-heat pattern of evil lodged in the lesser yáng. These were not cases that simply piled up or enumerated the symptoms such as joint pain, inability to walk, unilateral headache, agitation, intermittent pain on the head and face, pain in the lower right side of the abdomen, nausea and vomiting, high fever that does not abate, symptoms that worsen in the afternoon, poor appetite, chest oppression, slimy tongue fur, or a stringlike, slippery, sunken, or rapid pulse. These were, instead, examples of "determining treatment" based on the "pattern."

THE SIMILARITIES AND DIFFERENCES BETWEEN PATTERN, SYMPTOM, AND DISEASE

When we know what a "pattern" is, then the main problem is already solved. However, we must still understand the differences between "pattern," "symptom," and "disease." Some scholars hold the opinion that the written characters for symptom and for pattern may be used interchangeably. This opinion is based on the fact that in ancient times there was no character for symptom, only a character for pattern (证), so they believe there is no requirement to differentiate between them. This type of research based on a single character may certainly be correct, and I agree. Yet, topics such as these have greatly expanded since then. Some characters did not exist in ancient times, but we have other characters that we commonly use; for example, we customarily use the word "symptom" to indicate a certain physical condition. Therefore, I believe that if we grasp the explicit meaning given to symptom, pattern, and disease, and we gradually begin to see ways to unify these concepts, then we gain an advantage for further exploration of medical theory in the realm of observing and studying disease. This is my opinion.

Pattern: I have already discussed the definition of pattern in the text above, so it is not necessary to discuss it again. Some people use the word pattern as a substitute for "pattern condition (证候)," but this term pattern condition is different from "symptom (症状)."

Symptom: "Pathocondition" refers to "symptoms." The symptoms refer to the manifestation of an abnormal condition. In general, there are subjective symptoms, which are perceived only by the patient, and objective symptoms, which are detectable by others. Subjective symptoms include headache, aversion to cold, cough, fever, abdominal pain, diarrhea, chest oppression, abdominal fullness, dizziness, and flowery vision. Objective symptoms include scorching generalized fever, reversal cold of the limbs, abdominal tenderness, yellowing of the eyes, red eyes, halitosis, yellow and slimy tongue fur, abdominal distention, a stringlike pulse, rapid pulse, or an absence of pulse. These two categories of symptoms often appear simultaneously, and sometimes they are not clearly distinguished. For instance, abdominal distention, high fever, and accumulation lumps in the abdomen are both subjective and objective symptoms. In summary, during the course of disease, these manifestations of various abnormal conditions are comprehensively grouped together and generically referred to as "symptoms."

Disease: A "disease" refers to a comprised symptom set that possesses particular characteristics and embodies its own rules of transformation. Disease is an unhealthy state that has specific characteristics and its own specific laws of transformation, including different patterns appearing at different stages. There are many examples of the Chinese medical definition of "disease," such as cold damage disease, warm heat disease, malarial disease, dysentery, wind strike, and cholera. Here is another example:

Diagnostic Method	Chinese medical diagnosis and treatment	Integrated Diagnosis and Chinese Medical Treatment
Disease	Cold damage	Acute bacterial dysentery (damp-heat dysentery)
Symptoms	Headache and rigidity of the neck, fever and aversion to cold, spontaneous sweating, floating and moderate pulse	Abdominal pain, diarrhea, tenesmus, stool containing pus and blood with more blood than pus, generalized heat, heaviness, thirst with no desire for liquids, thick yellow slimy tongue fur, slippery and rapid pulse
Pattern	Greater yáng exterior vacuity pattern	Damp-heat accumulation and stagnation in the center burner
Treatment Method	Harmonize construction and defense	Clear heat, disinhibit dampness, and abduct stagnation
Formula	Modified *guì zhī tāng* (Cinnamon Twig Decoction)	Modified *sháo yào tāng* (Peony Decoction)

From the examples given above, we can see the essential idea of a "pattern," and from the pattern we establish the method, select a formula, and apply the needed medicinals. However, the determination of the pattern is dependent on the collection and analysis of many symptoms. To take this idea a step further, if the pattern belongs to a certain disease, then the identification and management of the pattern, as well as the analysis of its transformational tendencies, can be followed even more closely and more systematically.

Consider the patient in Case 4 as an example. By analyzing the symptoms, I arrived at a diagnosis of a lesser yáng pattern of cold damage disease, complicated by damp evil transforming into heat. This was enduring disease, and it presented a difficult recovery for the patient. According to the transformational laws of cold damage disease, a lesser yáng pattern may transform into a yáng brightness pattern. In Case 4, there were already more heat than cold symptoms (a yáng brightness pattern has only heat and not any cold symptoms), such as sweating, dry stools, and thick tongue fur. The appearance of these symptoms illustrated that the mechanism of yáng brightness transformation had indeed already occurred. Therefore, I eliminated the method of using *chái hú guì zhī tāng* (Bupleurum and Cinnamon Twig Decoction) to harmonize and resolve the lesser yáng, and I chose instead to use *bái hǔ tāng* (White Tiger Decoction) to clear heat that was shifting to the yáng brightness channel. By using this method, I was able to clear heat and prevent its transformation, and, at the same time, by following the pattern, I was able to coordinate the use of medicinals to transform damp turbidity. Thus, I pressed forward with the treatment method. The sweating had already disappeared at the time of the second visit, so I removed *guì zhī tāng* (Cinnamon Twig Decoction). By the third visit, the heat evil had been eliminated; thus, I removed *bái hǔ tāng* (White Tiger Decoction) and continued to prescribe *xiǎo chái hú tāng* (Minor Bupleurum Decoction) as the chief formula, modified with aromatic damp-transforming medicinals. The patient recovered.

In conclusion we can say that the symptom, the pattern, and the disease all reflect the unhealthy condition of the human body; these three concepts are related to each other yet distinct from each other. When applying the principle of pattern identification to determine treatment, you should always pay attention to this distinction.

DISTINGUISHING THE CHIEF PATTERN AND ITS SPECIFIC CHARACTERISTICS

The principal goal in pattern identification involves finding the chief pattern and identifying its special characteristics. Chinese medicine believes that during the emergence, development, and process of disease, the yīn-yáng, qì-blood, viscera and bowels, and channels and network vessels of the human body are all engaged in a struggle with disease evils. This struggle manifests various patterns at any given time. Some patterns are more predominant than others, and from all these patterns, the pattern that most aptly reflects the chief or principal problem will inevitably emerge. Chinese medicine refers to this emerging principal pattern as the "chief pattern." On the method of distinguishing the chief pattern, please refer to the section, "What is a pattern?" appearing earlier in this commentary. I will not give the details here. Simply to devise a treatment by identifying the chief pattern would not make a complete and accurate treatment possible. Therefore, after distinguishing the chief pattern, it is equally important to distinguish the special characteristics of that chief pattern. I give you the following example.

If we distinguish the chief pattern as liver-spleen disharmony, then the treatment should use the liver-spleen harmonization method. Although this is certainly a valid approach, should we not go a step further to ask if the underlying cause of the disharmony is liver effulgence? Or ask if the cause is perhaps spleen vacuity? If the disharmony is indeed due to liver effulgence and transverse counterflow of liver qì restraining the spleen-stomach, then it follows that the treatment method should suppress the liver and support the spleen. If severe, it would suffice to simply suppress the liver. However, if the disharmony is due to spleen-stomach vacuity weakness with the liver exploiting spleen vacuity and restraining the spleen-stomach, for this particular situation, the treatment method must support the spleen and suppress the liver. Thus, if we use the liver-spleen harmonization method in a generalized way, it is unlikely that we will obtain the most satisfactory results.

Consider the example from Case 1 in this chapter. The chief pattern involved the combination of wind, damp, and cold, which caused qì-blood impediment and unsmooth movement in the channels and network vessels. The joints were deprived of nourishment, and became deformed as a result. I could have used a treatment method focused on dispelling wind-damp, freeing the channels and network vessels, and disinhibiting the joints. If I had proceeded with such a treatment, it is unlikely that the results would have been very good, because I would have distinguished only the chief pattern and would not have investigated the specific characteristics of that pattern. The special characteristic of the chief pattern for this patient was kidney yáng vacuity. Cold evil had deeply invaded the kidney, and since kidney governs bone, cold evil entered the bones and caused bone impediment deformity. Sinew and bone lost their normal function, and the joints became deformed and painful. Consequently, the patient could not walk. The treatment therefore emphasized the kidney-supplementing cold-dispelling method and selected medicinals that were able to enter the kidney. Only when these medicinals were added to the prescription did the treatment obtain ideal results.

In Case 2, the chief pattern was liver yáng exuberance and liver wind harassing the upper body. If I had used only the liver-calming wind-extinguishing method, the results would have been less than ideal since I would not have distinguished the characteristics of this one specific chief pattern. This was an elderly patient who suffered a wind pattern, which is a yáng evil; when wind endures, it enters the blood aspect and damages yīn. As liver yīn became increasingly vacuous, liver yáng became more and more exuberant. Therefore, I selected a treatment method to nourish yīn and emolliate the liver while quickening the blood and extinguishing wind, and the results were very good. From these examples you can see that when identifying patterns, you should not only identify the chief pattern but also identify its specific characteristics, for only then can you proceed with the appropriate treatment. The chief pattern and its specific characteristics coincide with the transmutation and transformation of each circumstance. Nevertheless, when conducting pattern identification to determine treatment, you should always focus throughout the entire process on distinguishing the chief pattern and its specific characteristics.

This is a most important point because this process enhances the treatment efficacy, and is the ultimate key to restoring health and recovering from illness.

GIVE CONSIDERATION TO CONCURRENT PATTERNS

In disease onset and development, many different pathoconditions appear at the same time, and from these a chief pattern and concurrent patterns emerge. When diagnosing and treating disease, it is first of all important to decide which is the chief pattern and to distinguish the characteristics of the chief pattern, and then treat the disease with a resolution in mind. Generally, we say that once the chief pattern is resolved, then look to the concurrent patterns and follow through to resolution with these as well. Moreover, if some concurrent patterns are not resolved, they will have a reverse influence on the development and transformation of the chief pattern.

I prescribed *xiǎo chái hú tāng* (Minor Bupleurum Decoction) with added *cǎo guǒ* (tsaoko) and *bīng láng* (areca) for the patient in Case 4 to harmonize and resolve the lesser yáng and to transform damp turbidity with aromatics. This formula resolved the chief pattern, which was cold-damp transforming into heat evil and lodging itself in the lesser yáng. But at the same time, I prescribed *guì zhī tāng* (Cinnamon Twig Decoction) to address spontaneous sweating and aversion to wind and to resolve the concurrent pattern of construction-defense disharmony. I also prescribed *bái hǔ tāng* (White Tiger Decoction) for dry stools and for the symptom of more heat signs than cold. Thus, the second concurrent pattern, the shifting of disease to the greater yáng, was resolved. In this way, treatment of the chief pattern and the concurrent patterns is like a plan that considers all the factors, and in this fashion we obtain a satisfactory result. You accomplish good results by having a plan that considers all aspects. Do not treat this subject superficially, and do not treat each aspect equally at face value, for the result would be a method without priorities, with medicinals simply thrown together in a disorderly and unsystematic manner. If you practice medicine in this way, it is highly unlikely that you will obtain good therapeutic results.

CAREFULLY CONSIDER PATTERN TRANSFORMATIONS AND TRUE AND FALSE PATTERNS

When identifying patterns, besides focusing on distinguishing the chief pattern and its characteristics, you should also pay attention to pattern transformations and true and false patterns. Chinese medicine proceeds from the idea of "restraining and engendering transformation." It believes that the patterns of disease are unceasingly transforming. Do not think that a vacuity pattern will always remain a vacuity pattern, or that a repletion pattern will always be a repletion pattern. You should instead focus at all times on pattern transformation. For example, a yáng exuberant heat pattern manifesting with symptoms of high fever and clouded spirit may, under certain conditions, transform into a vacuity cold pattern of yáng desertion and yīn exuberance, with symptoms such as reversal cold of the four limbs, sudden decline of body temperature, dripping cold sweat, spiritlessness, and loss of speech. On the other hand, a pattern of yīn cold may, under certain conditions, also transform into a yáng heat pattern. Thus, it is also important to distinguish true cold–false heat and true heat–false cold patterns.

Generally speaking, a true cold–false heat pattern, in the elderly patient or the patient with enduring or serious illness, will manifest with symptoms such as fever and disquieted spirit, thirst with no desire for fluids, a red face as if dabbed with rouge, icy-cold feet and knees, heart vexation, wanting to cover with clothes and blankets, easy to fall asleep, and a sunken, fine, and weak pulse. However, the pattern is true heat and false cold if the patient presents with symptoms such as clouded spirit, counterflow cold of the limbs, sometimes fear of cold but no desire to cover with bedclothes, high heat in the chest, abdomen, and armpits but icy-cold limbs, thirst with the desire to drink cold water, vexation and agitation, inability to sleep, and a sunken, small pulse that is forceless upon heavy pressure.

Furthermore, you must pay attention to the situation of "major repletion resembling weakness and consummate vacuity producing signs of exuberance." For example, when a patient in robust health presents with symptoms such as fatigue and a desire to sleep, poor appetite, clouded heavy head and lack of spirit, lack of strength in the limbs and body, thick yellow tongue fur, constipation, and a large, replete, and forceful pulse, then the pattern is true repletion–false vacuity. Children most often exhibit this pattern. They are usually active and play every day, they enjoy eating, and they have abundant essence-spirit. If parents do not pay attention to the eating habits of their children and stagnation occurs due to food damage, then the following symptoms will emerge: no desire to play and be active, laziness and desire to sleep, poor appetite, fatigue and clouded head, poor essence-spirit, and a sunken, slippery, forceful pulse. In this case, the symptoms of fatigue, poor essence-spirit, and desire to sleep by no means indicate a pattern of vacuity, but rather indicate the emergence of false vacuity symptoms within a true repletion pattern.

Contrary to this is the example of the elderly patient or the patient with enduring or serious illness. If such patients exhibit symptoms such as a spirit-mind that is suddenly and completely active and alert, loss of speech that is suddenly very distinct, a voice that is suddenly more clear and resonant than before, suddenly sitting up and moving about with strength when previously bed-ridden, suddenly having total recollection of events and people that were previously forgotten, and a vacuous, weak, faint, or scattered, barely detectable pulse, it is often described as "the last radiance of the setting sun," when original spirit in extreme vacuity verges on desertion—the true vacuity false repletion pattern that is the most dangerous pattern of all—and you should take immediate emergency measures to save the patient. You must realize that there is only a small chance of saving such a patient.

Several problems concerning treatment determination

Treatment determination and pattern identification share a very close relationship with each other. Since a pattern is a prerequisite to treatment determination, pattern identification cannot be separated from treatment determination. However, for the convenience of discussion, in this section I will temporarily separate these two concepts and address several problems and issues concerning treatment determination.

WHY IS IT IMPORTANT TO "DETERMINE" A "TREATMENT?"

"Determining treatment" in Chinese medicine means working out which of the treatment options is qualitatively most suited to the pattern that has been identified. You have to investigate the pattern carefully, and consider appropriate action according to person, time, and place to choose the appropriate formula containing the right medicinals. In this way, you apply Chinese medical theory in extensive deliberation of the case at hand. This is called "determination of treatment."

In pattern identification, for example, when the pattern is greater yáng bowel repletion, then the treatment should use the precipitation method. However, there are many differences in the precipitation method alone, such as emergency precipitation, mild precipitation, warm precipitation, cold precipitation, moist precipitation, diffusion of the lungs and freeing of the intestines, increasing humor to push the ship, regulating the stomach to free the bowels, and nourishing blood to free the dark-gate. Furthermore, you should investigate other factors that influence the treatment, such as the strength or weakness of the patient's constitution, whether the patient lives in a northern or southern region, the season in which the disease occurred, the gender and age of the patient, whether the patient is overweight or underweight, or even the size of the selected formula and the application of medicinal dosages. These factors must be thoroughly considered and studied.

Yet even these considerations are not enough, for according to the requirements of pattern identification, the following factors must also be considered. Some patterns require treatment of the tip and then treatment of the root. Some first need treatment of the root then the tip, others require simultaneous treatment of root and tip. Some patterns require treating upper body disease through the lower body; others require treating lower body disease through the upper body. For some, it is essential to treat yīn for yáng disease or to treat yáng for yīn disease. Some need the attacking method more than supplementation, others need supplementation before attacking. Still others need attacking and supplementation methods equally. Some require straight treatment application of bitter cold medicinals, others require sweet cold medicinals that foster yīn, and still others require the return of fire to its origin. You must investigate thoroughly when treating extremely complicated conditions, for only then can you accurately determine the treatment method and associate it with the formula and medicinals. This is very simply the reason why you should "determine treatment."

Case 3 is a good example: the patient suffered intestinal welling-abscess disease with a pattern of qì-blood congestion and stasis brewing and transforming into heat. According to the characteristics of the chief pattern, this was a repletion heat pattern of congestion and stasis in the intestines. This patient was young in age and lived in Hénán province. Even though he had fallen ill in December, the southern region where he lived was still milder than the northern region. After considering these factors as well as the others, I finally selected medicinals that were bitter-cold and salty-cold and used the urgent-precipitation method to free the intestines and eliminate congestion, quicken blood and transform stasis, and clear heat and resolve toxin. This approach yielded satisfactory results.

There are other considerations as well. For example, for all other patients with abdominal welling-abscess, for elderly patients, for those living in Northwestern China, and for female patients, the treatment method and the application of medicinals will change according to the different circumstances of each patient. You must make the appropriate adjustments to accommodate these differences. It is clear that "determining treatment" is an especially important process.

"TREATMENT DETERMINATION" IS A TWO-STEP PROCEDURE

Treatment determination is a process that can be divided into a two-step procedure. The first step is the establishment of method; the second step is the selection of formulas and application of medicinals.

Establish the method

Establishing the method is the ultimate key to determining treatment based on pattern identification. The accuracy of the established method will directly affect the treatment. When establishing the method, you must first of all determine the treatment principle according to the requirements of the pattern identification. This principle is called the "therapeutic principle" and is also referred to as the fundamental treatment. The treatment principles resemble or convey the idea of a military operation or "strategy." The *Huáng Dì Nèi*

Jīng ("The Yellow Emperor's Inner Canon") has recorded a great deal of material concerning treatment principles, and these are some examples:

"Treat cold with heat; treat heat with cold; treat warmth by clearing; treat clear [discharge] with warmth; treat dissipation by contracting; treat repression by dissipating; treat dryness with moistness; treat tension by relaxing; treat hardness by softening; treat brittleness by hardening; treat debility by supplementing; treat strength with draining."

"Treat mild [disease] by counteraction (straight treatment); treat severe [disease] by co-action (paradoxical treatment); treat hardness by whittling; treat visiting [evil] with elimination; treat taxation with warmth; treat binds by dissipating; treat lodged [evil] by attacking; treat dryness with moistness; …treat detriment with warmth; treat straying by moving; treat fright by calming."

"Counteraction is straight treatment; co-action is paradoxical treatment."

"Treat heat by using cold; treat cold by using heat; treat the stopped by unstopping; treat the unstopped by stopping."

"When you apply cold treatment, and there are [still] heat signs, supplement yīn; when you apply heat treatment, and there are [still] cold signs, supplement yáng."

"For exterior signs from an interior condition, regulate the interior; for interior signs from an exterior condition, treat the exterior; for exterior signs arising from the interior with exuberance in the exterior, first regulate the interior and then treat the exterior; for interior signs arising from the exterior with exuberance in the interior, first treat the exterior and then regulate the interior; when the interior and exterior do not influence each other, then treat the chief disease."

"If disease is in the upper body, treat the lower body; if disease is in the lower body, treat the upper body; for disease in the center, treat the sides."

"Depressed wood is treated by outthrusting; depressed fire is treated by diffusing; depressed earth is treated by despoliating; depressed metal is treated by discharging; depressed water is treated by regulating."

"For great accumulations and great gatherings that may invade [the interior], stop treatment when they have been reduced by more than half; to proceed further will bring death."

"When urine and stool are inhibited, treat the tip; if urine and stool are disinhibited, treat the root. When disease arises with superabundance, use a root-to-tip treatment; first treat its root and then treat its tip. When disease arises with insufficiency, use a tip-to-root treatment; first treat its tip and then treat its root."

"When [the disease] is mild, raise [and effuse] it; when [disease] is severe, reduce it; when [qì and blood] are debilitated, strengthen them. When the body is insufficient, use qì to warm it; when the essence is insufficient, use flavors to supplement it."

In the past, physicians commonly believed that treatment principles were defined in eight fundamental categories: sweating, ejecting (vomiting), precipitating, harmonizing, warming, clearing, supplementing, and dispersing. These are called the "eight methods of treating disease." Determining the treatment, however, is only the first phase in the first step of this process, for this step is merely the consideration of the treatment principle and may also be referred to as the general direction of the treatment. You are still required to accomplish phase two, namely, the formulation and provision of the specific "treatment method" according to the requirements of the treatment principle. Once you have arrived at the specifics of the "treatment method," then you have accomplished the step of "establishing the method." The treatment method is more detailed and more specific than the treatment principle; therefore the treatment method is also more refined than the treatment principle. Moreover, there are more treatment methods than there are treatment principles, and it is difficult to quantify exactly how many there are.

For instance, within the sweating method, there are many sub-methods, such as sweating with warmth and acridity, sweating with coolness and acridity, sweating by enriching yīn, sweating by inducing ejection (vomiting), and sweating by boosting qì. Within the precipitation method, there are other methods as well, such as emergency precipitation to preserve yīn, moistening precipitation with salty, cold medicinals, precipitation by increasing humor to free the intestines, and precipitation by diffusing the lungs to free the intestines. The examples are endless, and it is not necessary to give details here.

The treatment method resembles a military tactic or "strategy." Therefore, it is said that the treatment method is the specific, concrete embodiment of the treatment principle. Among the Chinese characters for principle, method, formula, and medicinals, the character for "method" embodies within itself the concepts of treatment principle and treatment method. When the formulation of the treatment method is accomplished, then the first step of determining treatment, namely, the establishment of treatment, is completed.

Select the formula and apply the medicinals

The second step in "determining treatment" is the selection of formulas and the application of medicinals according to the requirements of the established method. Strictly speaking, this step is also divided into two phases. The first phase is formula selection. During this phase, you may select a formula from among antique or modern prescriptions that meets the requirements of the basic treatment method. The prescription should be skillfully organized, well-directed at the condition of the patient, and highly effective to serve as the foundation formula. This formula should yield itself easily to modifications according to the pattern. If you cannot find a set prescription that is appropriate, then you may, on the basis of organizational principles for prescription writing, simply organize a new prescription. At that moment, you enter into the second phase, namely, that of applying medicinals.

If you choose to use a set prescription, you should analyze each medicinal in that formula and remove any medicinal ingredients that may be detrimental to the patient. You may then choose to add certain medicinals that enable the set prescription to better conform to the treatment method and that are better suited to the condition of the patient; the added medicinals should further enhance the therapeutic effect. If you choose to organize a new formula, then you must carefully consider medicinals and organize a prescription according to the requirements of the treatment method. It should be based on the organizational principles of prescription writing and coordinated with the specific circumstances of the patient. In the selection of formulas and the application of medicinals, you may consult sources written by past physicians on the seven formula types: large, small, gentle, urgent, odd-numbered, even-numbered, and compound. You may also consult the ten prescription types, which are diffusing, freeing, supplementing, discharging, light, heavy, lubricating, astringent, dry, and moist. There are other principles to organizing a prescription and applying medicinals, such as sovereign, minister, assistant, and courier, which are also called chief, support, assistant, and courier, as well as the four qì, the five flavors, the eighteen clashes, the nineteen fears, mutual need, and mutual empowering. The *Huáng Dì Nèi Jīng* ("The Yellow Emperor's Inner Canon") records the following:

> "One sovereign and two ministers comprise an odd-numbered formula; two sovereigns and four ministers comprise an even-numbered formula. Two sovereigns and three ministers comprise an odd-numbered formula, but two sovereigns and six ministers an even-numbered formula. For proximal parts [upper body], use an odd-numbered formula; for distal parts [lower body], even-numbered. Use an even-numbered formula if the patient is sweating; use an odd-numbered formula if the

patient has diarrhea. Treat the upper body with gentle formulas; treat the lower body with urgent formulas. Use thick medicinals to treat acute conditions, and use thin medicinals for mild conditions."

When treating proximal [upper body] disease, whether using an odd or even-numbered [formula], it should be a small formula. When treating distal [lower body] disease, whether using an odd or even-numbered [formula], it should be a large formula. In a large formula, the dosages are small; in a small formula, the dosages are large. A large dose is nine; a small dose is two. If [the disease is] not eliminated with an odd-numbered formula, then [change the formula to] even-numbered; this is called a heavy formula. If [the disease is] not eliminated with an even-number formula, then assist with a paradoxical formula.

At the time of applying medicinals to the formula, it is certainly appropriate to include the findings of modern scientific research; you should be flexible, but follow the requirements of the treatment method. In summary, while it is important to focus on accomplishing the method and formula, you should also pay attention to flexibly adapting modifications according to the pattern. It is necessary to be completely attuned to the needs of the patient. Emphasize the formulas and medicinals directed at the chief pattern, and pay attention to the concurrent pattern, as well as the surrounding circumstances and lifestyle of the patient.

The treatment principle in Case 1 was "to treat debility with supplementation and to treat visiting (evil) by elimination." The treatment method was to supplement the kidney and dispel cold, quicken blood and free the network vessels, strengthen the sinews and bones, and disinhibit the joints. I selected two formulas, *guì zhī sháo yào zhī mǔ tāng* (Cinnamon Twig, Peony, and Anemarrhena Decoction) and *hǔ gǔ sǎn* (Tiger Bone Powder), and applied certain medicinal modifications according to the pattern.

In Case 4, the treatment principle was the "harmonizing and clearing method," assisted by transforming dampness with aromatic medicinals. The treatment method harmonized and resolved the lesser yáng, and also transformed dampness and cleared heat. Here I again selected two formulas, *chái hú guì zhī tāng* (Bupleurum and Cinnamon Twig Decoction) and *bái hǔ tāng* (White Tiger Decoction), and I added several aromatic medicinals to transform dampness. I will not present the details of these cases here.

At this point in the presentation, we have completed two steps of the "treatment method." Determining treatment on the basis of pattern identification means varying the treatment in accordance with the transmutation and transformation in the patterns presented by the patient.

Thus, pattern identification to determine treatment is not immutable; it is, instead, a process that is repeated again and again should any changes in the pattern itself occur. In acute cases, changes in the pattern may differ from morning to afternoon; this process can happen very quickly, so the treatment method reflects the changes. Even in chronic cases, it is necessary to continuously conduct the process of treatment based onpattern identification, and to investigate this process step by step to bring the patient to the final recovery. Do not under any circumstances take the maxim, "do not change an effective formula," to mean that you are spared the bother of reassessing the patient at each consultation. "Do not change an effective formula" is only applicable when you have reassessed the patient and are certain that the formula used before is still the right one for the patient.

Earnestly read medical literature to study and apply pattern identification to determine treatment.

Chinese medical literature is vast in scope, and you may feel truly inadequate and frustrated when attempting to read it. Therefore, you should know which books to focus on so you can thoroughly study, assimilate, and absorb the most important things. When you apply this knowledge in your clinical practice, you improve your ability to diagnose and treat. For physicians who have been working independently in a clinic for several years, reading the case studies of physicians of both the past and present is a great help. These medical case reports contain the clinical notes of skilled doctors who are diagnosing and treating disease, and the notes are the substantive embodiment of pattern identification to determine treatment. Although some case reports are written in a relatively brief and sketchy style, each one reflects the theory and practice of carefully integrated principles, methods, formulas, and medicinals, all flexibly combined in a variety of ways. For example, Huá Xiù-Yún wrote a guidebook to the volumes of Yè Tiān-Shì's *Lín Zhèng Zhǐ Nán Yī Àn* ("A Clinical Guide with Case Studies") and said:

> "If one case uses a certain method, then a similar case uses it as well; if one method uses a certain formula, then another case with that method uses it as well. Through this concept, complicated transformations are managed meticulously and easily. Furthermore, after careful consideration of the medicinals in the formula, and which are the sovereigns, ministers, assistants, and couriers, the cases coordinate the medicinals with the disease source. Where the ancient formula modifies with one or two ingredients, it is especially appropriate to understand why. Where the pattern is identified and treatment established, you

should mark it with red ink, then these sections will never be forgotten. Never make rash observations or satisfy yourself with a superficial understanding of a case without understanding its true essence, for this profits no one."

From this written text, you can learn how to study medical case reports; on the subject of pattern identification to determine treatment, they provide great insight and assistance. Everyone should also frequently consult the following books for medical case reports:

Míng Yī Lèi Àn ("Classified Case Histories of Famous Physicians")

Xuē Shì Yī Àn ("Master Xuē's Case Histories")

Liǔ Xuǎn Sì Jiā Yī Àn ("Case Histories of Four Masters Selected by Master Liǔ")

Lín Zhèng Zhǐ Nán Yī Àn ("A Clinical Guide with Case Histories")

Yù Yì Cǎo ("A Draft of Cherished Thoughts")

Wú Jū Tōng Yī Àn ("Wú Jū-Tōng's Case Histories")

Quán Guó Míng Yī Yàn Àn Lèi Biān ("Empirical Case Histories from Famous Physicians of the Nation, Classified and Compiled")

Qīng Dài Míng Yī Yàn Àn Jīng Huá ("The Essence of Empirical Case Histories of Famous Physicians from the Qīng Period")

Pú Fǔ Zhōu Yī Àn ("Pú Fǔ-Zhōu's Case Histories")

Yuè Měi Zhōng Yī Àn ("Yuè Mei-Zhōng's Case Histories")

Huáng Wén Dōng Yī Àn ("Huáng Wén-Dōng's Case Histories")

Lǎo Zhōng Yī Yī Àn Yī Huà Xuǎn ("Selected Discussion on Case Histories of Famous Physicians of the Past")

These books are fundamental reading for Chinese medical theory and doctrines of past physicians, and you can reap great benefits by reading them. As Huá Xiù-Yún said:

"To read these cases, you need to be a person who can understand the language and discourse. Have a lively and open mind, study the *Líng Shū* ("The Magic Pivot") and *Sù Wèn* ("Elementary Questions"), and the works of other worthy writers of the past."

If you have the desire to learn pattern identification to determine treatment using good examples, then I belive you should read from the following list of medical texts:

Sù Wèn Líng Shū Huì Zuǎn Yuē Zhù ("Compiled and Edited Notes on the Elementary Questions and Magic Pivot")

Líng Sù Jí Zhù Jié Yào ("Essential Collected Commentaries on the Magic Pivot and Elementary Questions")

Nèi Jīng Jí Yào ("Summary of the Inner Canon")

Nèi Nàn Xuǎn Shì ("Selected Explanations on the Inner Canon and the Canon of Difficult Issues")

First, choose one book from among these texts, and study and read it thoroughly. It would be even better, if possible, to read the entire *Huáng Dì Nèi Jīng* ("The Yellow Emperor's Inner Canon"). Next, read *Shāng Hán Lùn* ("On Cold Damage") and *Jīn Guì Yào Lüè* ("Essential Prescriptions of the Golden Coffer") and commence reading Chén Xiū-Yuán's *Shāng Hán Lùn Qiǎn Zhù* ("Easy Commentary on the Treatise on Cold Damage") and *Jīn Guì Yào Lüè Qiǎn Zhù* (Easy Commentary on the Essential Prescriptions of the Golden Coffer"). For several years, the Chinese medicine schools and universities have provided *Shāng Hán Lùn* and *Jīn Guì Yào Lüè* as printed class materials in vernacular style with annotations attached. In addition to the literature already mentioned, I would also recommend the following texts for everyone to examine and study:

Wēn Bìng Tiáo Biàn ("Systematized Identification of Warm Diseases")

Wēn Rè Jīng Wěi ("Warp and Weft of Warm Heat")

Gè Jiā Xué Shuō Jiǎng Yì ("Lecture Notes on Schools of Theory")

Yè Xuǎn Yī Héng ("The Level Line of Medicine Selected by Master Yè")

Bīn Hú Mài Xué ("Bīn-Hú's Pulse Theory")

Zhōng Yào Fāng Jì Xué Jiǎng Yì ("Lecture Notes on Chinese Pharmaceutics")

Zhōng Yī Zhěn Duàn Xué Jiǎng Yì ("Lecture Notes on Chinese Diagnostics")

Běn Cǎo Bèi Yào ("Essential Materia Medica")

Yī Fāng Jí Jiě ("Medical Formulas Gathered and Explained")

I integrate into each special field of research the selected writings that address that specialty. Thus, I learn and comprehend that specialty through a study of the medical cases. By doing so, I progressively advance more deeply into the subject and continuously improve my skills.

The study of medical cases is a sound endeavor and truly provides us enormous assistance for diagnosis and treatment. Below are two sections that I have extracted from the writings of our predecessors; these excerpts will conclude this chapter. The first section concerns the requirements for writing a medical case; the second section is the analysis of a medical case, or as we say today, a case history. The excerpts appear below.

The first excerpt is taken from the *Yù Yì Căo* ("A Draft of Cherished Thoughts"):

> "A medical case requires the following information: a certain day of a certain month (i.e., the date of consultation) and the age of the patient. Is the patient's physical appearance thin or fat; is the duration of illness long or short? Is the complexion dark or bright? Is the skin withered or lustrous? Is the voice distinct or unclear? Is the patient joyful or sorrowful in body and mind? On what day did the illness begin? Which medicinals were initially prescribed; which medicinals were later prescribed? Which medicinals had a slight effect and which ones had no effect?

> At the time of the examination, when is the disease more severe, during the day or at night? Which is greater, heat or cold? Is there a desire or an aversion to food and drink? Are the urine and stool smooth or rough, and do they occur or not? What are the three positions and nine indicators of the pulse; which indicator is different from the others? Of the twenty-four pulses, which one is predominant and which are concurrent?

> Is the illness due to internal damage or external contraction? Is it due to concurrent internal and external causes, or is it not concurrent? If the menses have stopped, what is the reason? What is the priority, the tip or the root? Which method of treatment to use: sweating, ejection, precipitation, harmonization, cooling, warming, supplementation, or draining? Which among the seven formula types is appropriate to use and which medicinals? Among the ten formula types, which formula type to use? Among the five qì, which qì is appropriate? Among the five flavors, which flavor?

> Each step must be completely clear, and the task must be accurate and free of error. Then you build a practice with many patients who come for treatment out of faith, and this you will never gain from literature." (Qīng: Yù Jiā-Yán [Yù Chāng])

The second excerpt concerns the empirical treatment of yáng collapse with excessive sweating from the *Wèi Shēng Băo Jiàn* ("Precious Mirror of Health"):

> "The patient was Xuē Lĭ, the thirteen-year-old second son of prefect magistrate Zhōng Shān-Wáng. On the thirteenth day of the sixth month, a torrential downpour occurred and the lakes

overflowed. The child played in the water, and his clothing was soaked. His mother scolded him for his carelessness. Later that evening, his essence-spirit was clouded and fretting, and he was fatigued and somnolent. On the next morning, he had fallen ill with a headache and generalized heat, and he complained of heaviness in the legs and feet. A female doctor treated him with a harmonizing, resolving, and diffusing method, closed the windows and doors, and covered the boy with a heavy quilt.

Because of this action, he suffered intolerably from the heat and began raving wildly. He wanted to remove the quilt, but could not. Consequently, he suffered night sweats and soaked through the quilt. The next morning, he was picking at his bedclothes and pulling invisible strings [a severe case of delirium]. He then received a precipitating treatment using *chéng qì tāng* (Qì-Infusing Decoction). Afterwards, his speech diminished, his limbs became uncoordinated, his neck became stiff, his extremities tugged and slackened repeatedly and were hypertonic, the white of the eye showed in his left eye, the flesh of his lips wriggled, eating and drinking decreased, and his body became emaciated. It was imperative that I treat the Life Gate (*mìng mén*), for the previous treatment had been in error. When I thought about the matter carefully, I realized that the problem was due to damage by dampness through excessive sweating.

The original qì of the human body is the stirring qì in the kidney that arises from below the umbilicus. It circulates throughout the entire body and passes through the hundred vessels. When this patient suffered exuberant heat, he was given a powerful sweating treatment. Since sweating was excessive, yáng collapsed, and the hundred vessels contracted. Therefore, qì of the triple burner could not bring luxuriance to the heart and lungs, so heart fire became exuberant and lung qì was parched. This condition was due to fright and fear amassing internally. The *Huáng Dì Nèi Jīng* ("The Yellow Emperor's Inner Canon") says, "Fear causes qì to precipitate, and yáng governs the voice; when yáng collapses, the patient has no voice. A person who possesses yáng qì has essence that nourishes the spirit and has emollients that nourish the sinews."

The *Huáng Dì Nèi Jīng* ("The Yellow Emperor's Inner Canon") also says, "When blood is despoliated, there is no sweat; when sweat is despoliated, there is no blood."

This young patient suffered excessive sweating, so both qì and blood were debilitated and the sinews were without nourishment. This is tetany disease with stiff neck and hypertonicity and tugging and slackening of the extremities. The eye is the passage to the liver; the person who has a sound liver has coordinated sinews. This patient had dry sinews without moisture, and the white of the eye showed in the left eye. The flesh is governed by the spleen; if there is spleen heat, the flesh wriggles, so the lips wriggled occasionally. The *Huáng Dì Nèi Jīng* ("The Yellow Emperor's Inner Canon") also says that flesh wilting is due to damp earth. If the patient suffers spleen heat, the flesh is numb; numb flesh becomes flesh wilting. The patient who suffers wilting has weakness without strength for physical movement, and has an enduring condition of numbness.

Yáng governs movement; in this case qì verged on exhaustion and heat was lodged in the spleen; therefore, the four limbs became useless. This case was a pattern of damage due to dampness and excessive sweating, and it was clear that the disease had become worse. To treat the heat pattern in this case, it was necessary to boost the source of water to stem counterflow, to supplement the upper body, and to raise and engender qì. The *Huáng Dì Nèi Jīng* ("The Yellow Emperor's Inner Canon") says, "When qì is insufficient in the upper body, push it and raise it upward."

This was such a case, so the treatment used *rén shēn yì qì tāng* (Ginseng Qì-Boosting Decoction). The *Huáng Dì Nèi Jīng* ("The Yellow Emperor's Inner Canon") also says, "heat overwhelms if it is excessive, so use cold, sweet medicinals and sour, contracting medicinals to treat." As sovereigns, sweet and warm *rén shēn* (ginseng) and *huáng qí* (astragalus) supplemented insufficient qì and relaxed the tension and the convulsions.

The kidney is averse to dryness; so acrid medicinals were immediately administered to moisten the kidney. As ministers, *shēng gān cǎo* (raw licorice), sweet in flavor and slightly cold in nature, and *huáng bǎi* (phellodendron), which is bitter, acrid, and cold, rescued kidney water and engendered fluids.

As assistants, acrid, warm *dāng guī* (Chinese angelica) harmonized the blood and vessels; bitter and acrid *chén pí* (tangerine peel), bitter and sweet *bái zhú* (white atractylodes), and sweet and warm *zhì gān cǎo* (mix-fried licorice) boosted the spleen and stomach and encouraged the appetite. The lung required contraction, so sour medicinals were urgently included to astringe the lung: *bái sháo yào* (white peony), sour in flavor and slightly cold in nature, contracted the dissipated qì and supplemented lung metal.

As couriers, *shēng má* (cimicifuga) and *chái hú* (bupleurum) are bitter in flavor and balanced in nature; thus, they raised and engendered qì that had been insufficient. This type of treatment is called "drawing out yáng from within yīn."

The ingredients and the dosages for *rén shēn yì qì tāng* (Ginseng Qì-Boosting Decoction) are as follows:

> *huáng qí* (黄芪 astragalus, Astragali Radix) 5 *fēn*
>
> *rén shēn* (人参 ginseng, Ginseng Radix) 3 *fēn*
>
> *huáng bǎi* (黄柏 phellodendron, Phellodendri Cortex) 3 *fēn* (remove the outer layer)
>
> *shēng má* (升麻 cimicifuga, Cimicifugae Rhizoma) 3 *fēn*
>
> *chái hú* (柴胡 bupleurum, Bupleuri Radix) 3 *fēn*
>
> *bái sháo yào* (白芍药 white peony, Paeoniae Radix Alba) 3 *fēn*
>
> *dāng guī* (当归 Chinese angelica, Angelicae Sinensis Radix) 2 *fēn*
>
> *bái zhú* (白术 white atractylodes, Atractylodis Macrocephalae Rhizoma) 2 *fēn*
>
> *zhì gān cǎo* (炙甘草 mix-fried licorice, Glycyrrhizae Radix cum Liquido Fricta) 2 *fēn*
>
> *chén pí* (陈皮 tangerine peel, Citri Reticulatae Pericarpium) 3 *fēn*
>
> *shēng gān cǎo* (生甘草 raw licorice, Glycyrrhizae Radix Cruda) 2 *fēn*

The above-mentioned ingredients were administered orally, all in one dose. First, the medicinals were soaked in two and a half cups water for four hours, and then decocted until the liquid was equal to one cup. The cooked ingredients were removed, and the decoction administered while hot, once in the morning after eating, and at noon before eating. Each time the ingredients were decocted with these instructions. Three days later, his voice had gradually improved, he took a few steps, his limbs were flexible, and his appetite had returned. By the following autumn, the patient had fully recovered." (Yuán: Luó Tiān-Yì)

I believe that we should meticulously study the cases of physicians from the past (such as the example above) and the essence of scholarly research without neglecting any details. At the same time, we should investigate every subject to find its root and consider all factors comprehensively. Our proficiency in determining treatments based on pattern identification will continuously improve by integrating this material with the achievements of modern scientific research whenever relevant, by carefully thinking through the evidence, by constantly summarizing of all the facts, and by thoroughly investigating all the details of a case.

CHAPTER EIGHT

It is important to constantly improve and develop pattern identification skills to determine treatment.

Over thousands of years of practice and application, Chinese medicine has been used innumerable times to prevent and cure disease. It has drawn upon perceptual knowledge, assembling, summarizing, and shaping it into rational knowledge. This process, together with standard of living improvements, has greatly contributed to the welfare of the public. Thus, I envision that when the empirical knowledge of past and contemporary physicians is properly compiled, we can improve the standard of Chinese medical theory.

I have learned over many years of clinical practice that Chinese medicine is a treasure house containing abundant empiricism and a profound philosophy of medical knowledge. I also believe that our own knowledge is insufficient and contains some errors or shortcomings. Therefore, I think that we should "understand disease by treating disease."

The Chinese character for "disease" actually has a double meaning: the first meaning is disease or illness, and the second meaning is a shortcoming, insufficiency, flaw, or error. When we have a profound understanding of disease, then we may also perceive the defects and shortcomings of our own knowledge of Chinese medicine and more properly advance our development. For this reason, I think that in treatment the process of "identifying patterns to determine treatment" must be constantly improved and developed. Following are five medical cases that succinctly illustrate several points based on my experience.

CASE STUDIES

CASE ONE
STONE STRANGURY (URINARY CALCULUS)
石淋 (泌尿系结石)

The patient, a 28-year-old male cook, was hospitalized at 2 PM on May 18, 1966.

CHIEF COMPLAINT

Pain in the lumbus on the left side, lesser abdominal pain on the left side, with pain radiating to the genitals.

INQUIRY EXAMINATION

The patient had experienced dribbling, difficult, and painful urination for the past nineteen hours. The left side of the lumbus had become painful four or five days before, and pain had also occurred in the lesser abdomen on the left side yesterday afternoon around 7 PM. Pain radiated to the genitals and the medial portion of the left thigh. The urination was urgent, frequent, difficult, inhibited, and painful; it was yellow in color. The stool was dry. He was constantly nauseous and took no pleasure in eating; he had a dry mouth and no desire to drink water.

INSPECTION EXAMINATION

His development and nutrition were good, but he presented with acute pain and suffering. The sides and tip of the tongue were red, and the tongue fur was slightly yellow.

LISTENING AND SMELLING EXAMINATION

His speech, voice, and respiration were all normal.

PALPATION EXAMINATION

Palpation of the lumbus and abdomen revealed no abnormalities. The pulse was slippery and slightly fine.

PATTERN IDENTIFICATION

Habitual consumption of fatty and sweet foods had caused the contents of the stomach to brew and form heat. Damp-heat poured downward and heat amassed in the bladder. By brewing over a prolonged period of time, water bound to form a stone, resulting in painful sand-stone strangury. In discussing stone strangury conditions, the text *Zhū Bìng Yuán Hòu Lùn* ("The Origin and Indicators of Disease") explains:

The kidney governs water; when water binds, it transforms into stone. Thus, sand-stone settles in the kidney. If there is kidney vacuity, then heat is overwhelming and strangury occurs. In this disease condition, there is pain in the penis upon urination and urine cannot easily exit; pain stretches into the lesser abdomen with urgency in the bladder, then sand-stone exits through the urinary pathway. In severe cases, congestion and pain cause oppression and expiry.

This patient had a tongue with red sides and tip and yellow tongue fur, so I knew this was a heat pattern; the slippery pulse was the chief indicator of damp evil. After correlating the four examinations, my diagnosis was stone strangury disease manifesting as a pattern of bladder damp-heat.

For diagnostic confirmation, X-rays were taken of the abdomen. One calculus measuring 1.0 x 0.8 cm was located at the third vertebra on the left side of the lumbus (L3).

TREATMENT METHOD

Clear and disinhibit damp-heat in the lower burner and lubricate the orifice, and quicken stasis and disperse stones.

PRESCRIPTION

I gave the patient one packet of the following prescription:

hǎi jīn shā (海金沙 lygodium spore, Lygodii Spora) 15 g (wrapped in cloth)

jīn qián cǎo (金钱草 moneywort, Lysimachiae Herba) 60 g

biǎn xù (萹蓄 knotgrass, Polygoni Avicularis Herba) 15 g

huá shí (滑石 talcum, Talcum) 15 g

chē qián zǐ (车前子 plantago seed, Plantaginis Semen) 12 g (wrapped in cloth)

lù lù tōng (路路通 liquidambar fruit, Liquidambaris Fructus) 9 g

shēng dà huáng (生大黄 raw rhubarb, Rhei Radix et Rhizoma Crudi) 6 g

yán hú suǒ (延胡索 corydalis, Corydalis Rhizoma) 1.5 g (powdered, divided and taken drenched)

FORMULA EXPLANATION

This prescription is based on *hǎi jīn shā sǎn* (Lygodium Spore Powder). As chief medicinals, *hǎi jīn shā* (lygodium spore) clears and disinhibits bladder damp-heat and *jīn qián cǎo* (moneywort) disinhibits urine and expels stones.

As support medicinals, *huá shí* (talcum) disinhibits dampness and lubricates the orifice and *biǎn xù* (knotgrass) clears heat and disinhibits urine.

As assistant medicinals, *chē qián zǐ* (plantago seed) disinhibits dampness and boosts the kidney, but does not injure yīn. *Shēng dà huáng* (raw rhubarb) quickens stasis and clears heat by removing the old to bring in the new, and *yán hú suǒ* (corydalis) quickens blood and simultaneously rectifies qì and stops pain.

As the courier medicinal, *lù lù tōng* (liquidambar fruit) frees and moves qì while quickening the blood and freeing the network vessels.

The entire prescription clears heat and disinhibits dampness, lubricates the orifice, quickens stasis, and disperses stones.

FOLLOWUP TREATMENT

<u>Second visit on May 19</u>: The symptoms remained unchanged although the patient had taken the prescription packet. I removed *yán hú suǒ* (corydalis), *shēng dà huáng* (raw rhubarb), and *lù lù tōng* (liquidambar fruit) and added the following medicinals to strengthen the kidney-boosting, blood-quickening, and tension-relaxing effect:

chuān niú xī (川牛膝 cyathula, Cyathulae Radix) 9 g

chǎo dù zhòng (炒杜仲 stir-fried eucommia, Eucommiae Cortex Frictus) 9 g

shēng gān cǎo (生甘草 raw licorice, Glycyrrhizae Radix Cruda) 5 g

<u>Third visit on May 23</u>: After four packets of this modified prescription, pain was alleviated in the lumbus and lesser abdomen. The volume of urine increased, but the patient still experienced pain in the urethra after urinating. The tongue and pulse signs had not changed. Again, I prescribed the above-mentioned formula, substituted *shēng gān cǎo shāo* (raw fine licorice root) for *shēng gān cǎo* (raw licorice), and gave the patient two more packets.

The patient took this prescription at 9 AM the following morning, but did not urinate at all. By 5 PM that afternoon, the lesser abdomen was distended, swollen, and painful. He was immediately rushed to the hospital for another X-ray which revealed that the stone, originally in the left urethra, had fallen to the mouth of the bladder. The urethra above this point had become blocked, so the patient could not even urinate. The lesser abdomen was severely distended and painful. I prescribed one packet of the following emergency prescription, to be decocted and administered immediately:

huá shí (滑石 talcum, Talcum) 30 g

dōng kuí zǐ (冬葵子 mallow seed, Malvae Semen) 15 g

chuān niú xī (川牛膝 cyathula, Cyathulae Radix) 9 g

I also recommended one injection each of dolantin and atropine. After this, the pain was at last relieved and the patient urinated approximately 50 ml.

<u>Fourth visit on May 24</u>:   Urination was still blocked on the night before this visit, so on the morning of the visit the patient received another injection of dolantin and atropine.   However, the lesser abdominal distention and pain was still not relieved. At 11:45 AM, the doctors performed a paracentesis of the bladder; afterwards the patient urinated 800 ml and the lesser abdominal distention and pain stopped. I then advised the patient to immediately decoct and take one packet of the following prescription:

huá shí (滑石 talcum, Talcum) 30 g

jīn qián cǎo (金钱草 moneywort, Lysimachiae Herba) 60 g

dōng kuí zǐ (冬葵子 mallow seed, Malvae Semen) 24 g

chuān niú xī (川牛膝 cyathula, Cyathulae Radix) 15 g

chì sháo yào (赤芍药 red peony, Paeoniae Radix Rubra) 15 g

At 3:30 PM, I referred him for another X-ray to see the location and position of the stone. I performed a rectal examination on the patient and gently massaged for 2–3 minutes along the urethra just above the mouth of the bladder. After that, the urethra discharged two drops of watery, pale blood. I advised him to continue with the decoction that was previously prescribed.

At 8:30 PM, the patient wanted to urinate; that is, he strained to urinate. The urethra discharged one oval-shaped stone that was similar in appearance to a shelled peanut, brown in color and slightly yellow. After discharging the stone, the patient immediately went to the radiology department for another X-ray. The X-ray revealed no image at all of the stone, and the bladder and urethra were normal.

<u>Fifth visit on May 25</u>: The urethral stone had been discharged, every symptom had disappeared, and the patient's essence-spirit was good. The tongue and pulse signs were balanced and normal, so I again gave the patient three packets of medicinals as a regulating therapy. I prescribed the following:

hǎi jīn shā (海金沙 lygodium spore, Lygodii Spora) 9 g

jīn qián cǎo (金钱草 moneywort, Lysimachiae Herba) 15 g

huá shí (滑石 talcum, Talcum) 15 g

niú xī (牛膝 achyranthes, Achyranthis Bidentatae Radix) 9 g

chǎo dù zhòng (炒杜仲 stir-fried eucommia, Eucommiae Cortex Frictus) 9 g

fú líng (茯苓 poria, Poria) 12 g

chǎo bái zhú (炒白术 stir-fried white atractylodes, Atractylodis Macrocephalae Rhizoma Frictum) 9 g

chén pí (陈皮 tangerine peel, Citri Reticulatae Pericarpium) 6 g

shēng gān cǎo (生甘草 raw licorice, Glycyrrhizae Radix Cruda) 6 g

The patient received an additional two packets to take with him when he returned home. On May 26th, the patient had recovered and was discharged from the hospital.

CASE TWO
HEADACHE AND HEART PALPITATIONS (LEVEL III ATRIOVENTRICULAR BLOCK)
头痛、心悸 (第 III 度房室传导阻滞)

The patient, a 38-year-old male from Shāndōng province, was initially examined on October 27, 1974.

CHIEF COMPLAINT

Cloudy head, headache, flusteredness, and slow heartbeat for more than ten years.

INQUIRY EXAMINATION

In the summer of 1961, the patient had experienced symptoms such as headache, dizziness, flusteredness, shortness of breath, and entire body fatigue, all of which gradually became more severe over time. In 1964, he had visited the local hospital in Shāndōng province, where he had received a diagnosis of level III atrioventricular block. He had received treatment at that time and gradually regained his health. Then, due to excessive overwork from 1965–1968, the symptoms started to return; the headache became more intense, he felt suffocated and flustered, and his heartbeat was 36 beats per minute. For the second time, he was admitted to the hospital for treatment, but this time he had no positive results.

In April 1969, he transferred to the China Medical Sciences Academy Hospital in Běijīng and was again diagnosed with level III atrioventricular block. Even though his treatment had obtained less than ideal results, he was discharged in September of the same year. From 1970 until the first half of 1974, the patient visited several hospitals, including his local hospital in Shāndōng province, the Shànghǎi People's Hospital, the Shànghǎi First Medical School Hospital, and the Chinese People's Liberation Army Hospital. He even received Chinese and Western integrated medical treatments, but all methods failed. In every hospital he visited, the attending physician recommended that the patient have a cardiac pacemaker installed to avoid the possibility of a terminal event.

However, the patient preferred to use Chinese medicine, so he was admitted to my hospital for consultation and diagnosis. I have extracted from his file the diagnosis and treatment opinions of physicians from several hospitals concerning the condition of the patient. The extracts are included in the text following the case itself.

At the time of the initial examination, the chief symptoms were cloudy head, dizziness, and a headache described as an empty pain in the head. When the pain was severe enough, it caused the patient to faint. His faculties had diminished; he was flustered and short of breath. He suffered chest oppression, slow heartbeat, and entire body fatigue. His essence-spirit had vanished, and he feared cold and had many dreams at night. However, his appetite was good and urine and stool were still regular.

INSPECTION EXAMINATION

His development and nutrition appeared normal. He presented with pain and suffering, his complexion was dark and gloomy without luster, and his essence-spirit was devitalized. The tongue body was slightly dark, and the root of the tongue had slightly thick white fur.

LISTENING AND SMELLING EXAMINATION

His speech was clear and distinct, but his voice was relatively low. When he spoke, he became short of breath.

PALPATION EXAMINATION

His extremities were quite cool, and his pulse was slow and weak.

PATTERN IDENTIFICATION

The heart governs blood vessels; its bloom is in the face. The heart resides above the diaphragm and governs yáng qì in the chest. The kidney holds the office of labor and stores essence; it engenders marrow (the brain is the sea of marrow) and is the place where the true yáng of the body resides. Yáng governs movement; yīn governs tranquility.

This patient had become ill due to overwork; his head was cloudy, dizzy, and felt empty. His body was fatigued and lacking strength, his essence-spirit was devitalized, and he feared cold; all these symptoms were manifestations of kidney yáng insufficiency. The symptoms of flusteredness, shortness of breath, slow heartbeat, and chest oppression were all signs of devitalized heart yáng. Both heart and kidney yáng were vacuous, and essence-blood could not ascend to provide luxuriance to the face. Thus, the patient felt that his head was empty, he had symptoms of cloudiness and dizziness in the head, he sometimes fainted, and his complexion was dark, gloomy, and without luster. The heart and kidney were unable to interact with each other, so the patient was forgetful and had many dreams. Since heart and kidney yáng were vacuous, blood vessel flow was inadequate; thus, the tongue body was dark and the pulse was slow and weak. After correlating the four examinations, I diagnosed heart and kidney yáng vacuity.

TREATMENT METHOD

Warm the yáng qì of the heart and kidney, and boost qì and quicken blood.

PRESCRIPTION

I prescribed six packets of the following:

zhì má huáng (炙麻黄 mix-fried ephedra, Ephedrae Herba cum Liquido Fricta) 5 g

zhì fù piàn (制附片 sliced processed aconite, Aconiti Radix Lateralis Praeparata Secta) 9 g

xì xīn (细辛 asarum, Asari Herba) 3 g

xiè bái (薤白 Chinese chive, Allii Macrostemonis Bulbus) 9 g

shú dì huáng (熟地黄 cooked rehmannia, Rehmanniae Radix Praeparata) 15 g

shān zhū yú (山茱萸 cornus, Corni Fructus) 9 g

shān yào (山药 dioscorea, Dioscoreae Rhizoma) 12 g

ròu guì (肉桂 cinnamon bark, Cinnamomi Cortex) 3 g

wǔ wèi zǐ (五味子 schisandra, Schisandrae Fructus) 6 g

mài mén dōng (麦门冬 ophiopogon, Ophiopogonis Radix) 9 g

fú shén (茯神 root poria, Poria cum Pini Radice) 9 g

hóng huā (红花 carthamus, Carthami Flos) 9 g

chuān xiōng (川芎 chuanxiong, Chuanxiong Rhizoma) 9 g

bái rén shēn (白人参 white ginseng, Ginseng Radix Alba) 1.8 g (powdered, divide in half and take drenched)

FORMULA EXPLANATION

This prescription uses *má huáng fù zǐ xì xīn tāng* (Ephedra, Aconite, and Asarum Decoction) with added *xiè bái* (Chinese chive). As the chief medicinal, *xiè bái* warms and assists heart yáng.

As support medicinals, *shú dì huáng* (cooked rehmannia), *shān zhū yú* (cornus), *ròu guì* (cinnamon bark), and *shān yào* (dioscorea) warm and supplement kidney yáng.

As assistant medicinals, *rén shēn* (ginseng), *mài mén dōng* (ophiopogon), and *wǔ wèi zǐ* (schisandra) boost heart qì, nourish heart blood, and regulate the blood and vessels. *Fú shén* (root poria) nourishes the heart and quiets the spirit; while *hóng huā* (carthamus) quickens blood and moves stasis.

Chuān xiōng (chuanxiong) is the courier medicinal. It is acrid and fragrant, mobile and penetrating; it travels upward to the head and chest and downward to the knees and abdomen. It also moves qì within blood. *Chuān xiōng* and *fù zǐ* (aconite) together warm the channels and dispel cold, and free the twelve channels by reinforcing the return of yáng to its origin.

The prescription warms and assists heart and kidney yáng, and simultaneously boosts qì and quickens blood.

FOLLOWUP TREATMENT

Second visit on November 4: Altogether, the patient took seven packets of
the prescription, but there were no significant changes in the symptoms and
no harmful side-effects. The tongue body was still dark and the pulse was still
slow. Consequently, I modified the previous prescription and gave him six
more packets as follows:

> *má huáng* (麻黄 ephedra, Ephedrae Herba) 5 g
>
> *fù piàn* (附片 sliced aconite, Aconiti Radix Lateralis Praeparata Secta)
>   6 g
>
> *bái jiè zǐ* (白芥子 white mustard, Sinapis Albae Semen) 5 g
>
> *shú dì huáng* (熟地黄 cooked rehmannia, Rehmanniae Radix Praeparata)
>   24 g
>
> *ròu guì* (肉桂 cinnamon bark, Cinnamomi Cortex) 5 g
>
> *lù jiǎo shuāng* (鹿角霜 degelatinated deer antler, Cervi Cornu
>   Degelatinatum) 12 g
>
> *zǐ sū zǐ* (紫苏子 perilla fruit, Perillae Fructus) 9 g
>
> *xìng rén* (杏仁 apricot kernel, Armeniacae Semen) 9 g
>
> *dǎng shēn* (党参 codonopsis, Codonopsis Radix) 12 g
>
> *xiāng fù* (香附 cyperus, Cyperi Rhizoma) 9 g
>
> *zhì gān cǎo* (炙甘草 mix-fried licorice, Glycyrrhizae Radix cum Liquido
>   Fricta) 6 g
>
> *chuān xiōng* (川芎 chuanxiong, Chuanxiong Rhizoma) 9 g

I also prescribed three bottles of *yún nán bái yào* (Yunnan White), to be
administered four times a day, each time one-eighth of a bottle.

Third visit on November 12: The symptoms remained unchanged even after taking eight packets of the prescription. The patient still experienced dizziness, reduced sleep, and chest oppression. The tongue and pulse had not
changed at all. This time, to stimulate the yáng qì of the entire body, I prescribed medicinals to loosen the chest and assist yáng qì and to boost the kidney and quicken stasis. The prescription was as follows:

> *quán guā lóu* (全栝楼 whole trichosanthes, Trichosanthis Fructus
>   Integer) 30 g
>
> *xiè bái* (薤白 Chinese chive, Allii Macrostemonis Bulbus) 15 g
>
> *guì zhī* (桂枝 cinnamon twig, Cinnamomi Ramulus) 12 g
>
> *ròu guì* (肉桂 cinnamon bark, Cinnamomi Cortex) 6 g

lù jiǎo shuāng (鹿角霜 degelatinated deer antler, Cervi Cornu
    Degelatinatum) 12 g

zhì gān cǎo (炙甘草 mix-fried licorice, Glycyrrhizae Radix cum Liquido
    Fricta) 6 g

dǎng shēn (党参 codonopsis, Codonopsis Radix) 15 g

hóng huā (红花 carthamus, Carthami Flos) 9 g

sū mù (苏木 sappan, Sappan Lignum) 12 g

chuān xiōng (川芎 chuanxiong, Chuanxiong Rhizoma) 12 g

zhēn zhū mǔ (珍珠母 mother-of-pearl, Concha Margaritifera) 24 g (pre-
    decocted)

gōu téng (钩藤 uncaria, Uncariae Ramulus cum Uncis) 15 g

tiān xiān téng (天仙藤 aristolochia stem, Aristolochiae Herba) 12 g

tiān xiān zǐ (天仙子 henbane seed, Hyoscyami Semen) 0.9 g

I gave the patient six packets of this prescription and changed the dosage
of *yún nán bái yào* (Yunnan White) to one-eighth of a bottle, three times a day.

Fourth visit on November 25: After taking twelve packets of the above-
mentioned prescription, the patient still had the following symptoms: dizziness, anterior headache, entire body fatigue and lack of strength, somnolence
and excessive dreaming, and forgetfulness. The tongue body was red, the fur
was yellow and slimy, and the pulse was slow (35 beats/minute). I conducted
another pattern identification and analysis, and as before I diagnosed the pattern as heart, chest, and kidney yáng vacuity with obstructed blood flow. Thus,
I administered the prescription as before, even though the symptoms had not
changed. I noticed that the tongue body color had changed from dark to red,
and this was an encouraging sign; it demonstrated that there had been a positive effect after all. Therefore, I again prescribed the previous formula, but
modified it slightly by using heavier dosages of several medicinals. The patient received six packets as follows:

quán guā lóu (全栝楼 whole trichosanthes, Trichosanthis Fructus
    Integer) 30 g

xiè bái (薤白 Chinese chive, Allii Macrostemonis Bulbus) 15 g

guì zhī (桂枝 cinnamon twig, Cinnamomi Ramulus) 24 g

lù jiǎo shuāng (鹿角霜 degelatinated deer antler, Cervi Cornu
    Degelatinatum) 12 g

ròu guì (肉桂 cinnamon bark, Cinnamomi Cortex) 5 g

bái jiè zǐ (白芥子 white mustard, Sinapis Albae Semen) 6 g

dǎng shēn (党参 codonopsis, Codonopsis Radix) 15 g

chuān xiōng (川芎 chuanxiong, Chuanxiong Rhizoma) 15 g

sū mù (苏木 sappan, Sappan Lignum) 15 g

hóng huā (红花 carthamus, Carthami Flos) 9 g

tiān xiān téng (天仙藤 aristolochia stem, Aristolochiae Herba) 12 g

bái zhǐ (白芷 Dahurian angelica, Angelicae Dahuricae Radix) 9 g

zhēn zhū mǔ (珍珠母 mother-of-pearl, Concha Margaritifera) 30 g (pre-
decocted)

zhì gān cǎo (炙甘草 mix-fried licorice, Glycyrrhizae Radix cum Liquido
Fricta) 6 g

This prescription was based on *guā lóu xiè bái bái jiǔ tāng* (Trichosanthes, Chinese Chive, and White Liquor Decoction) without *bái jiǔ* (white liquor), but with *guì zhī* (cinnamon twig) and *bái jiè zǐ* (white mustard). As chief medicinals, these assist chest yáng, open chest impediment, and downbear phlegm turbidity.

As support medicinals, *ròu guì* (cinnamon bark) and *lù jiǎo shuāng* (dege-latinated deer antler) supplement true yáng in the kidney and reinforce yáng qì in the entire body.

As assistant medicinals, *hóng huā* (carthamus), *sū mù* (sappan), and *tiān xiān téng* (aristolochia stem) quicken blood and free the network vessels; *dǎng shēn* (codonopsis) and *zhì gān cǎo* (mix-fried licorice) boost qì and har-monize blood; *zhēn zhū mǔ* (mother-of-pearl) nourishes heart yīn and quiets the spirit; and *chuān xiōng* (chuanxiong), important as a blood aspect medici-nal, promotes movement in the twelve channels to transform stasis and en-gender the new; thus, it rallies qì aspect medicinals to command the move-ment of blood.

Bái zhǐ (Dahurian angelica) is acrid in flavor and warm in nature; it is aromatic and penetrating. As the courier medicinal, its qì ascends and enters the greater yáng channel to treat anterior headache.

<u>Fifth visit on December 3</u>: The patient had taken eight packets of the pre-scription, and finally the headache and dizziness were alleviated. The slow heartbeat appeared to increase slightly and at one point had reached 38 beats per minute. The patient's complexion was beaming for he now had hope that his condition would improve. Yet, some symptoms still remained, such as generalized fatigue, excessive dreaming, forgetfulness, and poor appetite. The tongue was red and moist and the tongue fur was yellow and slimy. Further-more, the pulse was slow and the heart rate remained 35 beats per minute. I prescribed six more packets with the following modifications:

quán guā lóu (全栝楼 whole trichosanthes, Trichosanthis Fructus
Integer) 30 g

xiè bái (薤白 Chinese chive, Allii Macrostemonis Bulbus) 15 g

guì zhī (桂枝 cinnamon twig, Cinnamomi Ramulus) 30 g

bái jiè zǐ (白芥子 white mustard, Sinapis Albae Semen) 9 g

lù jiǎo jiāo (鹿角胶 deerhorn glue, Cervi Cornus Gelatinum) 9 g

ròu guì (肉桂 cinnamon bark, Cinnamomi Cortex) 5 g

shú dì huáng (熟地黄 cooked rehmannia, Rehmanniae Radix Praeparata) 15 g

má huáng (麻黄 ephedra, Ephedrae Herba) 3 g (crushed together with *shú dì huáng* (cooked rehmannia))

hóng huā (红花 carthamus, Carthami Flos) 9 g

sū mù (苏木 sappan, Sappan Lignum) 15 g

tiān xiān téng (天仙藤 aristolochia stem, Aristolochiae Herba) 15 g

dǎng shēn (党参 codonopsis, Codonopsis Radix) 15 g

zhēn zhū mǔ (珍珠母 mother-of-pearl, Concha Margaritifera) 30 g (pre-decocted)

chuān xiōng (川芎 chuanxiong, Chuanxiong Rhizoma) 15 g

bái zhǐ (白芷 Dahurian angelica, Angelicae Dahuricae Radix) 9 g

Besides increasing the dosage of *guì zhī* (cinnamon twig) and *bái jiè zǐ* (white mustard), this formula also used the method of crushing *shú dì huáng* (cooked rehmannia) and *má huáng* (ephedra) together. I used *bái jiè zǐ* (white mustard), *lù jiǎo jiāo* (deerhorn glue), and *ròu guì* (cinnamon bark), with *guā lóu xiè bái jiā guì zhī tāng* (Trichosanthes and Chinese Chive Decoction plus Cinnamon Twig) as the basis; this is rich in the spirit of *yáng hé tāng* (Harmonious Yáng Decoction) and strengthens the yáng-supplementing, stagnation-freeing, bind-dissipating, and stasis-quickening actions of the formula.

<u>Sixth visit on December 9</u>: The headache did not occur this week, and the remaining symptoms had all been alleviated. The heart rate at times reached 38–39 beats per minute. The patient had recently experienced pain in the lumbus, so I removed *bái zhǐ* (Dahurian angelica) from the formula, added 12 grams of *xù duàn* (dipsacus), and gave him six more packets. The patient informed me that he wished to return to Shāndōng province and wanted to continue taking the medicinals. I advised him to take this prescription long-term.

Two months later, in the middle of February 1975, I received a letter from the patient. He wrote that after he had returned home, he had taken one packet each day of the formula that had been prescribed for him on December 9. These, together with the decoctions that he received during his stay in Běijīng, numbered approximately 100 packets. The patient informed me that on one occasion shortly after the Chinese New Year, he suddenly experienced an increased heart rate of 80 beats per minute. He had immediately gone to the local hospital where he received both an electrocardiogram and an auscultation examination from his physician, but the results were normal. After that, although he sometimes had a heart rate that was less than 50 beats per minute, the rate would quickly change to 80 beats per minute. He had written in his letter that he was very happy about this situation. I replied in a letter to him that he was welcome to return to Běijīng sometime for a re-examination, and he did eight months later on October 9, 1975.

At the time of the re-examination, his essence-spirit was very good, he was radiant with happiness, he had gained some weight, and his body was healthy and strong. He had gone back to work long before, and since he was on a business trip to Zhāngjiākǒu (a city in northern China, west of Běijīng), he decided to come to my hospital for re-examination. He brought with him the electrocardiogram results from April 14, 1975 and the vector-cardiogram results from July 20, 1975. The results were respectively "normal electrocardiogram" and "generally normal vector-cardiogram (heart rate 76 beats per minute)." On the day of the examination, I immediately ordered another electrocardiogram, and it, too, was normal.

As a follow-up in June 1980, I received a reply to my letter. It read:

> Since my return home from the re-examination, my health has been very good continuously. My heart rate is quite normal, always remaining within the range of 60–70 beats per minute. Moreover, my other health problems have not relapsed even once. Currently, my workplace is near Mount Tài, and every day I get up early and climb to the mountain peak. The climb is 300 meters and takes an hour to climb and return. I feel strong and my diet is very good; at work I am constantly energetic. All subsequent electrocardiograms have been normal, and my blood pressure has also been normal.

CASE NOTES

(1.) Chinese Academy of Medical Sciences Hospital Běijīng: excerpt from medical case history summary.

Case history 171379: Hospitalized for treatment from April 26 to September 3, 1969. Examination upon admittance revealed that his condition was in general very good, body temperature normal, blood pressure 130/80 mmHg, heart rate 40 beats per minute, regular and forceful, cardiac apex not heard upon auscultation and no pathological murmur. Lung percussion was clear, the liver and spleen were not enlarged, and there was no puffy swelling in the lower limbs. The electrocardiogram revealed a Level III atrioventricular block. X-rays indicated ventricle enlargement, which indicated myocardial pathology. The ESR (erythrocyte sedimentation rate), liver and kidney functions, and electrolytes were all normal. During the time he was hospitalized on the evening of June 22, 1969, he suddenly had a fainting spell and was treated with oxygen inhalation and cardiac compression. After receiving an adrenaline drip, his heart rate dropped to 31 beats per minute, but was regular, and he regained consciousness.

Today his situation is relatively good, his condition stable, and he can return home and continue treatment. (September 2, 1969)

(2.) Summary of case study from Shāndōng Hospital dated April 25, 1973.

The patient was seen at the Běijīng Internal Medicine Hospital for treatment, but without success. The physicians in Běijīng recommended the installation of a pacemaker, but the patient did not consent. After he returned home to Shāndōng, the heart rate remained slow, and he had many incidences of fainting, so he again requested treatment.

The patient was chronically ill; his heart rate was 36 beats per minute, a cardiac apex systolic retraction murmur was present, blood pressure was 130/80 mmHg, but no abnormalities were seen in the lungs or abdomen. Moreover, there was no puffy swelling in the lower limbs. The diagnosis was complete atrioventricular block.

The electrocardiogram revealed that the electrocardial potential was half capacity; there was counter-clockwise rotation. P-wave was normal. The QRS interval was 0.08 of a second. Voltage was normal; ST section and T-wave were normal; and Q–T intervals were 0.52 of a second. The concluded diagnosis was Level III atrioventricular block and automatic ventricular regulation.

Since the patient had for many years received unsuccessful treatment with internal medicine pharmaceuticals, the recommendation is referral to another hospital to receive treatment outside Shāndōng province. He is referred to a Běijīng or Shànghǎi hospital for the installation of a heart pacemaker and requires a medical transport together with emergency medications.

(3.) Excerpt from the medical records at Shànghǎi People's Hospital dated December 18, 1973 to February 19, 1974.

Comments written on the last day of hospitalization: The patient was admitted with a diagnosis of complete atrioventricular block. Although taking symptomatic medication, he showed no improvement. He needed an implanted demand pacemaker, but the hospital did not have one, so it was not fitted. The patient was discharged today from this hospital and advised to continue with his medications. Under the care of his original physician, should the patient later require the pacemaker, he is welcome at any time to return here for installation. If, when taking the medication, the condition changes as a result of the absence of an implanted demand pacemaker, the patient can come to the hospital any time to have an external demand pacemaker fitted.

Furthermore, the patient still carries with him the medical records of his diagnosis and treatment at other hospitals, including Shāndōng Provincial Hospital, the Shànghǎi First Medical School Hospital, and the Chinese People's Liberation Army Hospital. The content, however, was fundamentally the same as the case histories from the three hospitals mentioned above, so I have omitted it here.

CASE THREE
SUSPENDED RHEUM (EXUDATIVE PLEURISY)
悬饮(渗出性胸膜炎

The patient was a 27-year-old male, an outpatient from Héběi Provincial Hospital. His initial examination date was June 16, 1972.

CHIEF COMPLAINT

Left-sided chest pain, suffocating sensation, and cough for more than ten days.

INQUIRY EXAMINATION

The patient suffered chest and rib-side pain on the left side with a suffocating sensation. When he coughed, the pain became severe. He could only lie on his left side, and he developed a fever in the afternoon. His appetite was still good, and urine and stool were normal.

INSPECTION EXAMINATION

He looked as if he was suffering from an acute disease, and his breathing was hasty and rapid. His development and nutrition were normal. The tongue fur was white. The chest x-rays revealed accumulated fluid in the thoracic cavity on the left side below the fourth intercostal space.

LISTENING AND SMELLING EXAMINATION

When the patient coughed, his voice was diminished. Auscultation of the chest area revealed that respiration was reduced on the left side, and percussion revealed a turbid sound in the lung.

PALPATION EXAMINATION

The pulse was slippery, but there were no other abnormalities.

PATTERN IDENTIFICATION

The lung governs qì; it is in charge of breathing. When lung diffusion and downbearing is impaired, there are symptoms such as cough, suffocation, chest and rib-side pain, and heat effusion. The lung is the upper source of water; it regulates the waterways and transports water to the bladder. In this case, since lung qì could not diffuse and its function lost regularity, water-rheum could not be diffused and transformed normally, so it accumulated in the chest and rib-side. White tongue fur and a slippery pulse both indicated the collection of water-damp. After correlating the four examinations, my diagnosis was suspended rheum disease.

TREATMENT METHOD

Diffuse and depurate lung qì, and disinhibit water and transform rheum.

PRESCRIPTION

I prescribed six packets of the following:

jiāo mù (椒目 zanthoxylum seed, Zanthoxyli Semen) 9 g

guā lóu (栝楼 trichosanthes, Trichosanthis Fructus) 30 g

dōng guā pí (冬瓜皮 wax gourd rind, Benincasae Exocarpium) 30 g

sāng bái pí (桑白皮 mulberry root bark, Mori Cortex) 9 g

zé xiè (泽泻 alisma, Alismatis Rhizoma) 9 g

fú líng pí (茯苓皮 poria skin, Poriae Cutis) 12 g

chē qián zǐ (车前子 plantago seed, Plantaginis Semen) 30 g (wrapped in cloth)

xìng rén (杏仁 apricot kernel, Armeniacae Semen) 9 g

zǐ wǎn (紫菀 aster, Asteris Radix) 9 g

guì zhī (桂枝 cinnamon twig, Cinnamomi Ramulus) 4.5 g

bǎi bù (百部 stemona, Stemonae Radix) 9 g

FORMULA EXPLANATION

This formula is a modified version of *jiāo mù guā lóu tāng* (Zanthoxylum Seed and Trichosanthes Decoction) from the *Yī Chún Shèng Yì* ("Enriching the Meaning of the Wine of Medicine"). As chief medicinals, *jiāo mù* (zanthoxylum seed) disinhibits water and eliminates rheum, while *guā lóu* (trichosanthes) loosens the chest and transforms phlegm.

As support medicinals, *sāng bái pí* (mulberry root bark), *fú líng pí* (poria skin), *dōng guā pí* (wax gourd rind), *zé xiè* (alisma), and *chē qián zǐ* (plantago seed) disinhibit water and transform dampness.

As assistant medicinals, *zǐ wǎn* (aster), *xìng rén* (apricot kernel), and *bǎi bù* (stemona) diffuse and depurate lung qì and while downbearing qì and transforming phlegm.

As the courier medicinal, *guì zhī* (cinnamon twig) warms yáng and transforms qì, reinforces qì transformation of water-rheum, and disinhibits water.

Followup Treatment

Second visit on June 30: The patient had taken twelve packets of this prescription, together with streptomycin injections and oral doses of isoniazid, and all subjective symptoms had disappeared. The chest x-ray revealed that the accumulated fluids in the thoracic cavity had been completely assimilated. I advised him to continue with several more packets of the prescription to consolidate the therapeutic effect.

This case is an example of the application of integrated Chinese-Western medicine. This approach promptly controlled the development of inflammation, promoted the assimilation of accumulated fluids, and reduced the treatment duration time.

Case Four
Chest impediment (coronary heart disease, angina pectoris)
胸痹(冠心病、心绞痛)

The patient, a 41-year-old male, was a regimental commander of the People's Liberation Army. His initial examination date was September 24, 1962.

Chief complaint

Oppressive chest pain and a feeling of oppression in the precordial area for the last eighteen months.

Inquiry examination

The patient also had the following symptoms: unstable sleep, susceptibility to fright, occasional heart palpitations and fearful throbbing, dizziness when climbing to high places, and occasional puffy swelling in the lower limbs. His appetite was still good, and urine and stool were normal. He had already visited two hospitals, the Shí Jiā Zhuāng City Hospital in Héběi province and the Běijīng Hospital. Electrocardiogram tests and the diagnoses at both hospitals were the same: coronary heart disease and angina pectoris.

Inspection examination

His development and nutrition were good, but his complexion was slightly dark. The tongue fur at the root area was grimy, thick, and slightly yellow.

Listening and smelling examination

His speech, voice, and respiration were normal.

Palpation examination

Palpation revealed a normal abdomen and limbs, and the pulse was slightly rapid.

PATTERN IDENTIFICATION

The chest is a region of yáng qì diffusion. When chest yáng is devitalized, the flow of qì and blood is depressed; where there is no free flow of qì and blood, there is pain. Since heart qì was obstructed, the patient felt constraint and oppression in the chest. Since heart blood was deprived of nourishment, he had symptoms such as susceptibility to fright, palpitations, and sleeplessness. After correlating the four examinations, my diagnosis was chest impediment caused by devitalized heart yáng.

TREATMENT METHOD

Loosen the chest and reinforce yáng while diffusing and freeing qì and blood, simultaneously assisted by quieting the spirit.

PRESCRIPTION

I prescribed six packets of the following:

quán guā lóu (全栝楼 whole trichosanthes, Trichosanthis Fructus Integer) 12 g

xiè bái (薤白 Chinese chive, Allii Macrostemonis Bulbus) 9 g

chǎo zhǐ qiào (炒枳壳 stir-fried bitter orange, Aurantii Fructus Frictus) 9 g

guì zhī (桂枝 cinnamon twig, Cinnamomi Ramulus) 3 g

hòu pò (厚朴 officinal magnolia bark, Magnoliae Officinalis Cortex) 4.5 g

shí chāng pú (石菖蒲 acorus, Acori Tatarinowii Rhizoma) 3 g

zhū yuǎn zhì (朱远志 cinnabar polygala, Polygalae Radix et Cinnabare) 6 g

zhū fú shén (朱茯神 cinnabar root poria, Poria cum Pini Radice et Cinnabare) 9 g

suān zǎo rén (酸枣仁 spiny jujube, Ziziphi Spinosi Semen) 9 g

jiāo shén qū (焦神曲 scorch-fried medicated leaven, Massa Medicata Fermentata Usta) 9 g

mù xiāng (木香 costusroot, Saussureae Radix) 1.5 g

FORMULA EXPLANATION

As chief medicinals, *guā lóu* (trichosanthes) loosens the chest and transforms phlegm, and moistens and downbears with its sweet and bitter flavor; *xiè bái* (Chinese chive) reinforces yáng and opens impediment, and dissipates qì and blood with acridity.

As support medicinals, *zhǐ ké* (bitter orange) frees stagnant qì in the chest, *guì zhī* (cinnamon twig) reinforces heart and chest yáng qì, and *hòu pò* (officinal magnolia bark) disperses distention and eliminates oppression.

As assistant medicinals, *yuǎn zhì* (polygala) promotes interaction between the heart and kidney and quiets the spirit, and *shí chāng pú* (acorus) frees the chest and diaphragm and opens the orifices. Sweet and sour *suān zǎo rén* (spiny jujube) contracts the spirit. Sweet and bland *zhū fú shén* (cinnabar root poria) quiets the heart, and *jiāo shén qū* (scorch-fried medicated leaven) disperses and transforms to harmonize the center.

As courier medicinal, the small dosage of *mù xiāng* (costusroot) moves cold stagnant qì. Pain stops because qì moves.

FOLLOWUP TREATMENT

Second visit on September 30: After taking the medicinals, the results were mediocre and the illness was neither better nor worse. The tongue fur was white, and the pulse was slightly sunken, so I prescribed three packets with the following modifications:

guā lóu pí (栝楼皮 trichosanthes rind, Trichosanthis Pericarpium) 12 g

chǎo zhǐ qiào (炒枳壳 stir-fried bitter orange, Aurantii Fructus Frictus) 9 g

qīng bàn xià (清半夏 purified pinellia, Pinelliae Tuber Depuratum) 6 g

běi shú mǐ (北秫米 sorghum, Sorghi Semen) 9 g

shí chāng pú (石菖蒲 acorus, Acori Tatarinowii Rhizoma) 3 g

zhū yuǎn zhì (朱远志 cinnabar polygala, Polygalae Radix et Cinnabare) 6 g

zhì rǔ xiāng (制乳香 processed frankincense, Olibanum Praeparatum) 3 g

zhì mò yào (制没药 processed myrrh, Myrrha Praeparata) 3 g

bái sháo yào (白芍药 white peony, Paeoniae Radix Alba) 9 g

bái jí lí (白蒺藜 tribulus, Tribuli Fructus) 9 g

huò xiāng gěng (藿香梗 patchouli stem, Pogostemi Caulis) 9 g

shēng suān zǎo rén (生酸枣仁 raw spiny jujube, Ziziphi Spinosi Semen Cruda) 12 g

chǎo suān zǎo rén (炒酸枣仁 stir-fried spiny jujube, Ziziphi Spinosi Semen Fricta) 9 g

chén xiāng fěn (沉香粉 aquilaria powder, Aquilariae Lignum Resinatum Pulveratum) 1.2 g (divided in half and taken drenched)

Third visit on October 5: After taking this prescription, the chest pain and oppression were relieved. Sleep was relatively good, but the fright palpitations remained. The symptoms of dizziness, puffy swelling in the lower limbs, and the oppressed feeling in the heart area had been alleviated. The yellow tongue fur that was previously grimy and thick had become thin. The pulse was still slightly rapid. Using the same method as before, I prescribed five packets with the following modifications:

guā lóu pí (栝楼皮 trichosanthes rind, Trichosanthis Pericarpium) 12 g

dāng guī shēn (当归身 tangkuei body, Angelicae Sinensis Radicis Corpus) 4.5 g

chǎo zhǐ qiào (炒枳壳 stir-fried bitter orange, Aurantii Fructus Frictus) 9 g

chǎo zhǐ shí (炒枳实 stir-fried unripe bitter orange, Aurantii Fructus Immaturus Frictus) 6 g

bái jí lí (白蒺藜 tribulus, Tribuli Fructus) 9 g

huò xiāng gěng (藿香梗 patchouli stem, Pogostemi Caulis) 9 g

shēng suān zǎo rén (生酸枣仁 raw spiny jujube, Ziziphi Spinosi Semen Crudum) 9 g

chǎo suān zǎo rén (炒酸枣仁 stir-fried spiny jujube, Ziziphi Spinosi Semen Fricta) 9 g

běi shú mǐ (北秫米 sorghum, Sorghi Semen) 9 g

fǎ bàn xià (法半夏 pro formula pinellia, Pinelliae Rhizoma Praeparatum) 7.5 g

bái sháo yào (白芍药 white peony, Paeoniae Radix Alba) 12 g

zhū yuǎn zhì (朱远志 cinnabar polygala, Polygalae Radix et Cinnabare) 6 g

lóng chǐ (龙齿 dragon tooth, Mastodi Dentis Fossilia) 12 g (pre-decocted)

chén xiāng fěn (沉香粉 aquilaria powder, Aquilariae Lignum Resinatum Pulveratum) 1.5 g (divided in half and taken drenched)

<u>Fourth visit on November 1</u>: After the patient finished the five packets, the chest oppression essentially disappeared, and only when he tired from walking or climbed to high places did the pain return. However, due to his work schedule and business travel, he had discontinued taking the medicinals; subsequently, the pain in the precordial area recurred 1–10 times a day, and even more frequently when he overworked. Whenever he rested, the pain was less frequent. Furthermore, when the pain appeared, it radiated into the left armpit. The patient was somnolent and had nightmares, and the stool had a tendency to be dry. The tongue fur was white and slightly slimy and the pulse was slightly rapid.

I again prescribed six packets of the medicinals, just as I had on October 5th. I also prescribed 3 pills of *sū hé xiāng wán* (Storax Pill), with directions to take a half pill twice a day after taking the decoction.

<u>Fifth visit on November 6</u>: Sleep became quiet and steady after taking the prescriptions. Heart pain was less frequent, and every symptom was alleviated. The tongue fur, which was once yellow and slimy, had become thin; the pulse was slightly slippery. The color of the urine was yellow. I again used the formula from October 5th. I removed *dāng guī* (Chinese angelica) and *zhǐ shí*

(unripe bitter orange), added 6 grams of *shí chāng pú* (acorus), and gave the patient three packets. Once more, I prescribed 3 pills of *sū hé xiāng wán* (Storax Pill), with directions to take a half pill twice a day after taking the decoction. These were the same directions as before.

Sixth visit on November 9: On this visit, it was clear that the heart and chest pain had been eliminated, and the remaining symptoms had basically disappeared. The tongue fur, however, was still yellow and thick, which may have been caused by excessive smoking. In addition, the stool was recently dry, the appetite was devitalized, and the pulse was slightly rapid and fine. Because of the demands of his work, he had to do some business travel, so he wanted to take his prescriptions with him.

I advised him to take this formula often to maintain the therapeutic effect, and I prescribed six packets for him as follows:

guā lóu pí (栝楼皮 trichosanthes rind, Trichosanthis Pericarpium) 12 g

xiè bái (薤白 Chinese chive, Allii Macrostemonis Bulbus) 6 g

dān shēn (丹参 salvia, Salviae Miltiorrhizae Radix) 9 g

chǎo zhǐ qiào (炒枳壳 stir-fried bitter orange, Aurantii Fructus Frictus) 9 g

chǎo zhǐ shí (炒枳实 stir-fried unripe bitter orange, Aurantii Fructus Immaturus Frictus) 9 g

bái jí lí (白蒺藜 tribulus, Tribuli Fructus) 9 g

huò xiāng gěng (藿香梗 patchouli stem, Pogostemi Caulis) 12 g

shēng suān zǎo rén (生酸枣仁 raw spiny jujube, Ziziphi Spinosi Semen Crudum) 9 g

chǎo suān zǎo rén (炒酸枣仁 stir-fried spiny jujube, Ziziphi Spinosi Semen Fricta) 9 g

běi shú mǐ (北秫米 sorghum, Sorghi Semen) 9 g

shí chāng pú (石菖蒲 acorus, Acori Tatarinowii Rhizoma) 3 g

tiáo qín (条芩 young scutellaria, Scutellariae Radix Nova) 9 g

tiān zhú huáng (天竹黄 bamboo sugar, Bambusae Concretio Silicea) 6 g

chì sháo yào (赤芍药 red peony, Paeoniae Radix Rubra) 12 g

chén xiāng fěn (沉香粉 aquilaria powder, Aquilariae Lignum Resinatum Pulveratum) 1.2 g (divided in half and taken drenched)

I also prescribed 6 pills of *sū hé xiāng wán* (Storax Pill), with instructions to take one pill whenever the pain occurred. I advised him to purchase a refill locally when he had finished these pills.

Seventh visit on July 13, 1963: Altogether, the patient had taken the above-mentioned prescription for approximately three months, and had taken more than 30 pills of *sū hé xiāng wán* (Storax Pill). The chest pain, chest oppression, and precordial oppressive feeling were eliminated. Although the symptoms had occurred once at random, the incident was very mild, so I did not prescribe the decoction any longer. After he discontinued the medicinals, his work schedule became normal. His complexion was moist and lustrous, and his essence-spirit and speaking voice showed much improvement. He had recently repeated an electrocardiogram test at a Běijīng Hospital, and the results were normal. His blood cholesterol level, however, was 240 mg/dL. His tongue fur was still yellow, again probably due to his excessive smoking, and his pulse was quite balanced. On this occasion, I paid particular attention to his facial features, and noticed a slight greenish color on both cheekbones and several stasis macules below the lips. Therefore, I used a treatment method to nourish blood and quicken stasis while reinforcing heart yáng.

PRESCRIPTION

The patient was instructed to take this prescription 3–4 times per week, and I advised him to persevere for at least three months. The medicinals were as follows:

> *guā lóu pí* (栝楼皮 trichosanthes rind, Trichosanthis Pericarpium) 9 g
> *xiè bái* (薤白 Chinese chive, Allii Macrostemonis Bulbus) 3 g
> *hóng huā* (红花 carthamus, Carthami Flos) 6 g
> *quán dāng guī* (全当归 whole tangkuei, Angelicae Sinensis Radix Integra) 4.5 g
> *dān shēn* (丹参 salvia, Salviae Miltiorrhizae Radix) 12 g
> *chì sháo yào* (赤芍药 red peony, Paeoniae Radix Rubra) 6 g
> *bái sháo yào* (白芍药 white peony, Paeoniae Radix Alba) 6 g
> *huà jú hóng* (化橘红 Huazhou pomelo rind, Citri Grandis Exocarpium Rubrum) 6 g
> *huáng jīng* (黄精 polygonatum, Polygonati Rhizoma) (processed) 9 g
> *huò xiāng gěng* (藿香梗 patchouli stem, Pogostemi Caulis) 6 g
> *zhū fú shén* (朱茯神 cinnabar root poria, Poria cum Pini Radice et Cinnabare) 6 g
> *chǎo zhǐ qiào* (炒枳壳 stir-fried bitter orange, Aurantii Fructus Frictus) 6 g

Follow-up visit on March 23, 1966: Almost three years had passed, yet the patient had experienced no relapse. The angina pectoris had not recurred, even though the patient had discontinued the Chinese medicinals nearly three years ago. In January 1966, he had revisited a Běijīng hospital for an electrocardiogram test, and the results were still normal.

CASE FIVE
DIZZINESS AND HEADACHE, SOFT TETANY (RENAL AND MALIGNANT HYPERTENSION)
眩晕、头痛，柔痉（肾性、恶性高血压）

The patient, a 30-year-old male from Shěnyáng, was admitted to a Běijīng hospital emergency ward on February 26, 1976.

CHIEF COMPLAINT
Renal and malignant hypertension.

INQUIRY EXAMINATION
On January 24, 1976, without any known provocation, the patient had suddenly suffered a headache. After recovering from a subsequent common cold, the pain was relieved. On February 3, the headache had occurred a second time; it was more intense than before and was accompanied by nausea and vomiting. After this, the headache grew progressively worse, and it became so intolerable that he wanted to beat his head against a stone wall. The vomiting would not stop, and on February 6–9, he was dripping sweat incessantly. Whenever the headache occurred, he dripped with great sweat, his complexion was pale, he had no desire to speak, and his spirit-mind was somewhat incoherent. At that time, his blood pressure was in the range of 190–210/110–130 mmHg, and urinary protein was (+++). He was admitted to a local hospital and the diagnosis was malignant hypertension, but the treatment he received there was unsuccessful. On February 12, he had suddenly fainted while urinating, and five days later, on February 17, he arrived in Běijīng. He was admitted to a Běijīng hospital on February 18, and was given Western drugs for his hypertension, which at that time was 170/110 mmHg. Two days later, his blood pressure abruptly dropped to 100/60 mmHg, and he had another fainting spell when he urinated (during this incident another person caught him before he fell down).

On February 23, he entered the observation ward for emergency treatment, and a renogram conducted at that time revealed extreme insufficiency in the function of both kidneys. A chest x-ray showed no abnormalities of the heart and lungs. He also consulted with a physician in the ophthalmology department, who informed him that both eyes suffered hypertensive retinal arteriole spasms. By February 24, his physicians generally agreed that the diagnosis was renal hypertension (malignant) and the possibility of medullary paraganglioma. The recommendation was the administration of anti-hypertensive drugs. But on February 25, the patient discontinued the drugs since he still experienced dizziness and had other symptoms such as numbness in the head, inadequate sleep, and poor appetite.

The dizziness was clearly related to the position of his body. When he was standing, he became dizzy, his eyes would dilate, and he would faint. But when he was standing, his blood pressure was low compared with his blood pressure when lying down. In the middle of the night when he got up to urinate, the dizziness was so intolerable that he quickly climbed back into bed and urinated in his pants. He was well aware of this incident, but because of the dizziness and discomfort, he could not help himself. There was discomfort at the back of his head, and the back of his neck was tense. He experienced vexing heat, had no fear of cold, and had long voidings of clear urine.

INSPECTION EXAMINATION

His development was normal, but his complexion was relatively pale. His tongue fur was white. He remained lying in bed and did not dare to stand up. His facial expression was anxious and fearful.

LISTENING AND SMELLING EXAMINATION

His speech was clear, but the tone of his voice was slightly low.

PALPATION EXAMINATION

Palpation of the chest and abdomen was normal, but both sides of the lumbus were painful when tapped. The pulse was stringlike, and the instep yáng pulse (*fū-yáng* pulse) was fairly good.

PATTERN IDENTIFICATION

The governing vessel (*dū mài*) travels up the back of the body to the head; the foot greater yáng (*tài yáng*) channel also travels from the back up to the head. The hand yáng brightness (*yáng míng*) channel travels to the shoulder, emerges at the collar bone and meets the greater yáng channel at GV-14 (*dà zhuī*). The *Huáng Dì Nèi Jīng* ("The Yellow Emperor's Inner Canon") says, "When illness affects the governing vessel, the backbone becomes rigid and arches backward." The *Jīn Guì Yào Lüe* ("Essential Prescriptions of the Golden Coffer"), in its discussion of tetany, says, "In diseases of the greater yáng, there is heat effusion and sweating with no aversion to cold; this is called soft tetany." The person with tetany disease has tension in the back and neck. This patient had symptoms such as headache, dizziness, and tightness and tension in the back and neck area. I therefore knew that the disease was in the governing and greater yáng channels, and the disease had also affected the yáng brightness channel.

The governing vessel manages the yáng qì of the body. In this case, yáng qì was devitalized, qì transformation was inhibited, the channels and network vessels were not harmonized, and construction and defense were in disharmony. Therefore, the patient was on the verge of soft tetany, and the back and neck had become rigid. Since yáng vacuity was present, the patient suffered long voidings of clear urine that he could not control. The governing vessel and the foot greater yáng channel are related to the kidney channel. Thus, with kidney vacuity present, there were symptoms such as dizziness when moving the head, discharge of urine, and pain in the lumbus. The *Jīn Guì Yào Lüè* ("Essential Prescriptions of the Golden Coffer") says, "The tetany pulse is tight like the stringlike pulse, but moves directly up and down." This patient had six stringlike pulses, so after correlating the four examinations, I concluded that the diagnosis was yáng vacuity of the governing and greater yáng channels verging on soft tetany disease.

TREATMENT METHOD

Reinforce yáng qì, harmonize construction and defense, and boost both the kidney and governing vessels.

PRESCRIPTION

I prescribed six packets of the following to be decocted in water:

guì zhī (桂枝 cinnamon twig, Cinnamomi Ramulus) 9 g

gé gēn (葛根 pueraria, Puerariae Radix) 30 g

qiāng huó (羌活 notopterygium, Notopterygii Rhizoma et Radix) 6 g

lù jiǎo shuāng (鹿角霜 degelatinated deer antler, Cervi Cornu Degelatinatum) 9 g

bái sháo yào (白芍药 white peony, Paeoniae Radix Alba) 12 g

sāng jì shēng (桑寄生 mistletoe, Loranthi seu Visci Ramus) 30 g

xù duàn (续断 dipsacus, Dipsaci Radix) 12 g

zhì fù piàn (制附片 sliced processed aconite, Aconiti Radix Lateralis Praeparata Secta) 3 g

gōu téng (钩藤 uncaria, Uncariae Ramulus cum Uncis) 15 g

tiān huā fěn (天花粉 trichosanthes root, Trichosanthis Radix) 15 g

mù tōng (木通 trifoliate akebia, Akebiae Trifoliatae Caulis) 6 g

FORMULA EXPLANATION

This prescription was a synthesis of three classical formulas: *guā lóu guì zhī tāng* (Trichosanthes and Cinnamon Twig Decoction), *guì zhī jiā gé gēn tāng* (Cinnamon Twig Decoction Plus Pueraria), and *guì zhī jiā fù zǐ tāng* (Cinnamon Twig Decoction Plus Aconite). These formulas use medicinals that ascend and reinforce the yáng qì of the governing vessel.

As chief medicinals, *guì zhī* (cinnamon twig) frees and reinforces yáng qì of the greater yáng channel and governing vessel, while *gé gēn* (pueraria) resolves neck and back rigidity and stiffness in the yáng brightness channel.

As support medicinals, *qiāng huó* (notopterygium) and *lù jiǎo shuāng* (degelatinated deer antler) ascend and reinforce yáng qì of the governing vessel. *Fù piàn* (sliced aconite) promotes the yáng qì of the entire body.

As assistant medicinals, *sāng jì shēng* (mistletoe) and *xù duàn* (dipsacus) supplement the kidney and boost the governing vessel. *Gōu téng* (uncaria) dispels wind and treats dizziness. *Bái sháo yào* (white peony) and *guì zhī* (cinnamon twig) together harmonize construction and defense, and *tiān huā fěn* (trichosanthes root) engenders liquids and nourishes the sinews.

As the courier medicinal, *mù tōng* (trifoliate akebia) diffuses the blood and vessels.

FOLLOWUP TREATMENT

<u>Second visit on March 4</u>: After taking the medicinals, the dizziness was clearly alleviated, the rigidity and tightness of the neck lessened, and the patient no longer wet his pants. However, he was still thirsty and liked cold drinks. He also complained of pain in the lumbus, weakness in the legs, and profuse urination. The tongue fur at the root was yellow and the pulse was slightly stringlike. The medicinals proved appropriate in this case since the condition of the patient had already improved. I knew this was a case of kidney vacuity because of the presence of pain in the lumbus, limp legs, and profuse urination. His thirst and desire for cold drinks did not really represent a pattern of repletion heat, but rather was the result of damage to fluids caused by profuse urination and the earlier identified symptom of dripping sweat. I continued to use the previously described treatment method. I removed *tiān huā fěn* (trichosanthes root) and *mù tōng* (trifoliate akebia) and changed the prescription to include *shēng dì huáng* (dried rehmannia) and *shí hú* (dendrobium); in this way, I strengthened the kidney-supplementing, fluid-nourishing action of the formula.

This was the prescription, to be decocted in water; the patient received six packets:

guì zhī (桂枝 cinnamon twig, Cinnamomi Ramulus) 9 g

gé gēn (葛根 pueraria, Puerariae Radix) 24 g

qiāng huó (羌活 notopterygium, Notopterygii Rhizoma et Radix) 6 g

lù jiǎo bàng (鹿角镑 flaked deerhorn, Cervi Cornu in Assula) 9 g

sāng jì shēng (桑寄生 mistletoe, Loranthi seu Visci Ramus) 30 g

xù duàn (续断 dipsacus, Dipsaci Radix) 15 g

zhì fù piàn (制附片 sliced processed aconite, Aconiti Radix Lateralis Praeparata Secta) 5 g

fù pén zǐ (覆盆子 rubus, Rubi Fructus) 12 g

shēng dì huáng (生地黄 dried rehmannia, Rehmanniae Radix Exsiccata) 12 g

shí hú (石斛 dendrobium, Dendrobii Herba) 12 g

bái sháo yào (白芍药 white peony, Paeoniae Radix Alba) 12 g

gōu téng (钩藤 uncaria, Uncariae Ramulus cum Uncis) 15 g

shēng mài yá (生麦芽 raw barley sprout, Hordei Fructus Germinatus
   Crudus) 12 g

ADDITIONAL NOTES

The following comments were taken from the patient's daily record:

March 5: When the kidney area was tapped, the pain had lessened, and the lumbar pain overall had improved. Blood pressure was stabilized, and the body position made no difference in blood pressure results (reclining blood pressure was 132/80 mmHg; blood pressure when standing was 130/84 mmHg). I advised his family members to prepare for his discharge from the hospital.

March 8: The lower back is no longer painful but still aching; tapping pain is not present in the kidney area on the right side.

March 10: His appetite has greatly improved since yesterday, and in one day he ate approximately 300 grams of food.

Third visit on March 11: The patient was able to walk as far as the main entrance of the hospital and return without dizziness and without discomfort at the back of the head or stiffness in the neck; in fact, these symptoms had disappeared. He had no subjective symptoms at all. His appetite had increased to 350–400 grams of food; his essence-spirit and complexion had greatly improved as well. The tongue fur, however, was still slightly yellow at the root, and the pulse was sunken and slightly stringlike. His blood pressure was steady at 140–150/90–100 mmHg. Since the medicinals were in harmony with the treatment method, his recovery was near; therefore, I used the original method again with just a slight modification.

PRESCRIPTION

guì zhī (桂枝 cinnamon twig, Cinnamomi Ramulus) 9 g

gé gēn (葛根 pueraria, Puerariae Radix) 24 g

qiāng huó (羌活 notopterygium, Notopterygii Rhizoma et Radix) 6 g

lù jiǎo bàng (鹿角镑 flaked deerhorn, Cervi Cornu in Assula) 9 g

sāng jì shēng (桑寄生 mistletoe, Loranthi seu Visci Ramus) 30 g

xù duàn (续断 dipsacus, Dipsaci Radix) 15 g

zhì fù piàn (制附片 sliced processed aconite, Aconiti Radix Lateralis
   Praeparata Secta) 5 g

fù pén zǐ (覆盆子 rubus, Rubi Fructus) 9 g

shēng dì huáng (生地黄 dried rehmannia, Rehmanniae Radix Exsiccata)
   12 g

bái sháo yào (白芍药 white peony, Paeoniae Radix Alba) 12 g

> *gōu téng* (钩藤 uncaria, Uncariae Ramulus cum Uncis) 15 g
> *shēng yǐ mǐ* (生苡米 raw coix seed, Coicis Semen Crudum) 15 g
> *chǎo shān yào* (炒山药 stir-fried dioscorea, Dioscoreae Rhizoma
>   Frictum) 15 g
> *shēng mài yá* (生麦芽 raw barley sprout, Hordei Fructus Germinatus
>   Crudus) 12 g

I prescribed six packets to be decocted in water, one packet every day for the next three days, and then one packet every other day until finished. The patient was discharged from the hospital. When he left the hospital the next day, the patient was overjoyed to be returning home to Shěnyáng. In the past, the patient had taken several Western antibiotic drugs such as nitrofurantoin and chloromycetin, but during the time of his treatment at my clinic, he had taken primarily Chinese medicinals.

EMPIRICAL KNOWLEDGE

The four examinations should strengthen objective knowledge. When four examinations are not enough, you should develop five or six examinations.

For several thousand years, physicians of past eras have resolved the problems of disease by using the four examinations to determine treatments based on pattern identification. Furthermore, their experience has contributed to an abundance of knowledge concerning the four examinations, so even in modern times, the four examinations method is still the primary weapon of Chinese medicine in the battle against disease. By modern standards, this method nevertheless has some drawbacks: the four examinations are difficult to master; they are not popular; and they are not objective.

For instance, when we inspect the color of the complexion, we may say it is "dark and gloomy," "without brightness or sheen," possibly with a "yellowish complexion" or "greenish complexion." When inspecting the tongue, we may say it is "red," "crimson," "purple," "dark," or "pale." At a time when scientific knowledge was not developed, students could only follow directions from a master physician to treat patients; in this way, they would gradually develop some empirical knowledge, but many years would be required before they could master the application of medicine.

By contrast, in the modern world where scientific knowledge flourishes, we can combine the research of Chinese medicine with the aspects of modern medicine whenever it is required. With so much technology available that can be used to monitor the patient's condition, we can now easily record any changes in the course of disease and classify and contrast any disease with greater detail. Modern education has made it easier to learn with visual aids and computers. Now when we conduct examinations, we record notes so that we can contrast the condition of the patient from one visit to the next. By doing so, we create a collective experience, raise the standard of proficiency, and promote the development of medical science; all of these provide great benefit to us.

Pulse diagnosis is another aspect of Chinese medicine that is extremely difficult to master. Physicians of the past have passed down 28 pulses, and some of these pulses are not easy to distinguish. During pulse diagnosis, it is very easy to become subjective, so unless you have had several decades of experience, this subject is extremely difficult to master. This is so true, in fact, that some doctors never completely grasp the concept of 28 pulses throughout their entire lives. Consequently, there is an extraordinary demand to create a pulse instrument that is capable of recognizing the characteristics of Chinese medical pulses. Such a device would improve not only the quality of pulse examination itself, but also the quality of teaching it.

In summary, inspection examination, listening and smelling examination, and palpation examination are all important subjects requiring improvements in objectivity. This constitutes a benefit to the development and enhancement of pattern identification and treatment determination. Even in the area of inquiry examination, you should follow the development of the case history and continually expand its content with new information. On the other hand, despite advances in science, Chinese medicine still uses only the four examinations to diagnose patients. Since the four examinations are clearly inadequate for the demands of modern technological medicine, we should follow historical trends and fill this gap.

Consider the condition of the patient in Case 1 of this chapter. If the patient had not received any X-rays at all, we would not have known about the urethral calculus. We would only have known that he suffered stone strangury, and we would not have had knowledge of the approximate location of the stone. Without the X-ray, we could only diagnose a pattern of bladder accumulated heat, gradually scorching and becoming a stone. During his treatment, if we had not known that the stone had traveled downward to the mouth of the bladder and had settled there to cause anuria, we would have adopted a treatment measure not aimed at this condition, but rather one which would have inevitably influenced the treatment effectiveness in a negative way and caused the patient more suffering.

Consider Case 2. If an electrocardiogram examination had not been performed repeatedly as many times as it was, and had the patient not visited so many different hospitals for diagnosis and treatment, we would not have comprehended the gravity of his disease or attached any importance to it, and we would have been unable to draw any useful conclusions. Also, if we could not contrast the electrocardiograms before and after treatment, we could never have confirmed the treatment results. As for Case 3, without the chest X-ray, we would not have known the extent or the amount of the thoracic cavity fluids; in fact, we would not have known that fluids existed in the lung at all. If the patient in Case 5 had not consulted with urologists and ophthalmologists, and had not received a renogram or had his blood pressure measured, then we would not have correctly diagnosed renal and malignant hypertension.

These modern examination methods and treatment measures supplement the deficits of Chinese medicine and endow new content for pattern identification and treatment determination. Thus, they enhance the benefit to collective experience and treatment results. Therefore, I hope that we all make an effort to explore the valuable legacy of Chinese medicine. I hope that we attempt to learn how to utilize modern scientific approaches such as optics, electricity, ultrasonic waves, infrared rays, computers, molecular biology, bionics, and meteorology. We will then produce new devices that can reflect objectivity in Chinese medical pattern identification. We should, at the same time, assimilate the strong points of Western medicine and attempt to utilize these points to improve the accuracy of pattern identification. If we augment the methods of examination and combine them with the characteristics of Chinese medicine, then we may develop a fifth, or even sixth, examination method.

Adopt another's strong points to supplement one's own weaknesses when further developing the process of determining treatment.

There are very many methods in the Chinese medical treatment of disease, and Chinese medicine has made a great contribution in the struggle against disease for several thousand years. Although the scientific methods of our modern world are wonderfully developed, science itself still embodies certain weaknesses. Nevertheless, we should still assimilate from Western science some of its strong points to supplement the shortcomings of Chinese medicine. There are many treatment methods in Western medicine that can be appropriately used and easily combined with the characteristics of Chinese medicine; these methods supplement the shortcomings of Chinese medicine and enhance the therapeutic effect. These methods include injection therapy, nasal feeding, oxygen therapy, blood transfusions, intravenous fluid infusions, artificial respiration, artificial alimentation, enema therapy, gastric lavage, vaccinations, and ion therapy.

A good example of this combined approach is the treatment method used in Case 1. When the calculus blocked the urethral opening and caused anuria, instead of using pain-relieving drugs alone, I used vesical perforation together with anal massage and prescribed urgent decoctions of Chinese medicinals. This approach produced good results.

For Case 2, Western medicine had no specific drug therapy for treatment, and the recommendation was the installation of a pacemaker. I conducted detailed pattern identification and decided on a bold treatment strategy. After the patient recovered, he continued to have many electrocardiograms and vector-cardiograms, although he had in fact already regained his health. Such an approach offers patients the possibility of treatment for this disease by the use of Chinese medicinals and provides the patient with a more promising future since the misgivings associated with the surgical installation of a pacemaker are eliminated. Certainly, if the condition of the patient requires that a pacemaker be installed, then such a procedure should be done and is the best approach. The pacemaker, in turn, supplements the medicinal therapy, which may not always be enough. The Chinese medical treatment of this particular case turns our attention specifically to the strong point of pattern identification to determine treatment. Moreover, this case also utilized special Western medical technologies such as electrocardiograms, vector-cardiograms, and heart auscultation, and the therapeutic effect was very good.

For the patient in Case 3, I used Western medical antibiotics to prevent tuberculosis and Chinese medicinals to treat water-rheum; the combined approach obtained excellent results. I used Western medical methods such as urinalysis, an ophthalmology exam, and a renogram to precisely diagnose "renal and malignant hypertension" for the patient in Case 5. Afterwards, I promptly used Chinese medicinals to treat tetany and dizziness. Furthermore, upon his return home, I advised the patient to continue with the treatments for nephritis based on the objective results that had been obtained.

We cannot, of course, regard each individual case as a general rule, but it is important to know that the specifics of each case are diverse. The specific circumstances of disease differ in a thousand ways, so you must analyze all the particulars. You cannot just copy mechanically and apply indiscriminately. Therefore, you must be a thorough clinical investigator, and you must study comprehensively and use pattern identification to determine a holistic Chinese medical treatment method. This method is, indeed, the specialty of Chinese medicine, and the use of it promotes recovery from illness.

There is a saying among doctors of Chinese medicine that has been passed to us from physicians of the past: "Being well-versed in Wáng Shū Hé is not as good as having clinical experience." When you encourage later generations to study Chinese medicine, you should urge them, of course, to be thoroughly versed in Chinese medical theory, but you should still advise them to engage in clinical practice. As already mentioned, you should take another's strong points to offset your own weaknesses, expand the four examinations into five or six examinations, create new devices and instruments, and assimilate new treatment methods. All of these things must be integrated with clinical practice to solve real clinical problems and to raise the standard of treatment based on pattern identification. Thus, you promote the further development of Chinese medicine.

Encourage subjective initiative, raise the standard of proficiency for pattern identification and treatment determination, and strive for the modernization of Chinese medicine and the integration of Chinese and Western medical modalities.

To be a Chinese medical practitioner at present, in addition to the need to be fully versed in traditional Chinese medical theory for increased proficiency in treatments based on pattern identification, you must also strive for close integration of theory and practice. You should summarize and collect experiences, and constantly raise the standard of proficiency for pattern identification and treatment determination.

The patient in Case 1 had a radiating pain along the ureter towards the external genitalia. According to Chinese medicine pattern identification, this type of pain is related to the lumbus and lesser abdomen, which are associated with the liver and kidney channels. Thus, besides using medicinals to clear heat, lubricate the orifice, and expel the stone, I also prescribed medicinals such as *xù duàn* (dipsacus), *dù zhòng* (eucommia), and *niú xī* (achyranthes) to boost the liver and kidney. This method obtained fairly good results. I have treated urinary tract calculi for many years, and very often I prescribe medicinals that boost the liver and kidneys, but I prescribe them according to the pattern, and when organizing the formula, I do not use clearing and disinhibiting medicinals alone. The therapeutic effect is always improved with this method.

The patient in Case 2 had symptoms of empty pain in the head, a slow heartbeat, bodily fatigue, and devitalized essence-spirit. Following Chinese medical theory, I identified the pattern by tracing it back to the root to seek the origin of the problem, and thus I theorized that this patient did not merely suffer from insufficient heart yáng, but also from insufficiency of chest yáng and kidney yáng (true yáng). Since this was an enduring disease, I also determined that the illness had entered the blood aspect. Thus, I used a method that physicians of the past have used: reinforce the yáng qì of the heart, chest, and kidney, and simultaneously quicken blood and free the network vessels while boosting qì. With this method, I obtained ideal results.

The patient in Case 5 suffered from serious dizziness and back of the neck rigidity. Following Chinese medical theory and analysis, my diagnosis identified the pattern as yáng vacuity of the kidney channel and governing vessel, and loss of regularity in construction-defense. The condition of the patient verged on "soft tetany" disease; thus, I used a treatment method that boosted the kidney and governing vessel, reinforced yáng qì, and harmonized construction and defense. Again, the results were very good.

As these three examples demonstrate, I have learned from experience how to apply the strong points of each medical modality and how to raise the standard of proficiency in diagnosis and treatment. This approach provides us with a key to solving the problem of a disease "without an effective drug" and offers the possibility of using Chinese medicinals for treatment and recovery. This is certainly a goal worthy of our effort. Even though physicians of the past reflected objective law in their theory, this is just one phase of collective experience in a long historical process of knowledge. We are still dependent on clinical examination and investigation, for the truth can never be fully revealed. Consequently, we should not regard the experience and theory of the past as an unsurpassable limit or as an immutable final conclusion. If we magnify relative things to the extreme, we will turn a correct conclusion into an incorrect one, which will become an obstacle to further understanding the truth. Therefore, we must recognize the objectivity of truth while knowing that it has a relative aspect. Present-day Chinese medical professionals need to study traditional Chinese medical theory in depth, and need to apply these theories properly and test them in practice. We must develop our self-motivation to better understand the objective laws of illness and draw timely conclusions so as to raise the standards of pattern identification and treatment determination. Yet, to meet the conditions of our colleagues, it is still necessary to study both modern science and medical science, to work with both medical modalities in collaboration, and to complete their integration.

I hope that I have met the requirements of the reader. I also hope that I have adequately presented the concepts of launching a multidisciplinary research approach, of endowing pattern identification and treatment determination with new content, of promoting the forward development of Chinese medicine, and of bringing to fruition the modernization of Chinese medicine.

This is the conclusion of *Cóng Bìng Lì Tán Biàn Zhèng Lùn Zhì*. I welcome all comments from my colleagues concerning the material in this book.

INDEX

Also published by Paradigm Publications

Ten Lectures on the Use of Medicinals from the Personal Experience of Jiāo Shù-Dé

This text comes from a popular lecture series first published in China's barefoot doctors' journal. Jiāo Shù-Dé describes over 300 medicinal substances in practical terms, providing copious detail

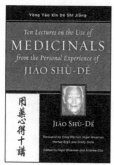

on clinical applications from his own personal experience. The lectures present medicinals grouped according to primary function: warm and hot medicinals, blood-quickening stasis-transforming medicinals, effusing and dissipating medicinals, and qi-rectifying medicinals. Within these categories individual medicinals are presented with discussions that include basic information such as taste, temperature, and entering channels, functions and indications, specific practical applications, and representative formulas for a given function. Each discussion also includes information about specific preparations and dosages, and comparisons with other medicinals having similar or related actions.

hardcover, 730 pp, 7x10"

This information about Chinese medicinals has not been previously available in an English-language materia medica. Jiāo's comparisons and contrasts of medicinals that have similar functions, and his discussions of a specific medicinal's actions in the context of well-known and frequently-used formulae, will help practitioners make better clinical decisions. His explications of fundamental theory allow all students and practitioners to gain increased understanding. His clear, practical, and comprehensive presentations of medicinals will cast the information in a new light and allow for better clinical agility.

Ten Lectures on the Use of Formulas from the Personal Experience of Jiāo Shù-Dé

In this subsequent volume over 200 major formulas and all their variations are detailed with remarkable cogency and clarity. Those who apply Jiāo's knowledge to their own patients find the results to be outstanding. His work is an essential guide for answering the questions and solving the problems that clinicians face in everyday practice.

Contents include lectures on relevant issues for the clinical application of formulas; qi-treating, blood-rectifying, and supplementing formulas; effusing and dissipating formulas; harmonizing and relieving formulas and formulas that treat exterior and interior; wind-dispelling, cold-dispelling, and dampness-dispelling formulas; fire-clearing, summerheat-dispersing, and dryness-moistening formulas; phlegm-eliminating, abductive dispersing, and offensive precipitating formulas; ejecting, securing-astringent, and worm-killing formulas; heavy settling, toxin-relieving, and anti-cancer actions formulas; commonly used gynecological and pediatric formulas; and Jiāo's empirical formulas.

hardcover, 640 pp, 7x10"

The lasting popularity of Jiāo's works in China is attributable to the fact that they have won the acclaim of practitioners and scholars as well as that of barefoot doctors. The clarity and practicality of presentation, and the comprehensiveness and depth of content, have assured Jiāo's works the lasting place in the West that they have already attained in China.

Order your copies through
Redwing Book Company, 202 Bendix Drive, Taos New Mexico USA 87571
www.redwingbooks.com